T0327699

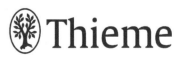

Pediatric Neuroradiology

Clinical Practice Essentials

Asim F. Choudhri, MD
Associate Chairman–Research Affairs and Education
Department of Radiology
Associate Professor of Radiology, Ophthalmology, and Neurosurgery
University of Tennessee Health Science Center
Director of Neuroradiology
Le Bonheur Neuroscience Institute
Le Bonheur Children's Hospital
Memphis, Tennessee

Thieme
New York • Stuttgart • Delhi • Rio de Janeiro

Thieme Medical Publishers, Inc.
333 Seventh Ave.
New York, New York 10001

Executive Editor: William Lamsback
Managing Editor: J. Owen Zurhellen IV
Editorial Assistant: Mary B. Wilson
Director, Editorial Services: Mary Jo Casey
International Production Director: Andreas Schabert
Vice President, Editorial and E-Product Development:
    Vera Spillner
International Marketing Director: Fiona Henderson
International Sales Director: Louisa Turrell
Director of Sales, North America: Mike Roseman
Senior Vice President and Chief Operating Officer:
    Sarah Vanderbilt
President: Brian D. Scanlan
Printer: King Printing Co., Inc.

Library of Congress Cataloging-in-Publication Data

Choudhri, Asim F., author.
    Pediatric neuroradiology : clinical practice essentials / Asim F.
    Choudhri.
        p. ; cm.
    Includes bibliographical references and index.
    ISBN 978-1-62623-096-5 –
    ISBN 978-1-62623-097-2 (eISBN)
    I. Title.
[DNLM: 1. Neuroradiography. 2. Central Nervous System Diseases–
diagnosis. 3. Child. 4. Head–radiography. 5. Infant. 6. Magnetic
Resonance Imaging. 7. Neck–radiography. WS 340]
RJ488.5.M33
618.92'8047548–dc23   2015026386

Copyright 2017 by Thieme Medical Publishers, Inc.
Typesetting by Thomson Digital, India

Also available as an e-book:
eISBN 978-1-62623-097-2

Important note: Medicine is an ever-changing science undergoing continual development. Research and clinical experience are continually expanding our knowledge, in particular our knowledge of proper treatment and drug therapy. Insofar as this book mentions any dosage or application, readers may rest assured that the authors, editors, and publishers have made every effort to ensure that such references are in accordance with **the state of knowledge at the time of production of the book.**

Nevertheless, this does not involve, imply, or express any guarantee or responsibility on the part of the publishers in respect to any dosage instructions and forms of applications stated in the book. **Every user is requested to examine carefully** the manufacturers' leaflets accompanying each drug and to check, if necessary in consultation with a physician or specialist, whether the dosage schedules mentioned therein or the contraindications stated by the manufacturers differ from the statements made in the present book. Such examination is particularly important with drugs that are either rarely used or have been newly released on the market. Every dosage schedule or every form of application used is entirely at the user's own risk and responsibility. The authors and publishers request every user to report to the publishers any discrepancies or inaccuracies noticed. If errors in this work are found after publication, errata will be posted at www.thieme.com on the product description page.

Some of the product names, patents, and registered designs referred to in this book are in fact registered trademarks or proprietary names even though specific reference to this fact is not always made in the text. Therefore, the appearance of a name without designation as proprietary is not to be construed as a representation by the publisher that it is in the public domain.

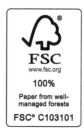

FSC
www.fsc.org
100%
Paper from well-
managed forests
FSC® C103101

This book is dedicated to all children with neurologic disorders, and to their families.

Contents

Part 3. Head and Neck Imaging

Part 4. Spine Imaging

Part 5. Appendices

Foreword

It is said, "Everyone has a book within them". The key is to write one that fulfills a niche and tells a good story. In this volume by Asim Choudhri, *Pediatric Neuroradiology: Clinical Practice Essentials*, one has the book that has been needed for a long time and that tells a good story. Let's face it, Jim Barkovich's *Pediatric Neuroimaging* is one of the bibles of Neuroradiology, but is not something that anyone can read cover to cover. It's more of a reference book that you consult, and it fulfills that niche. It is outstanding. What Dr. Choudhri has done is to write a book that captures 95% of what you will actually see in your clinical practice, distills it to an appropriate depth, and moves on to the next entity. The writing style is engaging and Asim's fund of knowledge is exceptional. He is a good "story-teller."

The book was designed with a carefully thought out table of contents, with 28 manageable chapters divided into sections for brain, head and neck, and spine. High quality images are supplemented with descriptive figure legends to allow the reader to extract maximum information. Beyond learning the information, it is important to clinically apply this knowledge, which is often the most difficult aspect to glean from a textbook. This is where the three appendices come in handy. An entire appendix is dedicated to protocolling studies, to allow the reader to learn how best (and when) to acquire the images that are most useful. A second appendix focuses on how to report studies, presenting templates and guidance for providing clinically helpful and consultative interpretations. The third appendix is a quick-reference for common pediatric neuroradiology indications/presentations, including condition-specific pertinent positive and negative studies for interpretation. It's all there!

I recommend this book to all trainees and practitioners that see a fair number of pediatric neuroradiology cases and/or patients. If you want an outstanding, practical, efficient read that does not get mired in the minutiae, buy this book.

I have known Dr. Choudhri since his year as a neuroradiology fellow at Johns Hopkins. In the time since his graduation from our program I have corresponded with him, collaborated with him, and also invited him to serve as a teacher at the American College of Radiology Education Center for its Neuroradiology Course. Asim has done a super job as a clinician, a researcher, and as an educator. I think that you are really going to enjoy this book from one of Neuroradiology's Triple Threats, Asim Choudhri. I tip my hat to him.

David M. Yousem, MD, MBA
Director of Neuroradiology, Vice Chairman of Program Development
Department of Radiology
Associate Dean for Professional Development
Johns Hopkins School of Medicine
Baltimore, Maryland

Preface

The idea for this book arose during my first few years of practice as a neuroradiologist in a pediatric hospital. During daily interactions with residents and fellows, as well as faculty members of various specialties, I was frequently asked to recommend a good resource for an individual to learn and review the fundamentals of pediatric neuroradiology. Extensive, and therefore appropriately expensive, resources exist, which are well served for the neuroradiologist and for reference libraries; however, there was no book which was light enough to carry around, practical enough to be used on a regular basis, detailed enough to be helpful while remaining accessible to those junior in training, and priced so that residents in radiology, neurology, and neurosurgery would consider it worth owning (not to mention residents and staff in otolaryngologyhead and neck surgery, ophthalmology, orthopaedics, neurosurgery, genetics, pediatrics, and other areas).

So from this came my working outline, which I added to and modified over several years. It became clear why the giants of the field wrote giant textbooks on this topic, and I realized that a 50-page all-encompassing text is not possible. I nevertheless believe that the book you are holding remains appropriately focused for the individual who wishes to learn the foundations of pediatric neuroradiology.

The content of this book come from cases I have seen during my first five years of practice. There are indeed many rare diseases I have seen that are not included in this book (e. g. melanocytic neuroectodermal tumor of infancy, methylmalonic academia, and others). I performed the imaging workup and preoperative planning for over 750 pediatric brain tumors while at Le Bonheur, but this is not meant to be a pediatric neuro-oncology textbook, therefore many of the esoteric entities I have encountered are not discussed. I also have performed a large volume of advanced imaging, including over 250 functional MRIs in children, and multi-delay ASL perfusion in dozens of children with moyamoya vasculopathy; however, this is not intended to be a textbook in advanced imaging techniques in neuroradiology.

This book is deliberately not kitchen-sink comprehensive, but is instead meant to be practical and focused on fundamentals. I am less concerned that the reader can identify a disease that has only been reported a few dozen times than I am to make sure they can confidently and safely interpret the common disorders of childhood. This book is meant to help reduce the over-diagnosis of normal pediatric conditions (such as mistaking a calvarial suture for a fracture), and reduce the under-diagnosis of conditions that present differently in children than in adults (such as mistaking a fracture for a calvarial suture). Another area of significant confusion I hope to clarify is the dandy-walker spectrum of malformations, and normal variants without pathologic significance that are confused with dandy-walker spectrum malformations. Accordingly, disease processes that I couldn't readily find examples of in my teaching files (and thus that I haven't knowingly encountered in the last five years) have been excluded, with rare exceptions. A few diseases I have not definitely encountered during my time at Le Bonheur Children's Hospital have been included some because they are common in other geographic locations, such as Lyme disease (which I saw multiple times when training on the East Coast), some because they have a very characteristic imaging appearance, despite their rarity, and others that are not commonly evaluated by radiologists today due to advances in clinical evaluation yet have historic importance, such as Coats disease, which is now confidently differentiated from retinoblastoma by ophthalmologists without the need for CT or MRI. Additionally, topics that have significant overlap with findings in adult neuroradiology are not covered in as comprehensive a manner as a general neuroradiology textbook does, in particular with entities that are much less common in children such as glioblastoma and acute stroke. Where possible, suggested readings are provided to learn more on given areas, typically review articles that further delve into a given topic. Many review articles arise from publications such as Radiographics, Neurographics, and the American Journal of Neuroradiology.

This book will not replace comprehensive reference texts in the field of pediatric neuroradiology, and it is not intended to do so. This book will serve as a foundation for a broader audience to understand the imaging appearance of neurologic diseases of childhood. With this foundation, readers may be in a position to further explore the details in sources such as reference textbooks and the peer-reviewed scientific literature. I hope and trust that the book has been structured to appropriately achieve this goal, and I look forward to feedback from readers about the impact this book has on your education and clinical care.

Acknowledgments

This book would not be possible without the guidance of my parents, Drs. Fiaz and Saleem Choudhri, who served as personal and professional role models. Each was the first physician in their families, showing a dedication to patient care that inspired my siblings and numerous cousins to pursue careers in medicine. My brothers, Drs. Haroon and Tanvir Choudhri, followed my father's footsteps into neurosurgery, and kept me apprised of their clinical thought processes along the way. They have served as a constant source of challenging consults and clinical feedback. To my loving wife Lauren, an academic pediatric neuro-ophthalmologist who is my collaborator, my supporter, and my perpetual cheering section. To my beautiful son Hilo, who joined us just as this book was going to print. To all of my in-laws, who are truly family members and supporters.

After family, I must acknowledge the significant efforts regarding proofreading this manuscript and serving as a source of ideas for improvement, often on exceedingly short deadlines, provided by Dr. Adeel Siddiqui and Dr. Zachary Abramson.

Thank you to my mentors within medicine, including Mehmet Oz who taught me to think critically, and helped me early in my career prior to entering medical school. To the memory of Theodore Keats, a spectacular radiologist, educator, and person. To Michael Dake, Bruce Hillman, Doug Phillips, Kiran Nandalur and other mentors and role models from my time at the University of Virginia. David Yousem, Thierry Huisman, Aylin Tekes, Ari Blitz, Dheeraj Gandhi, Nafi Aygun, Sachin Gujar, Jay Pillai, Bruce Wasserman, Mike Kraut, Izlem Isbudak, Dorris Lin, Marty Radvany, Philippe Gailloud, among other stellar physicians who trained me at Johns Hopkins.

Thank you to Harris Cohen who allowed me to convince him to hire a neuroradiologist to work at a pediatric hospital, and who throughout the last four and a half years has been a supportive Chairman, mentor, colleague, and friend. To James Wheless, Frederick Boop, Paul Klimo, and my collaborators at the Le Bonheur neuroscience institute, including Amy McGreggor, Stephen Fulton, Sarah Weatherspoon, Paras Bhattarai, Elena Caron, Ehab Dayyat, Masanori Igarashi, Swati Karmarker, Kathryn McVicar, Robin Morgan, Basan Mudigoudar, Namrata Shah, Stephanie Einhaus, Michael Muhlbauer, Lucas Elijovich, as well as Andy Papanicolaou, Roozbeh Rezaie, Shalini Narayana, and Abbas Babajani-Feremi. To Bruce MacDonald for giving me direct clinical feedback on skull base and temporal bone cases, and Jerome Thompson and Jennifer McLevy for their clinical collaborations on complex otolaryngology cases. To Dr. Chris Fleming of the department of Ophthalmology for his clinical collaborations and leadership. To Dr. Barrett Haik, a world class Ophthalmologist and role model in academic medicine, who has also been an important research and academic collaborator. To Zoltan Patay and the team at St. Jude, with whom we collaborate on pediatric neurooncology, not to mention Dr. Patay's ability to serve as the definitive resource on metabolic disorders.

Thank you to all of my radiology colleagues over the last four and a half years in at UTHSC and Le Bonheur; especially Matt Whitehead, a friend and stellar neuroradiologist who I have been lucky enough to work with at several stages of my career, and Adeel Siddiqui who has more recently joined our practice. To the team of pediatric radiologists who serve as colleagues, collaborators, and mentors, including Chandrea Smothers, Lynn Magill, Louis Parvey, Jeff Scrugham, Clint Teague, Nana Sintim-Damoa, Steve Miller (not *that* Steve Miller), Webster Riggs, and Thomas Boulden. To the many additional collaborators and teammates at Le Bonheur, including John Bissler, a collaborator on tuberous sclerosis as well as a leader in clinical and basic research, Eniko Pivnick, Karen Lakin, Jason Johnson, Nadeem Shafi, Regan Williams, Jie Zhang, and Royce Joyner. To the team of pediatric emergency specialists who I work with on a daily basis, led by Dr. Barry Gilmore, and the anesthesiologists who help us take care of patients, who work under the guidance of Dr. Joel Salzman.

Thank you to Tom Naidich, who has given me support and advice since I was in medical school, and served as an inspiration for how to develop as a pediatric neuroradiologist. Similarly, to Jeff Stone who has given me guidance since the start of medical school. To Mauricio Castillo, who served as an outstanding and inspiring leader and mentor during my AJNR editorial fellowship. To Jiro Ono, who has demonstrated that the pursuit of perfection is a never-ending goal requiring dedication, patience, and building an outstanding team. To Grant Achatz, for showing that effective use of technology can augment creativity and artistic expression.

Thank you to my classmates and co-residents throughout this process, in particular Eric von Johnson and Aaron Morrison (the other two musketeers). To Alan Levy, Gustavo Lozada, and others from medical school. To Trey Carr, Rourke Stay, Jimi Obembe, James Stone, Mike Meuse, and Chris Ho, a wonderful set of co-residents (with honorable mention to Jen Marler). To my co-fellows Muzammil Shafi, Sonia Ghei, Dan Hawley, Juan Gomez, Alper Acka, George Kuo, and Anna Nidecker, who helped make my time at Johns Hopkins such an eye-opening and life-changing experience. To all of the students and residents I have had the privilege to work with, teach, and also learn from, including Eric Chin, Chris Oh, and Zachary Abramson. To the technologists who I work with on a daily basis, who allow me to do the work that I do, including (but not limited to!) Will Boon, Lisa McAfee, Ratana Laurie, Megan Carroll, Stacy Pennington, Becky Cooper, Anita Young, Lori Bledsoe, Shawn Holliday, and Jeff Jenkins as well as the child life specialists who work closely with us. To Tracy Tidwell and Karen Butler who go above and beyond to make Le Bonheur such a special place to work. To the hard work and dedicated teammates Lai Brooks, Emily Johnson, Blakely Weatherford, Betsy Axente, and Geri Skelley, who allow Le Bonheur to work so efficiently.

Thank you to Nelson Strother, the dean of admissions at the University of Tennessee medical school who was willing to take a chance on me. To Dean David Stern who oversees the University of Tennessee College of Medicine. To Meri Armour, a hospital CEO who respects the role of radiologists, understands the value of clinician-researchers, and serves as the definition of a leader with vision. She has been responsible for building a world class hospital and pediatric neuroscience institute. I cannot thank her enough for her ever-constant encouragement and support.

Thank you to all of the patients I have had the honor to help care for, and their families. There are so many who have been special to me, including Lucy Krull (who graces the cover of this textbook). Yet, there are so many others whom I am likely anonymous to; hopefully our paths have crossed for the better. It is these children and their families, as well as all of the other children (and future children) out there, who in particular motivated me to write this book.

All of this would not be possible without God's guidance, which has been delivered through all of these wonderful people and the countless more who I would like to thank for helping me gain a skillset that hopefully can benefit others. Through this book, I hope the benefit spreads far beyond the walls of Le Bonheur Children's hospital and the University of Tennessee Health Science Center.

Part 1

Introduction to Pediatric Neuroradiology

1 Imaging Techniques

1.1 Introduction

Appropriate clinical interpretation of pediatric neuroradiologic studies requires an understanding of the imaging techniques they use. Only through this understanding can appropriate tests be performed and subsequently interpreted. A multitude of resources exist to provide this information, but a brief review follows, including several pediatric-specific considerations.

1.2 Radiographs (Plain-Film)

Plain-film evaluation is the foundation of radiology; however, it is not commonly used for modern evaluation of the central nervous system (CNS). Plain-film radiography is still used with shunt-series to detect discontinuity or atypical placement of cerebrospinal fluid (CSF) diversion tubing, such as a ventriculo-peritoneal shunt (▶ Fig. 1.1). In children, radiographs may still be appropriate for evaluation of the spine after trauma. Radiographic evaluation for skull fractures, craniofacial abnormalities, and calvarial suture development is sometimes performed, but its diagnostic performance is inferior to that of computed tomography (CT).

1.3 Ultrasonography

In the newborn period, sonographic evaluation of the intracranial contents can be performed through open fontanelles, most commonly the anterior fontanelle (▶ Fig. 1.2). Evaluation through the posterior fontanelle can also be performed. Ultrasonography is also the primary screening tool for fetal imaging. These techniques, and the pathology evaluated, are further discussed in Chapter 5.

Transcranial Doppler ultrasonography is a technique of interrogation of flow velocities in branches of the circle of Willis and is used to identify abnormal blood-flow patterns in patients with sickle cell disease to determine the timing of transfusions. Ultrasonography is helpful in evaluating the soft tissues of the neck, including muscles, lymph nodes, cystic lesions, and infectious collections.

Prior to ossification of the posterior spinal elements (typically the first 3 months postnatally), the spinal cord can be evaluated with ultrasound to determine the position of the conus medullaris, thickness of the filum terminale, and motility of the cauda equina. Sacral dimples can also be evaluated with ultrasound, to identify the presence of dermal sinus tracts/pilonidal sinus tracts.

1.4 Computed Tomography

Computed tomography is a cross-sectional imaging technique that uses ionizing radiation, is widely available, and provides excellent osseous detail (▶ Fig. 1.3). Soft tissue detail on CT is better visualized than with plain-film radiography but is limited in comparison to that provided by magnetic resonance imaging (MRI). Computed tomography is also the gold standard for detecting acute intracranial hemorrhage after trauma; however, modern MRI is more sensitive for detecting the chronic deposition of blood products/hemosiderin. Because CT is widely available and can be performed rapidly, usually without sedation, it is the mainstay imaging procedure for evaluating acute traumatic and infectious processes. Modern CT scanners can provide sagittal and coronal reformats, which significantly aid in the characterization of abnormalities in the pediatric head and are critical for imaging of the head and neck, as well as the spine. Three-dimensional (3D) reconstructions can be helpful in differentiating calvarial sutures from fractures, differentiating among craniofacial abnormalities, and characterizing complex dysraphisms of the spine.

The density detected on CT is related to the underlying electron density of the evaluated tissue. This is typically evaluated in a visual manner, but it can be evaluated quantitatively, with density values reported in Hounsfield units (HU); see ▶ Table 1.1. For CT, pure water is defined as having a density of 0 HU, and air is defined as having a density of –1000 HU.

1.5 Magnetic Resonance Imaging

Magnetic resonance imaging provides the best noninvasive characterization of the central nervous system (CNS) and soft tissues of the head and neck (▶ Fig. 1.4). Studies done with MRI must be tailored to the patient's specific clinical symptoms, with the selection of specific imaging sequences and acquisition

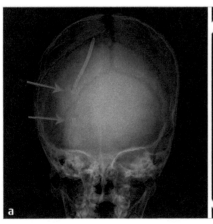
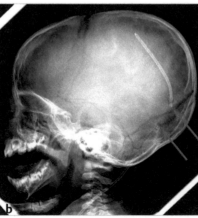

Fig. 1.1 Example of a plain-film image. (a) Anteroposterior and (b) lateral radiographs of the skull in a 9-month-old male show a ventriculostomy catheter, inserted through right parietal approach, with a discontinuity in its extracranial portion (between *red arrows*).

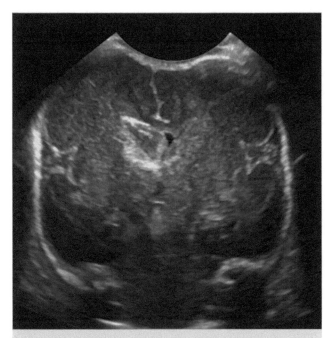

Fig. 1.2 Example of an ultrasound image. Coronal ultrasound image made through the anterior fontanelle in a 6-day-old female; a heterogeneous area of echogenicity in the expected location of the right caudate body, consistent with a focal hemorrhagic venous infarction (grade IV germinal matrix hemorrhage), is seen.

Table 1.1 Density of substances

Substance	Density (HU)
Air	−1000
Fat	−200 to −30
Water	0
Proteinaceous fluid	10 to 30
Acute blood	60 to 80
Muscle	~80
Bone	~600 to 1000
Metal	>1000

to a given sequence can be used; for instance, a hyperintense signal on T1 weighted (T1 W) imaging can be described as T1 shortening, and a hyperintense signal on T2 weighted (T2 W) imaging as T2 prolongation. A hypointense signal on T1 W imaging is T1 prolongation, and a hypointense signal on T2 W imaging is T2 shortening. Familiarity with these terms is helpful in understanding imaging reports produced by other persons, and in understanding journal articles and teaching resources, even if the reader does not choose to use "shortening" and "prolongation" in his or her reports (▶ Table 1.2).

Magnetic resonance imaging uses powerful magnetic fields to manipulate hydrogen protons for obtaining diagnostic information. The stronger the magnet, the better the information obtained. Modern clinical imaging is performed with scanners having a high field strength, with a static magnetic field of either 1.5 or 3.0 teslas. Scanners with higher field strengths than this exist, most commonly for research purposes. Older scanners with lower field strengths still exist, but should only be used if a high-field-strength alternative is unavailable. There also exist "open" MRI scanners, which use a lower field strength and do not circumferentially encompass the area being scanned. Although the concept of an open scanner is appealing from a marketing standpoint, such scanners provide limited diagnostic information in many circumstances and should be avoided unless there is an absolute contraindication to standard MRI.

planes to highlight the suspected pathology. Because MRI is probably the most important tool in evaluation of the pediatric CNS, the basics of different MRI sequences are discussed below. Note that although CT measures electron density, MRI evaluation has more to do with the molecular constituents and the percent of protons that are in free water, proteins, and lipids. A "bright" signal in a given sequence is most accurately described as having a "hyperintense" and not a "hyperdense" appearance. Likewise, a "dark" signal is "hypointense." Other terms related

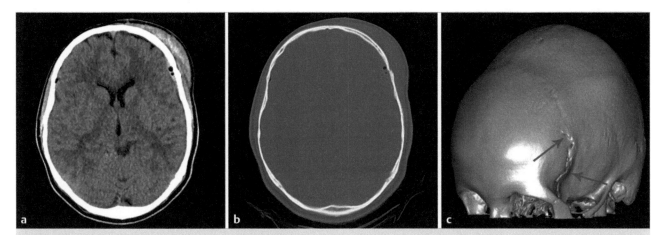

Fig. 1.3 Examples of CT images. (a) Axial CT image of the head, displayed in a soft tissue window, shows an extracranial hematoma overlying the left frontal region, with an intracranial extra-axial (epidural) hematoma. (b) An axial CT bone algorithm image of the head shows a punctate focus of pneumocephalus and an overlying fracture. (c) 3D reconstruction of the skull shows the left frontal fracture (*red arrows*) paralleling the coronal suture.

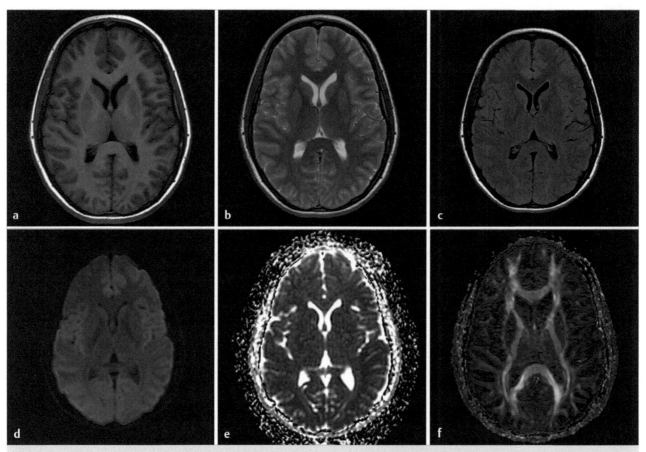

Fig. 1.4 Normal MRI image. (a) Axial T1 W image of the brain in a patient with a mature myelination pattern shows intermediate intensity of the peripheral cortex (gray matter) and relatively hyperintense signal of the white-matter structures. (b) Axial T2 W image of the patient shows a relatively hypointense appearance of the myelinated white matter, intermediate hyperintense appearance of the gray matter, and hyperintense appearance of CSF. (c) Axial FLAIR image shows suppression of the hyperintense signal of CSF as compared with that in the T2 W image. (d) Axial diffusion-weighted image and (e) ADC map. (f) Axial directionally encoded fractional anisotropy map shows the normal white matter anatomy of the brain of the patient, with transversely oriented fibers within the corpus callosum (red), anteroposteriorly directed fibers within the optic radiations (green), and cranio–caudally directed fibers in the posterior limb of the internal capsule, representing fibers of the corticospinal tract.

Table 1.2 Appearance on magnetic resonance imaging of various substances

Substance	T1 W	T2 W	FLAIR
Fat	Bright	Bright	Bright
Water/CSF	Dark	Bright	Dark
Proteinaceous fluid	Intermediate	Intermediate to bright	Intermediate
Methemoglobin	Bright	Dark (extracellular) Bright (intracellular)	Variable
Deoxyhemoglobin	Dark	Bright	Variable
Hemosiderin	Dark	Dark	Dark
Gray matter	Intermediate dark	Intermediate bright	Intermediate bright
White matter (myelinated)	Intermediate bright	Dark	Dark
White matter (unmyelinated)	Intermediate dark	Intermediate bright	Intermediate dark
White matter (incompletely myelinated)	Intermediate bright	Intermediate	Variable/bright

1.5.1 T1 Weighted Imaging

T1 weighted (T1 W) imaging is one of the two primary MRI sequences and is related to the longitudinal relaxation of hydrogen protons. Fat, protein, melanin, and gadolinium are among substances that demonstrate T1 shortening (or "bright" signaling).

1.5.2 T2 Weighted Imaging

T2 weighted (T2 W) imaging is the second of the two primary MRI sequences and is related to the transverse relaxation of hydrogen protons. Pure water is bright in T2 W sequences.

1.5.3 Fluid-attenuated Inversion Recovery

Fluid-attenuated inversion recovery (FLAIR) is an inversion recovery technique used in MRI in which the inversion pulse is timed to null the signal of pure water, and is typically applied to T2 W imaging. The result is a T2 W-like image with nulling of the water signal. This eases the detection of abnormalities in T2 signal (particularly abnormalities adjacent to the ventricles) and is most widely known for its utility in identifying abnormalities in white matter, such as multiple sclerosis. Because FLAIR nulls the signal of normal CSF, any contamination of the CSF, such as by blood products or infectious debris, will become more conspicuous. An absence of FLAIR suppression of the CSF signal within sulci raises concern for meningitis or subarachnoid hemorrhage, although in the pediatric setting it is noted that the two most common causes for this are artifactual. The first of these are heterogeneities in the magnetic field in patients with braces, which results in an artifactual lack of suppression of the CSF signal, most pronounced in the inferior frontal region and middle cranial fossae. Second, in the setting of supplemental oxygenation (usually related to sedation) (▶ Fig. 1.5), the paramagnetic effects of the high dissolved concentrations of oxygen in the CSF alter the properties of FLAIR and can result in decreased suppression of the CSF signal, typically in a posterior-predominant manner.

A FLAIR inversion pulse can also be applied to T1 W sequences, and this technique is used to address difficulties in T1 imaging in MRI at a field strength of 3 teslas. In this book,

and in most other books and journal articles, "FLAIR" means T2 FLAIR unless otherwise specified.

1.5.4 Short-tau Inversion Recovery

Short-tau inversion recovery (STIR) is an MRI technique that has T2 weighting (i.e., fluid is bright) but in which the signal in substances with a short T1 relaxation time (such as fat) is nulled. This is helpful in imaging of the head and neck, such as in infections of the neck, and of the spine, for seeking bone-marrow edema. Note that STIR is not a selective fat-saturation technique, because substances other than fat with short T1 relaxation times may suppress, and at times fat may not suppress. Accordingly, although STIR is helpful for identifying structures adjacent to fat, it should not be used as the means of definitively confirming whether or not something contains fat.

1.5.5 Fat Saturation

Fat-saturation, or fat-suppression, is a modification of a technique that can be applied to T1 W, T2 W, and FLAIR images, nulling the bright signal from fat. This is helpful in T2 W imaging for seeking edema within and around fat, such as in the orbits of the eyes, and in T1 postcontrast imaging for detecting enhancement in and around substances that have intrinsic T1 shortening.

1.5.6 Diffusion-weighted Imaging

Diffusion-weighted imaging (DWI) is an MRI technique that quantifies the Brownian motion of water. Any cause that reduces the ability of water to move will result in "restricted" diffusion, which will be manifested as a "bright" signal in DWI images and a corresponding "dark" signal on apparent diffusion coefficient (ADC) maps, which reflect the degree of diffusion of water molecules through different tissues. This is the gold standard for detecting acute cerebral infarction, but any DWI can detect any cause of reduced water diffusion. For instance, epidermoid cysts are inclusions with densely packed keratin that inhibits the movement of water, thick purulent material within an abscess will demonstrate reduced water diffusion, formed blood clots can have a restricted movement of water, and tumors with a high nuclear-to-cytoplasmic ratio will have

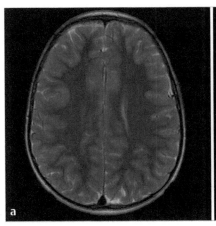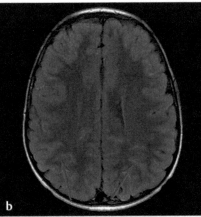

Fig. 1.5 Magnetic resonance image made with sedation. (a) Axial T2 W image of the brain in a 6-year-old male undergoing evaluation for seizures shows a normal appearance of the brain parenchyma and subarachnoid spaces. (b) Axial FLAIR image shows areas of incomplete suppression within the subarachnoid spaces (*red arrows*). The patient demonstrated no signs of meningitis or other possible causes for his seizures, and this incomplete suppression was attributed to the paramagnetic effects of supplemental oxygen administration.

reduced water diffusion because of a relatively lower quantity of cytoplasm in which water can freely move.

1.5.7 Diffusion Tensor Imaging

Diffusion tensor imaging (DTI) is a modified version of DWI that quantifies the degree of nonuniform diffusion of water along different axes. The extent of such nonuniform movement, or anisotropy, can range from zero for purely isotropic movement to 1 for purely unidirectional movement. The ratio of the isotropic movement of water along an axis of diffusion to the maximum value of 1 that represents unidirectional movement along that axis is known as fractional anisotropy (FA). In addition to detecting the degree of anisotropy, DTI can determine the predominant directions of water movement in an anatomic or tissue structure, providing the ability to directionally encode FA maps. The standard color convention for directional encoding of FA maps is to label transverse movement as red (as in the corpus callosum), anterior-posterior movement direction as green (as in the optic radiations), and craniocaudal movement as blue (as in the corticospinal tract in the posterior limb of the internal capsule). Diffusion tensor imaging can be processed to map individual fibers in diffusion tensor fiber tracking (DT–FT), also known as "tractography."

1.5.8 Susceptibility Weighted Imaging

Susceptibility weighted imaging (SWI) is a technique very sensitive to diamagnetic and paramagnetic substances, such as hemosiderin or areas of mineralization, and should be used in all cases in which trauma or hemorrhage may be suspected. T2-star (T2*) imaging, or "gradient" imaging, is an older technique that can be used if SWI is unavailable.

1.5.9 CSF Flow Study

Cerebrospinal fluid flow studies are phase-contrast MRI sequences that quantify the movement of cerebrospinal fluid (CSF). There are three main uses for CSF flow studies. One of them is for characterizing CSF flow dynamics through the foramen magnum in the evaluation of Chiari type I malformations. A second use for CSF flow studies is for evaluating the patency of the aqueduct of Sylvius in cases of suspected aqueductal stenosis. A third use for such studies is in evaluating the patency of an endoscopic third ventriculostomy. However, CSF flow study can also be used to evaluate CSF in other locations, including within arachnoid cysts. Phase contrast can also be used to evaluate blood flow in magnetic resonance angiography (MRA) and magnetic resonance venography (MRV).

1.5.10 Magnetic Resonance Angiography

Magnetic resonance angiography (MRA) is a technique for noninvasive evaluation of the intracranial vasculature. Magnetic resonance angiography of the brain typically does not require intravenous contrast agents, and the most common technique used is a three-dimensional (3D) time-of-flight (TOF) technique. Magnetic resonance angiography of the neck is done either with a 2D TOF technique or through contrast-enhanced MRA. Magnetic

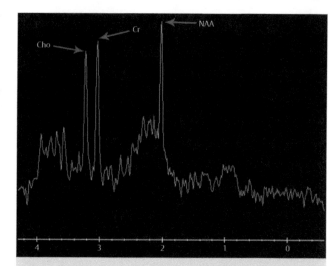

Fig. 1.6 Magnetic resonance spectroscopy. Single-voxel MR spectroscopy of the deep gray nuclei in a 1-year-old child shows the three dominant peaks of choline, creatine, and NAA. (In seismologic terminology, this might be described as a small earthquake with two small aftershocks.)

resonance venography (MRV) of the intracranial vasculature can be perforemd with 2D TOF, phase-contrast, and contrast-enhanced techniques. The spatial resolution of MRA is less than that of CTA and cerebral angiography, but the technique is noninvasive and typically does not require an intravenous contrast agent. Evaluation of vasculature near the skull base is easier with MRA than with CTA because dense bone in the base of the skull can complicate evaluation of this area with CTA.

1.5.11 Magnetic Resonance Spectroscopy

Magnetic resonance spectroscopy (MRS) is a technique that does not result in images but rather in spectroscopic profiles (▶ Fig. 1.6). The main role of MRS is in seeking the presence of normal neuronal substances and those involved in generating energy, including choline (Cho), creatine (Cr), and N-acetyl-aspartate (NAA). Other metabolites, including myoinositol (myoI), glycine, and glutamate (Glx), can also be detected with MRS, and in the presence of anaerobic metabolism, lactate can be detected. Lactate can be present in mitochondrial disorders, after stroke, and in high-grade neoplasms. The primary role for MRS is in suspected metabolic disorders, but it can at times also be used adjunctively in the characterization of tumors (or suspected tumor-like lesions). In tumors, a choline-to-NAA ratio exceeding 2:1 tends to be associated with high-grade neoplasms, as does the presence of lactate. A mild elevation in choline concentration and mild decrease in that of NAA can be seen with a low-grade neoplasm, gliosis, cortical dysplasia, and demyelinating lesions, among other abnormalities (▶ Table 1.3).

1.5.12 Gadolinium

Gadolinium is a T1-shortening agent with seven unpaired valence electrons that does not cross the intact blood–brain barrier (BBB). After its administration, areas of injury to the

Table 1.3 Common peaks of various substances seen on magnetic resonance spectroscopy and the commonly used abbreviations for these substances

Substance	Peak (ppm)	Clinical implications	Comments
Choline (Cho)	3.2	Marker of cellular proliferation, elevated in high-grade tumors	
Creatine (Cr)	3.0	Marker of cellular energy usage, relatively preserved peak height (internal control)	
N-Acetyl-aspartate (NAA)	2.0	Marker of neuronal integrity, decreased in tumors, also decreased at birth, elevated in Canavan disease	
Glutamate/glutamine (Glx) and γ-aminobutyric acid (GABA)	2.2–2.4		
Myoinositol (myoI)	3.5		Best seen at short TE (e.g., 35 msec)
Glycine (Gly)	3.5	Elevated in glycemic encephalopathy	Overlays with myoI, does not fade at long TE
Lactate (Lac)	1.33	Present in the setting of anaerobic metabolism (such as stroke/hypoxic–ischemic encephalopathy, mitochondrial disorders)	Doublet peak, inverted at long echo
Lipid	1.3	Will be present if bone marrow from adjacent calvarium is included by accident	

BBB (such as in the setting of infection) will show T1 shortening. Enhancement following the administration of gadolinium can be seen with many tumors as well as with leaky capillaries or injury to the BBB, but this does not necessarily mean that there is hyperemia, as is further discussed in Chapter 8. Post-gadolinium enhancement is seen on T1 W imaging; however, gadolinium has no appreciable effect on T2 W imaging (except at very high concentrations). It is worth noting that the use of gadolinium chelates is contraindicated in acute, severe, and dialysis-dependent renal failure because of the risk of nephrogenic systemic fibrosis.[1]

1.6 Other

1.6.1 Nuclear Medicine

Nuclear medicine in pediatric neuroradiology is predominantly related either to the evaluation of seizures or of cerebral blood flow during assessments of brain death. In patients with seizures, imaging via single-photon emission computed tomography with a tracer consisting of 99m-technetium-containing hexamethyl propylene amine oxime (HMPAO SPECT) (see Chapter 9) characterizes cerebral perfusion. When the injection of HMPAO is done during an interictal period, epileptogenic cortex is commonly hypoperfused in comparison to normal parenchyma. When the injection is done shortly after the onset of a seizure, there is ictal hyperemia, which can help confirm the location of the epileptogenic cortex. If SPECT is available both ictally and interictally, subtraction imaging can be done, in addition to fusion with CT or MRI data to help in treatment planning. Positron emission tomography (PET) can also be used for interictal seizure evaluation, as well as in the neuro-oncology setting.

1.6.2 Angio/Interventional

Image-guided procedures may be required in children, just as in adults, for both diagnosis and treatment. Endovascular procedures, image-guided biopsies and drain placements, and image-guided lumbar punctures can all be performed. Despite advances in noninvasive vascular imaging, digital subtraction angiography (DSA) remains unsurpassed in spatial and temporal resolution for the evaluation of dissections, occlusions, vasospasm, and vasculopathies. Computed tomography-guided biopsies and drainages may reduce the need for open surgical procedures, including those done for vertebral and paravertebral lesions, and for infectious collections in the head and neck.

1.6.3 Sedation

Depending on the age and clinical condition of the patient, the imaging modality being used, and the required level of detail, sedation may be required during an imaging procedure. Plain films are very rapid and rarely require sedation. Computed tomographic scans may require sedation, especially if detail is required for a study, such as a CT angiogram. Magnetic resonance imaging scans can take from 20 to 60 minutes, or even longer, and young children will nearly always require some sedation during these procedures. Interventional procedures, whether vascular, biopsies and drainages, or image-guided lumbar punctures, will also commonly require sedation. Sedation for young children is not something to be taken lightly, and its use requires appropriate training; readers who are unsure about having the appropriate training and availability of resources are unlikely to be in a position to sedate a child.

1.6.4 Braces

Braces and other dental hardware are commonly encountered in pediatric (adolescent) neuroradiology, often when the latter is related to the evaluation of seizures and/or headaches; in contrast, such hardware is rarely encountered in adult neuroradiology. Braces may result in signal loss (▶ Fig. 1.7), spatial distortion, and banding artifacts in MRI, and may alter the magnetic field, with the result being a heterogeneous application of inversion–recovery pulses or fat-suppression techniques. In patients with brain tumors, it is occasionally necessary to have dental braces removed to optimize surgical planning and disease surveillance.

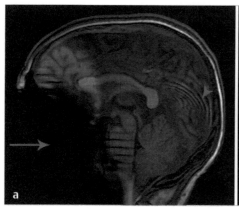 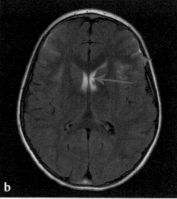

Fig. 1.7 Magnetic resonance image of a patient with braces. (a) Sagittal T1 W image in a 10-year-old female with headaches shows marked signal dropout in the region of the face (*red arrow*) related to braces. A banding artifact (*red arrowhead*) is also seen away from the braces as the result of distortion of the posterior banding. (b) Axial FLAIR image at the level of the body of the lateral ventricles shows incomplete FLAIR suppression of signal within the frontal horns and anterior body of the lateral ventricles (*red arrow*) and in the subarachnoid space (*red arrowhead*).

1.6.5 Functional Magnetic Resonance Imaging

Functional MRI (fMRI) is a technique that detects areas of cortical activation during a task, typically either a motor or language task. It is a helpful technique in surgical planning for patients with tumors or focal/lesion-based epilepsy. The proper performance of fMRI requires patient cooperation, which can be difficult with adolescents and is typically impossible with infants and young children. Functional MRI can be done on sedated patients for motor mapping in young children[2] through passive movement. Recent work has also shown the ability to perform receptive language mapping in sedated children through passive listening tasks.[3,4]

1.7 Radiation Safety and Dose Optimization

Radiation exposure carries a risk of cellular damage and the possible induction of neoplasia. The neoplastic risks of radiation exposure are difficult to exactly calculate but are known to be higher in children because of the more active cell division in their bodies (with cell division being the time when cells are most susceptible to damage to their DNA) and to a typically longer postscan life span during which tumors may arise. Accordingly, the use of ionizing radiation must be carefully considered before any radiologic study is done, and, when possible, alternative imaging modalities, such as ultrasound and MRI, should be considered. When the use of ionizing radiation is deemed appropriate, or is otherwise unavoidable, dose settings optimized for the size of the patient must be used. Because young children are smaller than adults, lower radiation settings may

be required for appropriate imaging in this patient population. Recognition of the potential risks of radiation, and the benefits of pediatric-specific radiation dose profiles, attempts to reduce or avoid modalities with ionizing radiation, and increased use of modalities with low or no ionizing radiation are the central themes of the Image Gently campaign.[5]

1.8 See the Patient in Person

At times, the most important imaging technique for a pediatric patient is seeing the patient in person. This can clarify a clinical question for which imaging is being considered, particularly if it is to be used for evaluating a superficial lesion or palpable finding. Despite the allure of advanced imaging technology, it should be remembered that the patient, and the patient's family, may hold more information than the most complex MRI scan, or at least facilitate the greatest information to be obtained from imaging studies.

References

[1]   Yang L, Krefting I, Gorovets A et al. Nephrogenic systemic fibrosis and class labeling of gadolinium-based contrast agents by the Food and Drug Administration. Radiology 2012; 265(1):248–253

[2]   Choudhri AF, Patel RM, Whitehead MT, Siddiqui A, Wheless JW. Cortical activation through passive-motion functional MRI. Am J Neuroradiol 2015 Sep;36(9):1675-1681. doi: 10.3174/ajnr.A4345

[3]   Suarez RO, Taimouri V, Boyer K et al. Passive fMRI mapping of language function for pediatric epilepsy surgical planning: validation using Wada, ECS, and FMAER. Epilepsy Res 2014; 108(10):1874–1888

[4]   Rezaie R, Narayana S, Schiller K et al. Assessment of hemispheric dominance for receptive language in pediatric patients under sedation using magnetoencephalography. Front Hum Neurosci 2014; 8:657

[5]   Goske MJ, Applegate KE, Boylan J et al. The Image Gently campaign: working together to change practice. AJR Am J Roentgenol 2008; 190(2):273–274

Part 2

Brain Imaging

2 Anatomy and Development

2.1 Introduction

Neuroradiology requires a detailed understanding of neuro-anatomy and its associated functions. The relationship between function and structure in neuroradiolopgy is less intuitive than, for instance, in musculoskeletal or cardiac imaging. With an appreciation for neuroanatomy, in conjunction with an understanding of pathophysiology and imaging technology (and its limitations), most neuroradiologic diagnoses can be approached in a logical manner. Within pediatric neuroradiology, the embryologic underpinnings of neuroanatomy become important, as does the process of normal myelination. This chapter addresses the basics of brain development and anatomy to serve as the foundation for additional chapters in this book. Further discussion of neuronal proliferation, migration, and organization is addressed in Chapter 3, and neurovascular anatomy is addressed in Chapter 12. Anatomy of the skull bones is presented in Chapter 15, and anatomy of the pituitary gland is addressed Chapter 13.

2.2 Basics of Embryology

The brain develops from the rostral neural tube first as a three-part structure during week four of gestation, and then as a five-part structure in week six of gestation (▶ Table 2.1). In the transition from a brain of three parts to a brain of five parts, the most rostral aspect (the prosencephalon) of the brain differentiates into the telencephalon and diencephalon. The mesencephalon remains the mesencephalon, and the more caudal rhombencephalon differentiates into the metencephalon and myelencephalon.

2.3 Basics of Neuroanatomy: Hemispheres, Lobes, and Gyri

The largest part of the human brain is the two cerebral hemispheres, which are divided into four lobes; frontal, parietal,

temporal, and occipital (▶ Fig. 2.1). The brainstem, including the midbrain, pons, and medulla, connects the cerebral hemispheres to the cerebellum and spinal cord. The cerebellum is separated from the cerebral hemiheres by a thick layer of connective tissue (dura) known as the tentorium cerebelli. The two cerebral hemispheres are separated by the falx cerebri and are connected by several commissures. Commissures are bundles of white matter that connect the hemispheres, with the largest commissure being the corpus callosum (▶ Fig. 2.2). Additional commissures include the anterior commissure, posterior commissure, habenular commissure, and hippocampal commissure.

The frontal lobes are commonly stated to be associated with emotion; however, the posterior aspect of the frontal lobes (the precentral gyrus) represents primary motor cortex. The precentral gyrus is along the anterior margin of the central sulcus (▶ Fig. 2.1), and the postcentral gyrus of the parietal lobes is along the posterior aspect of the central sulcus. The postcentral gyrus represents the location of primary sensory cortex. Collectively, the pre- and postcentral gyri are known as the peri-rolandic cortex, a highly eloquent area of the brain.

The frontal lobes anterior to the precentral gyrus can be divided into the superior, middle, and inferior frontal gyri (▶ Fig. 2.3). Along the inferior margin of the frontal lobe are anteriorly–posteriorly directed gyri, of which the gyrus rectus is the most medial (adjacent to the olfactory bulb), and lateral to this are the medial and lateral orbital gyri. The orbital gyri may be difficult to uniquely identify, depending upon the location. The orbital gyri are best seen on coronal images; however, they may be difficult to identify, as their appearance is different anteriorly than posteriorly.

The segments of the temporal lobe are best depicted on a coronal image, with the superior, middle, and inferior temporal gyri forming the lateral margin of the temporal lobe, and with the occipitotemporal (a.k.a. fusiform) gyrus and parahippocampal gyrus being located inferiorly. The parahippocampal gyrus is adjacent to the hippocampus. Along the anterior aspect of the temporal horn of the lateral ventricle is the amygdala, and the medial projection of the temporal lobe is the uncus (▶ Fig. 2.3). An additional gyrus is the transverse temporal gyrus, also known as Heschl's gyrus, which courses between the posterior insula and the superior temporal gyrus. Heschl's gyrus is involved in auditory processing, and language reception (Wernicke's area) is typically located within the posterior aspect of the left superior temporal gyrus. The capacity for expressive language (Broca's area) is typically located within the left inferior frontal gyrus, particularly in portions of this gyrus known as the pars opercularis and pars triangularis. Receptive and expressive language are connected by a bundle of white matter known as the arcuate fasciculus.

Behind the postcentral gyrus, the parietal lobe can be divided into the superior and inferior parietal lobules. Within the inferior parietal lobules are subareas known as the angular and supramarginal gyri (▶ Fig. 2.1). Located posteriorly and inferiorly to the parieto-occipital sulcus, as seen on a midsagittal image, is the occipital lobe. Within the occipital lobe is the calcarine fissure (▶ Fig. 2.4), which is lined by primary visual cortex. The wedge-shaped area between the parieto-occipital sulcus and calcarine fissure is known as the cuneus.

Table 2.1 Embryologic origins of structures

Three-part	Five-part	Mature
Prosencephalon	Telencephalon	Cerebral cortex and white matter, caudate nucleus, putamen, globus pallidus
	Diencephalon	Thalamus, hypothalamus, subthalamus, epithalamus (pineal gland)
Mesencephalon	Mesencephalon	Midbrain tectum (superior and inferior colliculi), substantia nigra, red nuclei, cranial nerves III and IV
Rhombencephalon	Metencephalon	Pons, cerebellum, cranial nerves V–VIII
	Myelencephalon	Medulla, cranial nerves IX–XII (and parts of VIII)

Data from Gilroy A, MacPherson B, Ross L. Neuroanatomy: Brain. In: Gilroy A, MacPherson B, Ross L, eds. Atlas of Anatomy. 2nd ed. New York, NY, Thieme, 2012, p 625.

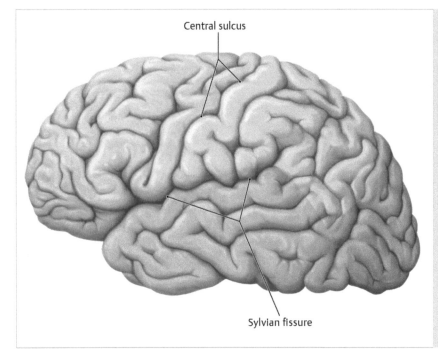

Central sulcus

Sylvian fissure

Fig. 2.1 Lobes of the brain. This lateral projection image shows the relationship of the lobes of the brain. The frontal lobe (green) is separated from the parietal lobe (yellow) by the central sulcus. The frontal and parietal lobes are separated from the temporal lobe (light blue) by the sylvian fissure. Posteriorly is the occipital lobe (red). (From Atlas of Anatomy, © Thieme 2012, Illustration by Karl Wesker.)

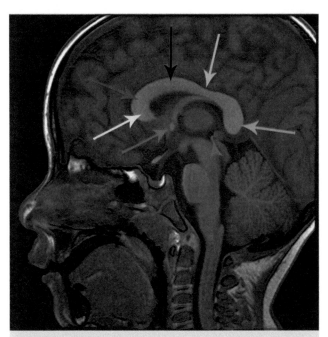

Fig. 2.2 Commissural anatomy of the brain. This sagittal T1 W image shows the corpus callosum, including its subparts, consisting of the rostrum (*yellow arrow*), genu (*purple arrow*), body (*black arrow*), isthmus (*green arrow*), and splenium (*blue arrow*). The anterior commissure (*red arrow*) and the posterior commissure (*red arrowhead*) are visible. The hippocampal commissure is inseparable from the splenium of the corpus callosum, resulting in focal thickening. Between the posterior commissure and the splenium of the corpus callosum is the pineal gland.

The deep gray nuclei include the caudate nuclei, the putamina, and the globi palladi. The putamen and globus pallidus are collectively referred to as the lentiform nuclei. The lentiform nuclei and the globus pallidus are separated from one another by the anterior limb of the internal capsule, a set of white-matter bundles (albeit with internal gray-matter bridges). The lentiform nucleus is posteriorly bounded by the posterior limb of the internal capsule (PLIC), behind which is the thalamus (▶ Fig. 2.5). Beneath the globi palladi are the hypothalami (▶ Fig. 2.6). The hypothalami join at the midline at the level of the infundibular stalk, which continues inferiorly to the pituitary gland. Posterior to the medial aspect of the thalami and projecting posteriorly into the interhemispheric fissure is the pineal gland, above the posterior commissure (▶ Fig. 2.7).

The PLIC carries the corticospinal tracts, which are primary motor tracts of the body. The posterior portion (retrolenticular portion) of the PLIC contains the optic tracts. The corticospinal tracts descend into the brainstem through the cerebral peduncles, a part of the midbrain. From there, they descend into the pons and medulla. Within the ventral medulla, fibers of the corticospinal tracts decussate within the medullary pyramids, after which they descend to the spinal cord.

The cerebellum is connected to the brainstem by three pairs of peduncles, the superior, middle, and inferior peduncles. The middle cerebellar peduncle is the largest white-matter bundle in the body, with more fibers than the spinal cord or the corpus callosum. The two cerebellar hemispheres are separated in the middle by the vermis, which forms the posterior margin (or "roof") of the fourth ventricle. A normally developed vermis has an appearance similar to the "Pac-Man" video game character when viewed on sagittal images.

The posteriormost portion of the midbrain is the tectal plate, comprising the two superior colliculi (involved in visual coordination) and the two inferior colliculi (involved in auditory processing). Because there are four colliculi in total, the tectal plate is sometimes known as the quadrigeminal (i.e., "four brothers") plate.

Within the cerebral hemispheres, the periphery is composed of gray matter, also known as the cerebral cortex. Gray matter

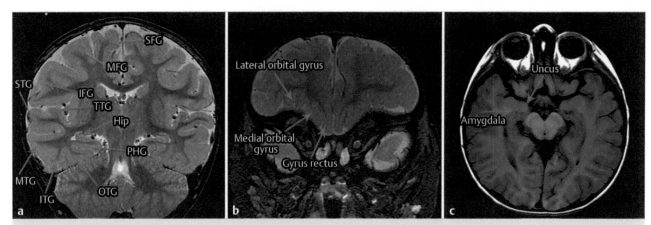

Fig. 2.3 Frontal and temporal anatomy of the brain. (a) A coronal STIR image shows the anatomy of the frontal and temporal lobes. Within the frontal lobes are the superior, middle, and inferior frontal gyri (SFG, MFG, and IFG, respectively). Within the temporal lobe are the the superior, middle, inferior, and transverse temporal gyri (STG, MTG, ITG, and TTG respectively), followed by the occipitotemporal gyrus (OTG) and parahippocampal gyrus (PHG), adjacent to the hippocampus (Hip). (b) A coronal STIR image of the anterior frontal lobes shows the gyrus rectus (GR), and the medial and lateral orbital gyri. (c) An axial T1 W image shows the uncus of the temporal lobe and the amygdala.

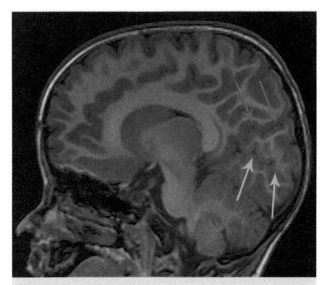

Fig. 2.4 Occipital anatomy of the brain. Parasagittal T1 W image shows the parieto-occipital sulcus (*red arrows*), which separates the parietal lobe from the occipital lobe. Within the occipital lobe is the calcarine fissure (*green arrows*). Between these two landmarks is a wedge-shaped area known as the cuneus.

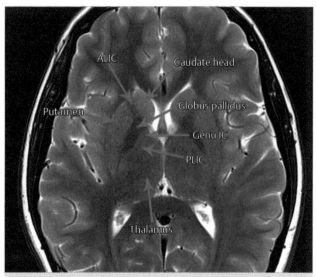

Fig. 2.5 Deep gray matter of the brain. Sagittal T2 W image shows the substructures of the deep gray nuclei, including the head of the caudate nucleus, globus pallidus, putamen, and thalami. These are separated by the anterior limb, genu, and posterior limbs of the internal capsule (ALIC, Genu IC, and PLIC, respectively).

represents neurons and cell bodies that perform the functions of the brain. Deep to this there is white matter, which represents the connections to different parts of the brain and body. White-matter fibers include commissural fibers, which travel to the opposite hemisphere; association fibers, which travel within a given hemisphere; and projection fibers, which extend to the deep gray nuclei, the brainstem/cerebellum, or the spinal cord.

The white matter of the brain can be approximately subdivided into juxtacortical and deep white matter, with periventricular white matter forming a subset of deep white matter. Some sources state that the white matter can be divided into subareas known as the centrum semiovale and corona radiata on the basis of its relationship to the level of the lateral ventri-

cles; however, this is incorrect. Formally speaking, the corona radiata represents the white-matter fibers that extend superiorly from the internal capsule, regardless of their relationship to the level of the lateral ventricle. The centrum semiovale is synonymous with cerebral white matter, which is also independent of the relationship with the lateral ventricle.

2.3.1 Ventricles and Cerebrospinal Fluid Spaces

The ventricular system is a collection of ependyma-lined CSF spaces within the brain. The two lateral ventricles communicate

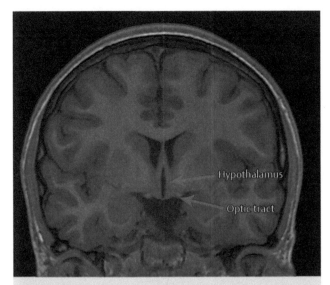

Fig. 2.6 Anatomy of the hypothalamus. Coronal T1 W image shows the hypothalamus along the lateral margin of the third ventricle. Infero-lateral to the hypothalamus are the optic tracts.

with the third ventricle through the foramina of Monro, which communicate with the fourth ventricle through the aqueduct of Sylvius. Outflow of CSF from the fourth ventricle can occur inferiorly through the foramen of Magendie, and laterally through the foramina of Luschka (▶ Fig. 2.8). This is further discussed in Chapter 11.

The superficial CSF space, the subarachnoid space, overlies the pia-lined brain surface. The areas within the subarachnoid space where the pia mater and arachnoid membrane are not closely approximated with one another can be subdivided at times to provide improved anatomic description, and they are often referred to as cisterns (collections of fluid). Superior to the sella turcica is the suprasellar cistern. Around the midbrain are the

perimesencephalic cisterns, including the anterolateral crural cisterns, the ambient cisterns laterally, and the quadrigeminal cistern posteriorly. Between the pons and the internal auditory canals, and anterior to the cerebellum, is the cerebellopontine angle cistern, and ventral to the pons is the prepontine cistern. Along the lateral aspect of the medulla are the lateral medullary cisterns, and below the cerebellar vermis is the cisterna magna.

2.3.2 Development and Anatomy of the Corpus Callosum

The corpus callosum is the dominant forebrain commissure in humans, and it is a white-matter structure containing fibers connecting the cerebral hemispheres. The anatomy and function of the corpus callosum are often misunderstood, but a summary of their key points does not have to be overly complicated. The corpus callosum is a hook-shaped structure that can be subdivided into different parts, including the rostrum, genu, body, isthmus, and splenium (▶ Fig. 2.2). A common misconception is that the rostrum forms last during development, but this is incorrect. The fibers within the corpus callosum are homotopic commissural fibers, meaning that they connect areas of one hemisphere with the identical points in these areas in the contralateral hemisphere. The rostrum contains fibers of the inferior frontal lobes, and the genu contains fibers from the frontal poles. The body of the corpus callosum is predominantly composed of fibers from the frontal lobes. The isthmus of the corpus callosum contains perirolandic and parietal fibers, and the splenium carries fibers from the occipital lobes. The white-matter tracts within the corpus callosum also have other names, and the fibers connecting the frontal poles of the hemispheres through the genu are known as the forceps minor, and the fiber bundles connecting the occipital poles through the splenium are known as the forceps major. The splenium of the corpus callosum also carries fibers of the hippocampal commissure.

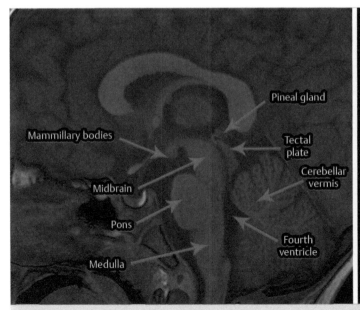

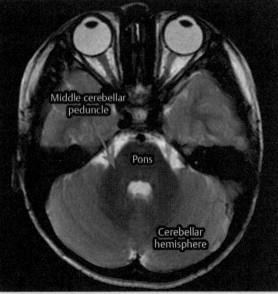

Fig. 2.7 Brainstem anatomy. (a) Sagittal T1 W image shows the structure of the brainstem, including the midbrain, pons, and medulla. Anterior to the midbrain are the mammillary bodies, and the posterior portion of the midbrain is the tectal plate. Behind the pons is the fourth ventricle, and posterior to that is the cerebellar vermis. (b) Axial T2 W image shows the pons connected to the cerebellar hemispheres by the middle cerebellar peduncles.

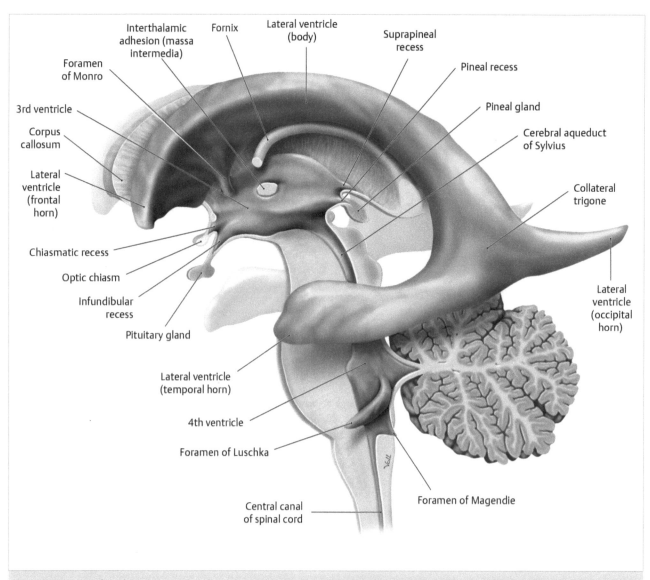

Fig. 2.8 Ventricles of the brain. (From Atlas of Anatomy, © Thieme 2012, Illustration by Karl Wesker.)

Anyone with an interest in learning more about the corpus callosum is directed to an excellent review article by Professor Raybaud.[1]

2.4 Myelination

Understanding myelination does not have to be as complicated as it is often made out to be. Myelination is often taught and assessed in a pattern-matching approach, or through tables. However, the easiest way to appropriately understand the imaging appearance of ongoing myelination is probably to first discuss the structure and function of myelin, and then the anatomy and function of the various white-matter pathways.

Unmyelinated white matter has a very high water content, and its signal characteristics on MRI are therefore dominated by the appearance of water, which is hypointense on T1 W and hyperintense on T2 W images (T1 and T2 prolongation). Myelin is a proteolipid, composed approximately of (70%) lipid and (30%) protein. Both protein and lipids tend to have intrinsic T1

shortening, and the presence of the myelin proteolipids in a given pathway is accompanied by T1 shortening. Mature myelin forms tightly wrapped hydrophobic layers around axons (▶ Fig. 2.9), decreasing the relative percent of the extracellular space that is occupied by water, and for this reason (among others) mature myelin has a hypointense T2 W signal (T1 and T2 shortening). More than 80% of unmyelinated white matter in the neonate consists of water, which declines to approximately 70% in maturely myelinated white matter.

In the transition between unmyelinated axons (T1 and T2 prolongation) to maturely mylinated axons (T1 and T2 shortening), there is a phase marked by the presence of immature myelin and myelin proteolipid precursors, which result in T1 shortening. Because the immature myelin proteolipids do not have a markedly decreased water content, the T2 W hyperintense signal remains. For this reason, T1 W hyperintense signal in a given location (representing the presence of myelin proteolipids) occurs approximately 3 months prior to the T2 W hypointense signal (representing the reduced water content of

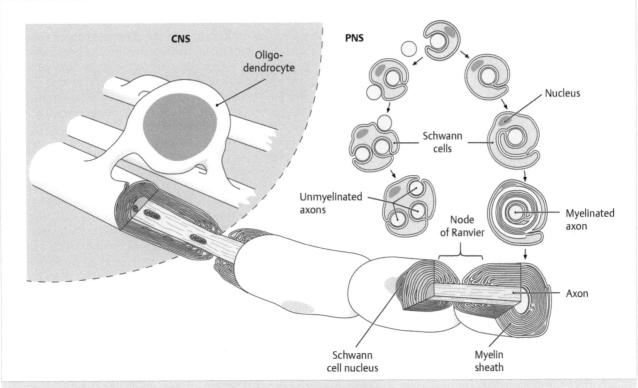

Fig. 2.9 Myelination. (From Atlas of Anatomy, © Thieme 2012, Illustration by Karl Wesker.)

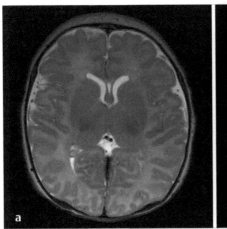
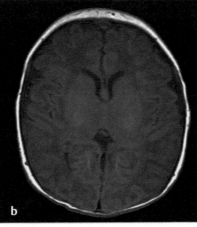

Fig. 2.10 Newborn myelination. (a) Axial T2 W image in a newborn shows a focus of hypointense signal in the posterior aspect of the PLIC, as well as in the VPL of the thalamus, and a mildly hypointense signal in the posterior lentiform nucleus. (b) T1 W image shows a similar pattern, minimally more progressed than the T2 W image.

mature myelin). It is relevant to note that the T2 W hypointense signal, indicating mature myelin, corresponds with an increase in fractional anisotropy related to decreased movement of water perpendicular to the long-axis of nerve fibers (radial diffusion) rather than along the long-axis (axial diffusion).

Once it is known why signal changes occur, it is only necessary to know where to look.[2]

A full-term infant will have T2 hypointense signal within the posterior aspect of the PLIC, and in the posterior lentiform nucleus and ventroposterolateral nucleus (VPL) of the thalamus (▶ Fig. 2.10). During the next few months after the infant's birth, the T2 hypointense signal extends anteriorly toward the genu of the internal capsule, and then toward the anterior limb of the internal capsule. At approximately 3 months of neonatal age, the splenium of the corpus callosum begins to myelinate, predominantly in a posterior to anterior manner, until approximately 9 months of age (▶ Fig. 2.11). Age-related sequential myelination in the first 2 years of life, the time of most active myelination, can be seen in ▶ Fig. 2.12, ▶ Fig. 2.13, ▶ Fig. 2.14, ▶ Fig. 2.15, ▶ Fig. 2.16, ▶ Fig. 2.17, and ▶ Fig. 2.18.

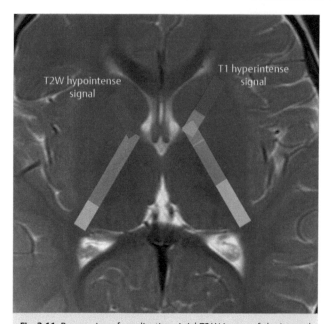

Fig. 2.11 Progression of myelination. Axial T2 W image of the internal capsule with overlays, showing the approximate time course of a T2 hypointense appearance (right side) and T1 hyperintense appearance (left side). The colors represent the approximate appearances of the signal changes for a term newborn (white), at 3 months of age (blue), at 6 months of age (green), and at 9 months of age (red).

The fibers within the PLIC, largely related to the corticospinal tracts, can be followed superiorly to the perirolandic cortex. Along the lateral margin of the occipital horns of the lateral ventricles, myelination can be seen within the optic radiations.

The occipital deep white matter begins to myelinate in the first few months of life, progressing anteriorly to the parietal and then to the frontal lobes over the first 2 to 3 years of life. Within a given region, the deep white matter myelinates before the juxtacortical white matter.

Myelination within given areas corresponds to associated developmental milestones. For instance, the progression of myelination in the PLIC is associated with motor control of the face, and then of the upper extremities (crawling) and later the body and lower extremities (walking). Myelination in the occipital lobe is related to the developing capacity for visual processing. This is followed by myelination in the temporal lobe and the development of language and memory skills. Later, the frontal lobes myelinate, which corresponds to the development of a personality and social awareness. Myelination in the corpus callosum occurs predominantly in a posterior-to-anterior manner (▶ Fig. 2.19), with the maturation of this myelination corresponding to the pattern of myelination in the lobes from which the fibers of the corpus callosum originate. For instance, the fibers in the splenium of the corpus callosum are predominantly fibers connecting the occipital lobes. The body and isthmus of the corpus contain fibers that connect the parietal

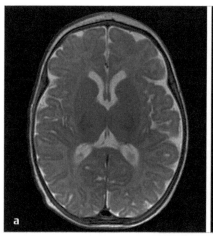
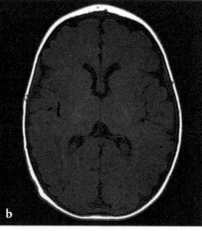

Fig. 2.12 Extent of myelination at 2 months of age. (a) Axial T2 W image shows hypointense signal in the posterior half of the PLIC, with some hypointense signal seen along the optic radiations. (b) T1 W image shows hyperintense signal involving most of the PLIC, as well as the optic radiations.

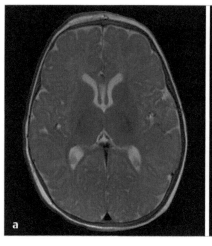
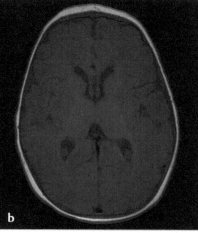

Fig. 2.13 Extent of myelination at 4 months. (a) Axial T2 W image shows hypointense signal along the entire PLIC, and early hypointense signal in the ALIC. (b) T1 W image shows hyperintense signal throughout the internal capsule.

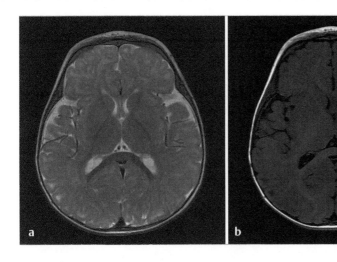

Fig. 2.14 Extent of myelination at 6 months. (a) Axial T2 W image shows hypointense signal throughout the entire internal capsule and within the splenium of the corpus callosum. (b) T1 W image shows hyperintense signal throughout the PLIC and in the occipital deep white matter, and early changes in the frontal white matter.

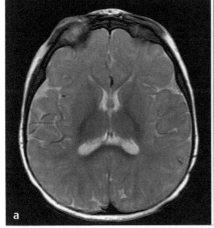 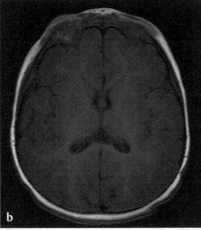

Fig. 2.15 Extent of myelination at 9 months. (a) Axial T2 W image shows early hypointense signal in the lateral aspects the genu of the corpus callosum and in the occipital deep white mater. Note that the occipital juxtacortical white matter remains hyperintense. (b) Axial T1 W image shows hyperintense signal in the frontal deep white matter and in the deep and juxtacortical white matter of the occipital lobes.

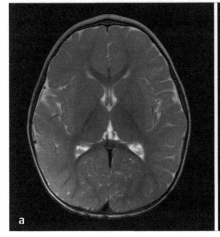 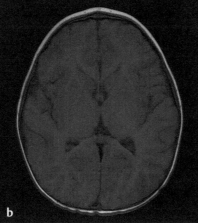

Fig. 2.16 Extent of myelination at 12 months. (a) Axial T2 W image shows hypointense signal in the occipital juxtacortical white matter and frontal deep white matter, and the genu of the corpus callosum has hypointense signal corresponding with myelination. (b) T1 W image shows early myelination of the frontal juxtacortical white matter.

and posterior frontal lobes. The genu of the corpus callosum contains fibers that connect the anterior frontal lobes.

Recognizing the normal pattern of myelination can aid in determining whether myelination in a particular patient is age-appropriate. It is important to be aware of a patient's gestational age when assessing myelination, because, for example, a pre-mature infant born at 28 weeks' gestation (i.e., 12 weeks early) and on whom an MRI is done at 3 months of age will have a myelination pattern that is likely to closely resemble that expected of a term infant. The myelination pattern in this patient is therefore delayed for the patient's chronologic age, although it is appropriate for the patient's corrected gestational age.

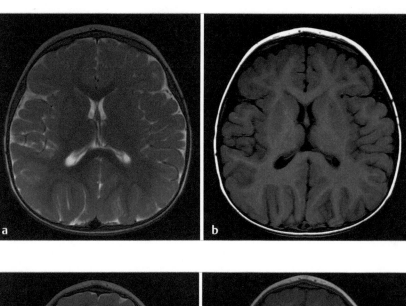

Fig. 2.17 Extent of myelination at 18 months. (a) Axial T2 W image shows hypointense signal throughout the cerebral hemispheres, but close attention reveals that the gray–white differentiation in the frontal lobes is less clear than in the occipital lobes, owing to incomplete frontal juxtacortical myelination. (b) T1 W image shows a nearly complete myelination pattern.

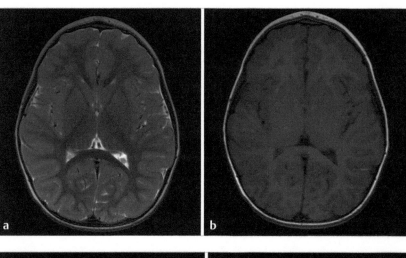

Fig. 2.18 Extent of myelination at 24 months. (a) Axial T2 W image shows improved definition of the frontal gray–white differentiation and a nearly mature myelination pattern, as is also seen in (b) the T1 W image. Note that with very-high-resolution imaging, the frontal juxtacortical white matter will continue to mature until 8 to 10 years of age, and histopathologic studies show subtle maturation continuing into adolescence.

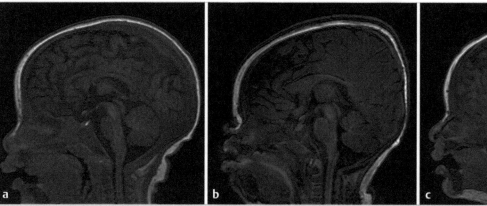
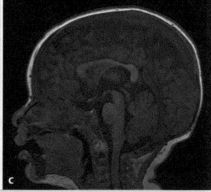

Fig. 2.19 Myelination of the corpus callosum. Midsagittal T1 W images of the corpus callosum in three different patients at 2, 4, and 6 months of age. (a) At 2 months of age the corpus callosum is hypointense and a majority of the brainstem is hypointense. (b) At 4 months the isthmus and posterior body of the corpus callosum are hyperintense, as are portions of the splenium. Note that there is a transient midsplenial area of incomplete myelination at approximately 4 months of age. (c) At 6 months the corpus callosum is nearly completely myelinated, as is the brainstem.

References

[1] Raybaud C. The corpus callosum, the other great forebrain commissures, and the septum pellucidum: anatomy, development, and malformation. Neuroradiology 2010; 52(6):447–477.

[2] Guleria S, Kelly TG. Myelin, myelination, and corresponding magnetic resonance imaging changes. Radiol Clin North Am 2014; 52(2):227–239.

3 Supratentorial Malformations

3.1 Introduction

Multiple malformations of development of the supratentorial parenchyma constitute some of the fundamental, as well as challenging and possibly confusing, aspects of pediatric neuroradiology. Understanding these entities requires some appreciation of embryology and genetics.

The mature cerebral cortex has six neuronal layers, which are formed through a complex developmental process. Cells originate within the germinal matrix of the cerebral cortex, which is located along the margins of the lateral ventricles ("neuronal proliferation"), after which time they move to the periphery ("neuronal migration") and then form an organized cortex ("neuronal organization"). Abnormalities in each of these stages of cortical development can result in characteristic abnormalities. Although the sequence of proliferation, migration, and organization of cortical neurons is stepwise for a given neuron, each of these three processes will at most times and to some degree be taking place simultaneously with the others.

3.2 Malformations from Abnormalities in Neuronal Proliferation

Neuronal proliferation occurs early in gestation, with the three-part brain from week 4 differentiating into five secondary vesicles during week 6, with subsequent histogenesis. In the most simplistic manner of description, abnormalities in proliferation can result in too many cells, too few cells, or abnormal cells.

The prototype abnormality with the occurrence of too many cells is hemimegalencephaly, a condition in which there is hamartomatous/dysplastic overgrowth of an entire cerebral hemisphere (▸ Fig. 3.1). The lateral ventricle in the abnormal hemisphere is typically larger than the ventricle in the contralateral hemisphere, and the abnormal hemisphere has altered blood flow resulting in accelerated myelination. Other abnormalities, including heterotopia and polymicrogyria, can also occur in hemimegalencephaly. Hemimegalencephaly can present with intractable seizures, and may require functional hemispherectomy for seizure control. Although the overgrowth in the condition typically involves an entire hemisphere, subhemispheric variants can occur. Furthermore, because the areas of overgrowth have many cells that are dysplastic, hemimegalencephaly overlaps with cortical dysplasia.

A focal area of proliferation of abnormal cells will result in cortical dysplasia. Focal cortical dysplasia (FCD) is divided into three types, each of which is further subdivided. Type I cortical dysplasia involves abnormal radial lamination (type IA), abnormal tangential lamination (type IB), or both (type IC).[1] Type II cortical dysplasia has dysmorphic neurons.[1,2] Subtype IIB (also called Taylor-type dysplasia) has dysmorphic neurons with balloon cells, with a characteristic transmantle sign with a T2/fluid-attenuated inversion recovery (FLAIR) signal abnormality that tapers as it extends inward from the blurred cortex toward the superolateral margin of the lateral ventricles (▸ Fig. 3.2). The abnormality is pathologicaly identical to that of the tubers in tuberous sclerosis complex. A less well-defined T2/FLAIR signal abnormality is seen in type IIA FCD. Although there are always exceptions, type I FCD shows up best on T1 W imaging and type II FCD shows up on T2 W and FLAIR images. Type III cortical dysplasia is associated with another lesion, which can be hippocampal sclerosis (IIIA), a tumor (IIIB), a vascular injury (IIIC), or an early-acquired parenchymal injury (IIID).

3.3 Malformations of Neuronal Migration

If a developing neuron fails to migrate appropriately to the periphery of the brain, the result is a heterotopic focus of gray matter. The area of heterotopia is most commonly seen as a nodular focus (or foci) of gray matter along the lateral margin of one of the lateral ventricles (▸ Fig. 3.3), an entity known as periventricular nodular heterotopia (PVNH). This heterotopia is most common along the margins of the trigones of the lateral ventricles, and next most common in the anterior body/frontal horns. The lesions of PVNH can be multifocal and are commonly bilateral. Isolated PVNH is commonly an incidental finding, perhaps in patients with headaches or trauma, but the ectopic gray matter of PVNH can be the source of seizures. PVNH is often best seen on T1 W imaging, although any imaging sequence may show abnormalities in contour along the margin of the lateral ventricles. Isolated foci of PVNH may be most conspicuous on DWI because it follows the diffusion characteristics of gray matter, in contrast to the adjacent white matter and CSF.

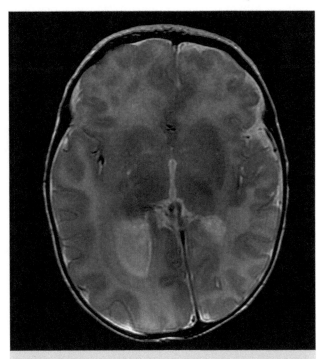

Fig. 3.1 Hemimegalencephaly. Axial T2 W image in a 1-month-old child shows enlargement of the right cerebral hemisphere, with cortex that is thickened and dysplastic.

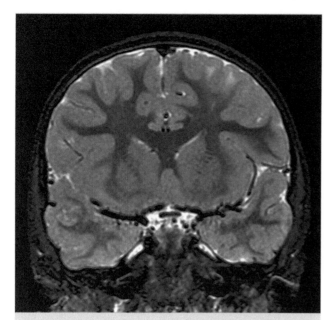

Fig. 3.2 Focal cortical dysplasia type IIB. Coronal STIR image in a 3-year-old child with seizures shows a juxtacortical hyperintense signal involving the left middle frontal gyrus, with a signal abnormality that tapers as it extends inferomedially. This represents an area of type IIB focal cortical dysplasia.

If the heterotopic gray matter of PVNH migrates partway toward the periphery of the brain, it will produce a visible subcortical deposit (▶ Fig. 3.4). Subcortical heterotopia often occurs in conjunction with areas of PVNH. At times, multiple foci of subcortical heterotopia form a confluent to near-confluent path of gray matter from the ventricular margin to the periphery of the brain, representing transmantle heterotopia, which can be difficult to distinguish from a closed-lip schizencephalic cleft.

A continuous rim of heterotopic gray matter can sometimes be seen paralleling the cortex of the cerebral hemispheres, representing band-type heterotopia (▶ Fig. 3.5). Band-type heterotopia is typically bilaterally symmetric and can involve the entirety of the cerebral hemispheres or only portions of them (most commonly, posteriorly if the heterotopia is incomplete). Band heterotopia can occur with lissencephaly-spectrum disorders (▶ Fig. 3.6).

3.4 Malformations of Neuronal Organization

If developing neurons successfully migrate to the periphery of the brain, they must still appropriately organize into a six-layered cortex with a characteristic sulcation pattern. The signaling pathways guiding this organizational process can be impaired by any injury to the parenchyma, such as an in-utero infectious or ischemic process, or by genetic abnormalities.[3] If there is a peripheral parenchymal injury before the completion of neuronal migration and organization, the developing brain will be unable to form the appropriate pattern of gyration and sulcation. The resultant attempts at organization yield multiple smaller gyri (▶ Fig. 3.7), whence the name polymicrogyria. Symmetric patterns of polymicrogyria tend to have genetic causes (▶ Fig. 3.8), but some infections (including in-utero infections, such as with cytomegalovirus [CMV]) can result in bilateral polymicrogyria. Infectious etiologies of polymicrogyria may have associated dystrophic mineralization, with this particularly being true for toxoplasmosis/other/rubella/cytomegalovirus/herpes (TORCH) infections.

If a transmantle (from ventricle to periphery) parenchymal injury occurs before the completion of neuronal migration and organization, the margins of the parenchymal injury may be lined with gray matter. A cleft will form connecting the subarachnoid space with the ventricular system in an entity known as schizencephaly (▶ Fig. 3.9). The schizencephalic cleft will commonly be lined with polymicrogyric tissue. If the transmantle injury that led to a cleft involved only a small amount of tissue, the margins of the cleft may be directly apposed, yielding the condition referred to as closed-lip schizencephaly.

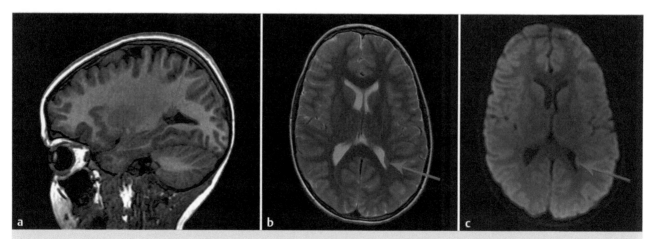

Fig. 3.3 Periventricular nodular heterotopia. (a) Sagittal T1 W image shows nodular areas of gray-matter signal along the superolateral margin of the posterior body of the left lateral ventricle, representing periventricular nodular heterotopia (PVNH, *red arrows*). (b) Axial T2 W image shows subtle signs of the PVNH. (c) Axial diffusion-weighted image shows slightly hyperintense signal associated with this gray matter, similar in appearance to cortex, and easier to identify than on a T2 W image alone.

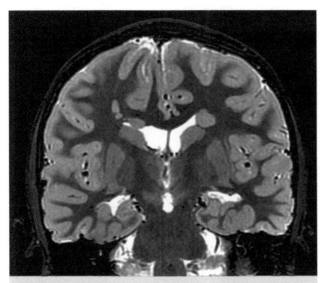

Fig. 3.4 Subcortical heterotopia. Coronal STIR image in a 5-year-old male with seizures shows several nodular areas of gray-matter heterotopia along the margins of the bodies of both lateral ventricles, with two right-sided foci of subcortical heterotopic gray matter.

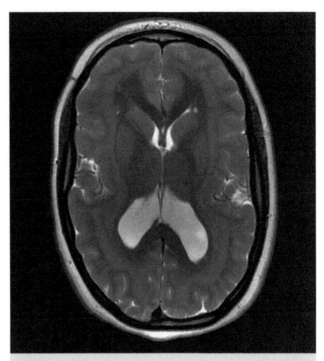

Fig. 3.5 Band heterotopia. Axial T2 W image in a 13-year-old female shows a band of gray-matter-like signal in the deep white matter. Accordingly, there is a zone of juxtaventricular white matter from the ventricles out to the periphery, followed by the band heterotopia, with a juxtacortical zone of white matter and the cortex. There is additionally pachygyria, most evident in the frontal lobes, representing a lissencephaly spectrum disorder of Dobyns grade 5.

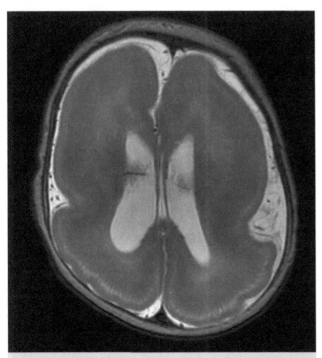

Fig. 3.6 Lissencephaly. Axial T2 W image in a 2-month-old male shows a relatively featureless brain with rudimentary sylvian fissures, but without any additional significant sulcation. There is additionally band heterotopia. The severity is nearly of Dobyns grade 1, or pure lissencephaly (agyria).

Closed-lip schizencephaly can be difficult to detect, and once detected can be difficult to differentiate from transmantle heterotopia, but there will commonly be a contour irregularity along the margin of the lateral ventricle, serving as a clue to the presence of a cleft. If a large area of parenchyma is injured, the margins of the schizencephalic cleft that are lined with gray matter are not in contact with one another, a condition called open-lip schizencephaly. At times radiologists agonize over whether a given defect is a closed-lip schizencepaly or an open-lip schizencephaly with a very narrow channel; this differentiation is arbitrary and probably has little clinical significance. A narrow channeled open-lip schizencephaly has a small amount of parenchymal injury similar to that of a closed-lip schizencephaly, and accordingly these entities are more similar in prognosis and extent of neurologic sequelae than are two patients each with an open-lip schizencephalic cleft, of which one is very narrow and the other is large. Schizencephalic clefts can be bilateral and do not have to be symmetric, so when a first cleft is detected, close attention is warranted for detecting a possible additional occult closed-lip schizencephaly. Schizencephaly is often an isolated finding, although it is seen with increased frequency in septo-optic dysplasia.

3.5 Other Supratentorial Entities

3.5.1 Agenesis of the Corpus Callosum

The corpus callosum is the largest forebrain commissure and connects the cerebral hemispheres. The absence of callosal

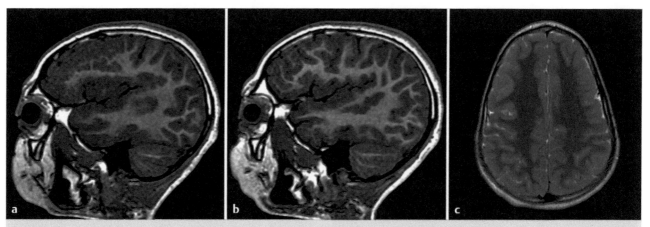

Fig. 3.7 Polymicrogyria. (a,b) Sagittal T1 W images of the left hemisphere. (a) Multiple small gyri in the left inferior and middle frontal gyri, as compared to the more normal sulcation pattern in the right hemisphere (b). (c) Axial T2 W image also shows more subtle signs of polymicrogyria, including lack of visualization of the subcortical U fibers in this region. On the axial image alone, the polymicogyria could be mistaken for pachygyria.

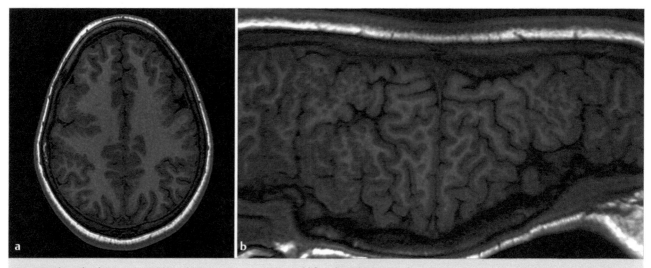

Fig. 3.8 Bilateral polymicrogyria. (a) Axial T1 W image in a 15-year-old female with seizures shows bilateral polymicrogyria. (b) A curved-plane reformat of the surface of the cerebral hemispheres makes it easier to identify multifocal areas of polymicrogyria.

development results in characteristic cerebral abnormalities and findings (▶ Fig. 3.10). A midline sagittal image in such a situation shows absence of the corpus callosum, absence of the cingulate gyrus, with parasagittal gyri radiating outward from the third ventricle, and a low position of the distal branches of the anterior cerebral artery. The bodies of the lateral ventricles have a parallel configuration, and the atria and occipital horns of the lateral ventricles are enlarged, in what is called colpocephaly. On coronal images, there is a high-riding appearance of the third ventricle, which is in direct continuity with the interhemispheric fissure. Interhemispheric arachnoid cysts/cystic meningeal dysplasia is not uncommon. In utero, colpocephaly can be mistaken for hydrocephalus. The fibers that would have traversed the corpus callosum instead have an anteroposteriorly directed course along the medial margins of the bodies of the lateral ventricles, and are known as Probst bundles. In a female with agenesis of the corpus callosum, particularly in the presence of arachnoid cysts, attention should be paid to the orbits, because agenesis of the corpus callosum with coloboma in a female is a feature of Aicardi syndrome.

3.5.2 Dysgenesis of the Corpus Callosum

Between a normal corpus callosum and complete agenesis of the corpus callosum is a broad spectrum of callosal dysgenesis. It is possible to have partial absence, abnormal morphology, a shortened anteroposterior dimension, and generalized thinning of the corpus callosum (▶ Fig. 3.11). Generalized thinning of the corpus callosum is most commonly related to cerebral white matter injury/volume loss and corresponding Wallerian degeneration. Congenital remnants of the meninx primitiva (neural crest mesenchyme) can result in a midline lipoma, which can

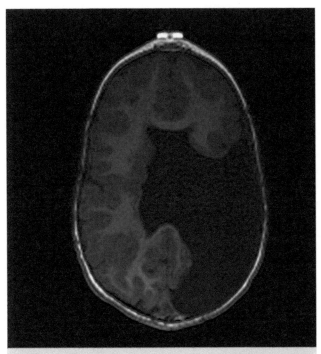

Fig. 3.9 Schizencephaly. Axial T1 W image in a 15-month-old female shows a large left-sided, open-lip schizencephalic cleft. There is also a right-sided closed-lip schizencephalic cleft, identified by a focal irregularity in contour along the lateral margin of the right lateral ventricle, with a gray-matter-lined cleft extending to the periphery.

be associated with the dorsal surface of the corpus callosum (▶ Fig. 3.12). Posterior callosal dysgenesis is more common than anterior dysgenesis and is a common feature of disorders like Chiari type II malformation.

3.5.3 Holoprosencephaly Spectrum

The prosencephalon is the embryologic forebrain, and it cleaves into the two cerebral hemispheres. Incomplete cleavage results in the spectrum of holoprosencephalic disorders. The most severe disorder in this spectrum is called alobar holoprosencephaly (▶ Fig. 3.13) and is marked by a dysmorphic monoventricle, absence of the interhemispheric fissure, a single anterior cerebral artery (azygous anterior cerebral artery), and fused thalami (▶ Table 3.1). A patient with more normally formed lateral ventricles, separate thalami, and partial presence of the interhemispheric fissure is referred to as having lobar holoprosencephaly. Between these two abnormalities is a variant known as semilobar holoprosencephaly (▶ Fig. 3.14). All patients with a disorder in the holoprosencephaly spectrum are at risk for pituitary/endocrine abnormalities, cleft palate, and other midline anomalies.

It is important to note that alobar, semilobar, and lobar holoprosencephaly are not three separate entities but are instead varying degrees of severity of the holoprosencephaly spectrum (▶ Fig. 3.15). Accordingly, most cases of holoprosencephalic disorders encountered clinically will not match the formal description of any of these entities. It is perfectly acceptable to describe the specific features of a case, and summarize it, for instance, as

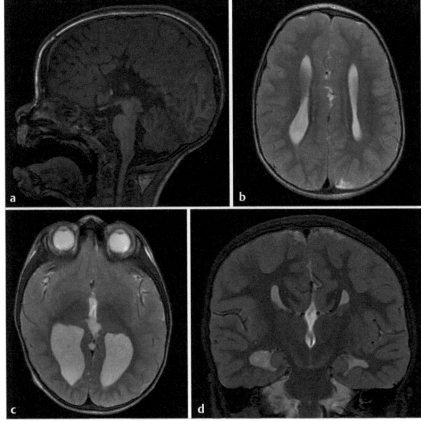

Fig. 3.10 Agenesis of the corpus callosum. (a) Sagittal T1 W image shows absence of the corpus callosum and cingulate gyrus. There are radiating gyri extending from the superior aspect of the third ventricle toward the periphery. The anterior commissure is present. (b) Axial T2 W image shows a parallel configuration of the bodies of the lateral ventricles. (c) Axial T2 W image at a lower level shows enlargement of the atria and occipital horns, known as colpocephaly. (d) Coronal STIR image shows a vertically oriented third ventricle that is in direct communication with the interhemispheric fissure. The relationship between the third ventricle and the lateral ventricles is sometimes known as the "longhorn" sign.

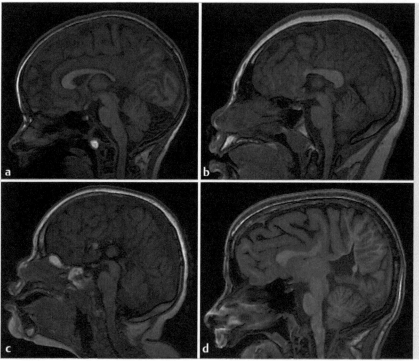

Fig. 3.11 Miscellaneous abnormalities of the corpus callosum. (a) Sagittal T1 W image shows mild dysplasia of the corpus callosum, with posterior thinning. (b) Sagittal T1 W image shows a foreshortened dysplastic corpus callosum. (c) Sagittal T1 W image shows nearly complete absence of the corpus callosum, with only a small portion in the expected location of the genu. A separate anterior commissure is seen inferior to this. (d) Sagittal T1 W image shows severe posterior dysplasia of the corpus callosum.

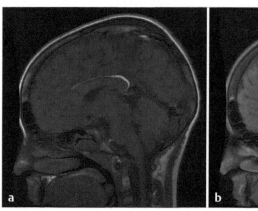
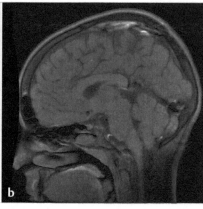

Fig. 3.12 Lipoma of the corpus callosum. (a) Sagittal T1 W image shows a hyperintense rim of material along the superior margin of the body of the corpus callosum, wrapping around the splenium. (b) This becomes hypointense on sagittal T1 W fat-saturation imaging, confirming that this is a lipoma of the corpus callosum.

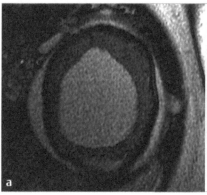
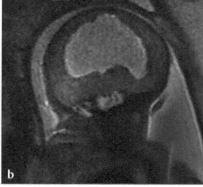

Fig. 3.13 Alobar holoprosencephaly. (a) Image made with fast imaging employing steady-state acquisition (FIESTA) from a fetal magnetic resonance (MR) scan in the axial plane relative to the fetal head shows a monoventricle and a peripheral contiguous rim of parenchyma without an interhemispheric fissure. (b) Single-shot T2 W sequence from a fetal MR scan in the coronal plane relative to the fetal head shows fusion of the thalami and midline structures. This represents alobar holoprosencephaly.

Table 3.1 Spectrum of holoprosencephaly

Type of holoprosencephaly	Interhemispheric fissure	Thalami	Corpus callosum	Ventricles	Septum pellucidum	Other
Alobar	None/minimal	Fused	Dysplastic/absent	Dysmorphic monoventricle	Absent	Azygous anterior cerebral artery, often with a single central incisor
Semilobar	Minimally present	Variable degree of fusion vs dysmorphia	Dysplastic	Dysmorphic monoventricle	Absent	
Lobar	Partially present	Separate, typically normal	Mildly dysplastic	Dysmorphic ventricles	Absent	
Syntelencephaly	Mostly present	Normal	Mostly normal, possible mid-callosal dysplasia	Mildly dysmorphic	Absent	Vertically oriented sylvian fissures ("middle interhemispheric variant")
Septo-optic dysplasia	Present	Normal	Normal/mostly normal	Relatively normal	Absent	Optic nerve hypoplasia, ± ectopic neurohypophysis, ± schizencephaly

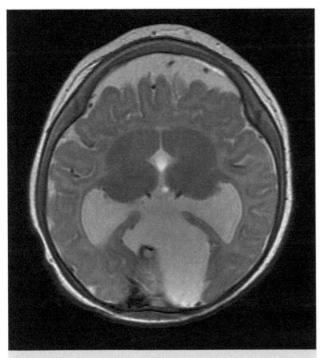

Fig. 3.14 Semilobar holoprosencephaly. Axial T2 W image shows anterior midline continuity of the cerebral hemispheres, with posterior separation, including a posterior midline arachnoid cyst. The anterior portion of the ventricular system is absent, and there is poor differentiation between the caudate nuclei and lentiform nuclei. The thalami are separated. This represents a disorder of mild to moderate severity within the holoprosencephaly spectrum, closest to what is typically defined as semilobar holoprosencephaly.

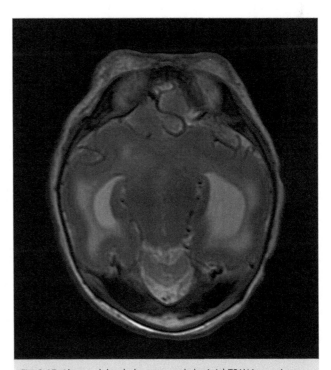

Fig. 3.15 Almost alobar holoprosencephaly. Axial T2 W image in a 1-day-old infant shows anterior absence of the interhemispheric fissure but presence of the posterior interhemispheric fissure. There is additionally fusion of the thalami, indicating that this is a moderate to severe disorder within the holoprosencephaly spectrum, with a severity between that of semilobar and alobar holoprosencephaly. The partial presence of the posterior interhemispheric fissure and partially formed temporal horns of the lateral ventricles prevent this from being classified as alobar holoprosencephaly.

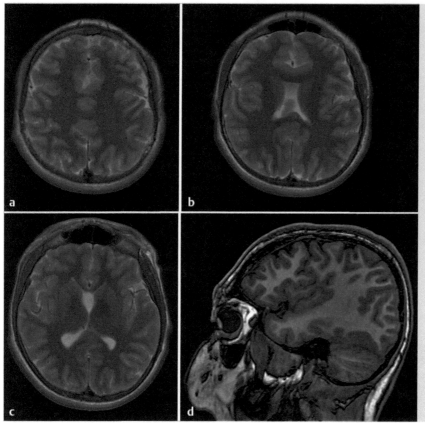

Fig. 3.16 Syntelencephaly. (a) Axial T2 W image above the level of the lateral ventricles shows midline gray-matter connections between the cerebral hemispheres (syntelencephalic bridges), but the interhemispheric fissure is present anteriorly and posteriorly. (b) An axial T2 W image at a lower level than the image in (a) shows a nearly normal morphology of the ventricular system, although with absence of the septum pellucidum, and at the periphery there is an atypical position of the sylvian fissure. (c) An additional T2 W image at a level lower than that in (b) shows separated deep gray nuclei that have a slightly atypical orientation. (d) Sagittal T1 W image shows a vertical extension of the sylvian fissure. Collectively, the images illustrate the mild disorder within the holoprosencephaly spectrum known as syntelencephaly.

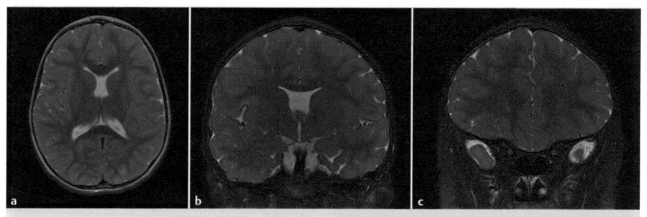

Fig. 3.17 Septo-optic dysplasia (SOD). (a) Axial T2 W image and (b) coronal T2 W fat-suppressed (FS) image show absence of the septum pellucidum in an otherwise normal-appearing brain. (c) Coronal T2 W FS image at the level of the posterior orbits shows diminutive optic nerves. This constellation of findings is characteristic of SOD.

a disorder within the holoprosencephaly spectrum of moderate severity with an appearance closest to that of semilobar holoprosencephaly.

An even more mild abnormality in the holoprosencephaly spectrum is one that involves only telencephalic abnormality, with normal diencephalic (thalamic) development. This is syntelencephaly, also known as the "middle interhemispheric variant" of holoprosencephaly. Patients with syntelencephaly will have a fully formed corpus callosum, but with possible mid-callosal dysplasia, and have an interhemispheric bridge of parenchyma connecting the cerebral hemispheres ("telence-

phalic bridge") (▶ Fig. 3.16). Another characteristic feature of syntelencephaly is a vertically oriented extension of the sylvian fissure that reaches the midline near the vertex.

3.5.4 Septo-optic Dysplasia

A developmental abnormality that some sources consider to be the most mild end of the spectrum of holoprosencephalic disorders is septo-optic dysplasia (SOD, also known as de Morsier syndrome) (▶ Fig. 3.17). The main clue to the presence of SOD is absence of the septum pellucidum, a feature (or lack thereof)

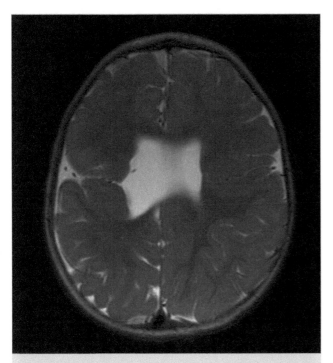

Fig. 3.18 Septo-optic dysplasia (SOD) with schizencephaly. Axial T2 W image in a 1 year old female with SOD shows a right-sided closed-lip (or very narrow open-lip) schizencephaly. There is a deep sulcus on the left side that does not reach the lateral ventricle.

that can be difficult to identify if one seeks only symmetry. Septo-optic dysplasia involves hypoplasia of the optic nerves, which may be the indication for the examination for this disorder (particularly if the examination is requested by an ophthalmologist). Some patients with SOD have an associated schizencephaly (▶ Fig. 3.18). In an evaluation for SOD, close attention should be paid to the pituitary gland, because SOD is frequently associated with ectopic neurohypophysis.

3.5.5 Lissencephaly/Pachygyria/Agyria Spectrum

A cortical developmental abnormality with a smooth, relatively featureless contour is an abnormality in the lissencephaly/pachygyria/agyria spectrum. Lissencephaly means "smooth brain," and it is marked by an immaturely formed cortex with only four cell layers instead of the typical six layers. Pachygyria means "thickened, relatively featureless gyri," and agyria is the absence of gyri, and it can be a milder, more focal malformation in the lissesencephaly spectrum. It is important to be extremely cautious before suggesting a diagnosis of lissencephaly in a premature or immature brain. The most severe form of lissencephaly is agyria, in which there is no appreciable sulcation throughout the cerebral hemispheres other than possibly a rudimentary indentation corresponding to the sylvian fissure (▶ Fig. 3.6), giving a "figure 8" appearance to the cerebral hemispheres on axial imaging. Agyria is also marked by a thickened, primitive cortex that has only four layers of cells and commonly has an associated band-type heterotopia. Milder forms of lissencephaly have more gyri (▶ Fig. 3.19) and blend into the spectrum of pachygyria disorders. Dobyns has proposed a six-level grading scale for disorders within the lissencephaly/pachygyria/agyria spectrum, ranging from agyria (grade 1) to diffuse pachygyria (grade 4) and band heterotopia without appreciable pachygyria (grade 6). More severe disorders in the lissencephaly spectrum (i.e., grades 1 and 2) can be associated with Miller–Dieker syndrome, in which there are associated developmental abnormalities of the kidneys and gastrointestinal tract. Agyria is associated with deletion of the *LIS-1* gene, and the milder forms of disorders within the lissencephaly/pachygyria/agyria spectrum have varying degrees of abnormalities of this gene, partial deletions of the gene, or missense mutations of it. Manifestations of partial deletions of *LIS-1* tend to have more of a posterior predominance, with relative frontal sparing of the cortex. Anteriorly predominant lissencephaly, with relative posterior sparing of the cortex, is seen with abnormalities of the *DCX* gene.[4]

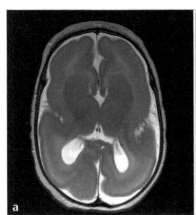
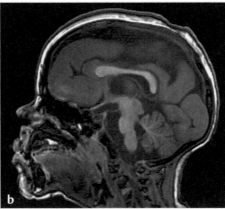

Fig. 3.19 Lissencephaly 2. (a) Axial T2 W image in a 3-month-old female shows a lissencephalic appearance slightly less severe than the example shown in ▶ Fig. 3.6. There is still band heterotopia, but the sylvian fissures are more formed. (b) Sagittal T1 W image of the same patient at 3 years of age shows a dysplastic corpus callosum, with a parieto-occipital fissure and calcarine sulcus posteriorly and partial visualization of the cingulate gyrus; however, no additional sulcation has taken place. This is closest to a Dobyns grade 2 lissencephaly.

References

[1] Blümcke I, Thom M, Aronica E et al. The clinicopathologic spectrum of focal cortical dysplasias: A consensus classification proposed by an ad hoc Task Force of the ILAE Diagnostic Methods Commission. Epilepsia 2011; 52(1): 158–174

[2] Barkovich AJ, Guerrini R, Kuzniecky RI, Jackson GD, Dobyns WB. A developmental and genetic classification for malformations of cortical development: Update 2012. Brain 2012; 135(Pt 5):1348–1369

[3] Stutterd CA, Leventer RJ. Polymicrogyria: A common and heterogeneous malformation of cortical development. In Mirzaa GM, Paciorkowski AR (eds). Am J Med Genet C Semin Med Genet 2014;166(2):227–239

[4] Leventer RJ. Genotype-phenotype correlation in lissencephaly and subcortical band heterotopia: The key questions answered. J Child Neurol 2005; 20(4):307–312

4 Posterior Fossa Malformations

4.1 Introduction

A wide variety of malformations of the posterior fossa can occur, including well-known characteristic conditions, misunderstood conditions, and missed (or misdiagnosed) conditions. Attention to the cerebellum in every imaging study is helpful, for detecting abnormalities that cannot be detected by a gestalt method, and for familiarizing oneself with normal anatomic appearances and development patterns of the cerebellum.

4.2 Chiari Type I Malformation

It is hard to know whether it is easier to miss or to overdiagnose a Chiari type I malformation in a child because both are easy to do. A Chiari type I malformation can be defined according to the two different criteria, either by anatomic features or physiologic alterations.

The anatomic description of a Chiari type I malformation is that of elongated cerebellar tonsils extending a specific distance below the plane of the foramen magnum (as approximated by a line connecting the basion to the opisthion on midsagittal images) (▶ Fig. 4.1). In adults it is said that tonsils extending 5 mm below the plane of the foramen magnum reflect a Chiari type I malformation, but in children less stringent criteria are used because ectopia of up to 6 mm (or even 7 mm) below the plane of the foramen magnum can be normal (▶ Fig. 4.2).

The term "peg-like" tonsils is sometimes used in the literature to describe the appearance of the cerebellar tonsils in a Chiari type I malformation, but this does not make sense to me and I do not use this term; I find "elongated" to be a sufficiently appropriate description for such tonsils. Making this determination requires familiarity with "normal" tonsillar morphology, which can be obtained only by attention to tonsillar morphology in every study of the cerebellum.

The other way of defining a Chiari type I malformation is a physiologic one, wherein there is a symptomatic impairment of the dynamics of cerebrospinal fluid (CSF) flow through the plane of the foramen magnum, resulting from effacement of the CSF space surrounding the cervicomedullary junction (junction of the brainstem and the spinal cord) as a consequence of cerebellar tonsillar ectopia. This definition is probably the more correct of the two, but it requires more than measurement of a single anatomic feature. Impaired transit of CSF traversing the plane of the foramen magnum can result in clinical symptoms, typically consisting of headaches, but also including dysphagia, vertigo, tinnitus, and other brainstem-related symptoms.

Ultimately, the diagnosis of a Chiari type I malformation is not a binary assessment, as 4.9 mm and 5.1 mm of ectopia are for all practical purposes identical, and the difference does not suddenly constitute a Chiari malformation.

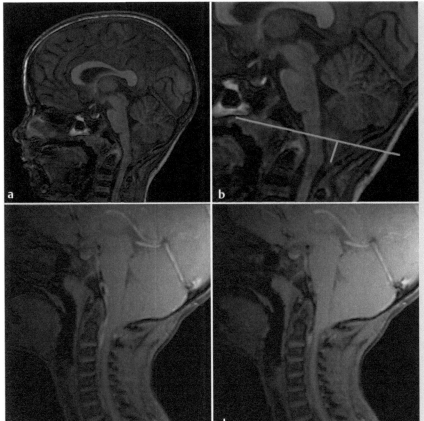

Fig. 4.1 Chiari I malformation. (a) Sagittal T1 W image shows elongation of the cerebellar tonsils, which extend below the level of the foramen magnum. (b) Magnified sagittal T1 W image of this region with an overlay of a line extending between the tip of the clivus (basion) and the posterior aspect of the foramen magnum (opisthion), and a perpendicular measurement showing the tip of the cerebellar tonsils extending more than 10 mm below the level of the foramen magnum. (c) Sagittal cardiac-gated CSF flow study in systole demonstrates caudally directed flow of CSF ventral to the brainstem and cervicomedullary junction across the foramen magnum, demonstrated by a hyperintense signal. (d) Sagittal cardiac-gated CSF flow study in diastole shows hypointense signal ventral to the brainstem and cervicomedullary junction across the foramen magnum, confirming flow in the superior (cranial) direction and confirming patent bidirectional flow of CSF.

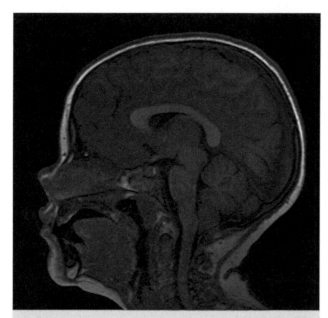

Fig. 4.2 Mild Chiari I malformation. Sagittal T1 W image shows mild caudal extension of the cerebellar tonsils to 8 mm below the plane of the foramen magnum, with patent CSF spaces around the brainstem. Although this formally meets the criteria for a Chiari type I malformation, it is unclear whether it will have symptomatic consequences, and accordingly no surgical procedure was performed in the case shown here.

Table 4.1 Findings on cerebrospinal fluid (CSF) flow study

	Dorsal CSF flow	Ventral CSF flow	Ventrolateral CSF flow
Normal	Pulsatile, minimal, or absence of flow can be normal	Pulsatile, bidirectional	Normal
Mild	Minimal to no flow	Pulsatile, bidirectional	Normal
Moderate	Typically no flow	Hyperdynamic, bidirectional	Normal to hyperdynamic
Severe	Typically no flow	None	Hyperdynamic

A syrinx in the absence of a Chiari type I malformation mandates a contrast-enhanced MRI scan of the entire neural axis (brain and total spine). Some sources advocate for a contrast-enhanced evaluation of the neural axis at baseline, even in the presence of a Chiari malformation, to ensure that a concomitant neoplasm is not the true cause of a syrinx.

Surgical treatment of a Chiari type I malformation involves enlarging the foramen magnum through a suboccipital decompressive craniectomy. If there is hypoplasia of the posterior neural arch of C1, it may be decompressed as well. After osseous decompression, there may still be effaced CSF spaces due to the configuration of the dura, and duraplasty may be performed to remodel the cisterna magna. Postoperative imaging of a patient with a Chiari type I malformation must include study for a restoration of pulsatile CSF flow across the foramen magnum and decrease and/or resolution of hydromyelia when the latter is present. Additionally, the site of duraplasty must be evaluated for a possible pseudomeningocele. Extradural fluid in the early postoperative period is not uncommon; it is probably related to the surgical decompression of the cerebellum done through craniectomy and does not necessarily indicate a pseudomeningocele.

As many as 50% of patients with a Chiari type I malformation will have associated craniocervical osseous abnormalities. Among the most commonly found abnormalities of this type are a retroflexed odontoid process (▶ Fig. 4.3) and a hypoplastic clivus. There may also be hypoplasia of one or both occipital condyles, assimilation of an occipital condyle with the lateral mass of C1, and basilar invagination. Attention should be given to these areas in all studies of patients with a Chiari type I malformation because the presence of these abnormalities can alter surgical management.

4.3 Chiari Type II Malformation

A Chiari type II malformtion is not a severe version or variant of a Chiari type I malformtion, and for those who are confused by the terminology it is at times unfortunate that the two malformations do not have different names. A Chiari type II malformation, for all practical purposes, is always associated with an open myelomeningocle (nearly always lumbosacral). Because of the loss of CSF from the open myelomeningocele, the pressure within the subarachnoid space remains low, and there is slumping of the contents of the posterior fossa through the foramen magnum. This results in cerebellar ectopia, including ectopia of the cerebellar tonsils and vermis

Alterations of CSF flow dynamics can result in an enlargement of the central canal of the spinal cord, with this enlargement commonly referred to as a syrinx. Dilation of the central canal of the spinal cord, with an intact ependymal lining, is more appropriately called hydromyelia. A fluid accumulation within parenchymal tissue of the spinal cord that lacks an ependymal lining represents syringomyelia. When the fluid collection becomes sufficiently large, it cannot be differentiated from syringomyelia, and the catchall term "syringohydromyelia" is used to describe it.

A phase-contrast magnetic resonance imaging (MRI) study of CSF flow across the plane of the foramen magnum can be used to evaluate CSF flow dynamics. Appropriate levels of encoding for fluid-flow velocity must be selected, typically with a value of approximately 10 cm/sec for evaluating a Chiari type I malformation. Midsagittal imaging is most commonly used for such evaluation, with flow ventral to the brainstem being characteristically decreased as the result of effacement of the CSF space. Note that narrowing of the CSF space will result in increased flow velocities before there is a loss of flow. Axial CSF flow imaging can help in seeking turbulent and/or hyperdynamic flow ventrolateral to the cord at the level of the foramen magnum, which presents as aliasing at appropriate levels of velocity encoding, helping to further confirm the altered CSF flow dynamics caused by a Chiari type I malformation (▶ Table 4.1). This is of particular interest in presurgical planning for borderline Chiari type I malformations in patients without syrinx/hydromyelia. A patient who has a syrinx can be assumed to have evidence of altered CSF flow physiology regardless of the findings in a CSF flow study. A pre-existing shunt catheter may alter CSF dynamics.

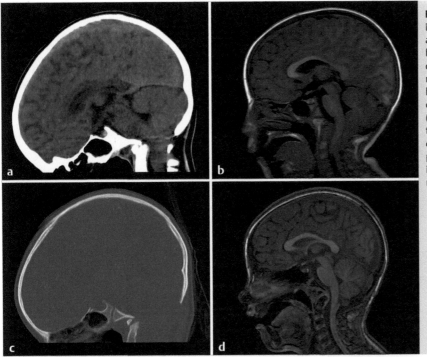

Fig. 4.3 Preoperative and postoperative imaging in Chiari type I malformation. (a) Sagittal brain algorithm CT scan in a 4-year-old female with headaches and a disorder of eye movement demonstrates a Chiari type I malformation, a retroflexed odontoid process, and a relatively hypoplastic basiocciput. (b) Sagittal T1 W image confirms the Chiari type I malformation. (c) Sagittal bone algorithm CT after surgical treatment shows findings of suboccipital decompressive craniectomy and removal of the posterior neural arch of C1. (d) Sagittal T1 W image made postoperatively shows a patent neo-foramen magnum.

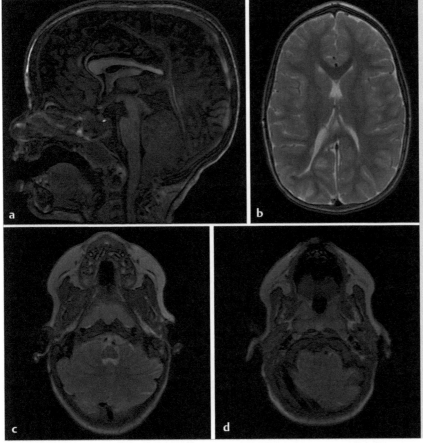

Fig. 4.4 Chiari type II malformation. (a) Sagittal T1 W image shows cerebellar ectopia (tonsillar and vermian) and a small fourth ventricle. There is a pointed appearance of the inferior colliculi, giving a "beaked" appearance to the tectal plate. There is a prominent massa intermedia, and posterior dysgenesis of the corpus callosum. (b) Axial T2 W image at the level of the septum pellucidum shows parieto-occipital loss of white-matter volume and partial visualization of a shunt catheter. (c,d) Axial T2 W images of the posterior fossa show cerebellar tonsillar and vermian ectopia through an enlarged foramen magnum, and the cerebellar tonsils wrapping around the cervicomedullary junction.

(in contrast to a Chiari type I malformation, in which there is only cerebellar tonsillar ectopia), and may induce a kink in the upper cervical cord. There is an enlarged foramen magnum as a result of the tonsillar and vermian ectopia, and a small posterior fossa. Additionally, there is abnormal development of the tectal plate, with a horizontal configuration of the inferior colliculi and a characteristic "beaked" appearance of the tectum on sagittal imaging (▶ Fig. 4.4). Other abnormalities in Chiari type II

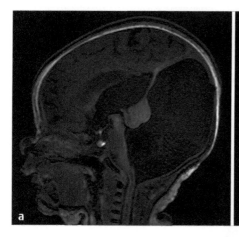
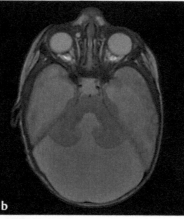

Fig. 4.5 Dandy–Walker malformation. (a) Sagittal T1 W image shows an uplifted hypoplastic cerebellar vermis, with the fourth ventricle in direct communication with a massively enlarged and cystically dilated posterior fossa. This results in uplifting of the torcula. (b) Axial T2 W image shows splaying of the cerebellar hemispheres without intervening vermis.

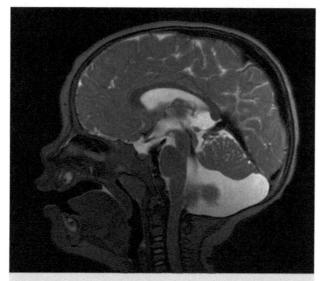

Fig. 4.6 Moderate Dandy–Walker spectrum. Sagittal T2 W image demonstrates inferior vermian hypoplasia, with mild cystic dilation of the infravermian CSF space, which is in communication with the fourth ventricle. This represents a moderate severity malformation within the Dandy–Walker spectrum.

malformation are enlargement of the massa intermedia; fenestration of the falx cerebri, with resultant interdigitation of gyri across the interhemispheric fissure; and a parieto-occipital-predominant loss of white matter volume and corresponding dysgenesis of the posterior corpus callosum. As the result of low CSF volume in utero, Chiari type II malformation is also marked by gyral impressions on the inner table of the skull, and after closure of the myelomeningocele there is hydrocephalus that typically requires shunting.

Recent work has involved attempts to close myelomeningoceles in utero to prevent the development of intracranial hypotension from the leakage of CSF, and early results with this have shown a decreased phenotypic severity of meningomyelocele and decreased incidence of the need for shunting, and possibly improved outcomes in neural development.

Although a Chiari type II malformation is nearly always secondary to a lumbosacral myelomeningocele, an open dysraphism in the thoracic or cervical spine can have a similar result. An occipital meningocele/encephalocele that results in a

Chiari type II-like phenotype is referred to as a "Chiari type III" malformation.

4.4 Cystic Lesions of the Posterior Fossa

4.4.1 Dandy–Walker Spectrum

The Dandy–Walker malformation is characterized by hypoplasia and malrotation of the cerebellar vermis with cystic dilation of the fourth ventricle, resulting in enlargement of the posterior cranial fossa (▶ Fig. 4.5). Dandy–Walker malformations may occur in isolation or be associated with other abnormalities. Further understanding of the classic Dandy–Walker malformation requires understanding of its variants as well as of conditions that mimic it.

Partial vermian development with a normal to mildly enlarged posterior fossa is a variant of the classic Dandy–Walker malformation (▶ Fig. 4.6). However, this represents a spectrum of abnormalities, and "Dandy–Walker variant" is not a discrete entity. Consequently, it is possible to have an abnormality of mild severity within the mild severity Dandy–Walker spectrum and a more severe abnormality that are not appropriately differentiated from one another by the single term "Dandy–Walker variant."

Some patients have a normally developed vermis with a cystic dilation of the cisterna magna; as long as the vermis is present in its entirety, such a dilation does not represent an abnormality within the Dandy–Walker spectrum. A prominence of the infravermian CSF space, with a normal vermis and normal foramen of Magendie, is commonly referred to as a "mega cisterna magna," but in fact probably represents an infravermian arachnoid cyst. Nevertheless, this is a normal variant and not a Dandy–Walker variant (▶ Fig. 4.7). An enlarged infravermian CSF space with a normal vermis but widened foramen of Magendie is probably related to a persistent Blake's pouch cyst, which is probably also a normal variant when seen in isolation, although it can be seen in the setting of peripartum obstructive hydrocephalus if the cyst has no fenestrations. A normal vermis and normal cisterna magna with a prominent retrovermian CSF space is likely to reflect a retrovermian arachnoid cyst, which is also a normal variant (▶ Fig. 4.8). More recent genetic analyses have shown variable origins of

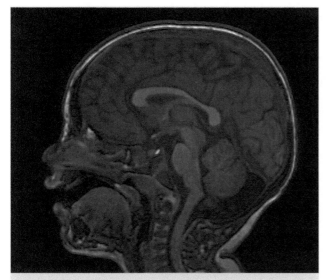

Fig. 4.7 Mega cisterna magna. Sagittal T1 W image shows a normal cerebellar vermis with a prominent infravermian CSF space. This represents an entity known as a mega cisterna magna, which may in fact be related to an infravermian arachnoid cyst.

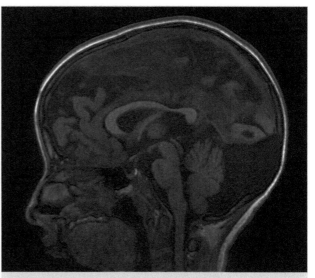

Fig. 4.8 Retrovermian arachnoid cyst. Sagittal T1 W image shows a normal cerebellar vermis with a prominent retrocerebellar CSF space and uplifting of the torcula. This represents a retrovermian arachnoid cyst, and does not represent a malformation within the Dandy–Walker spectrum.

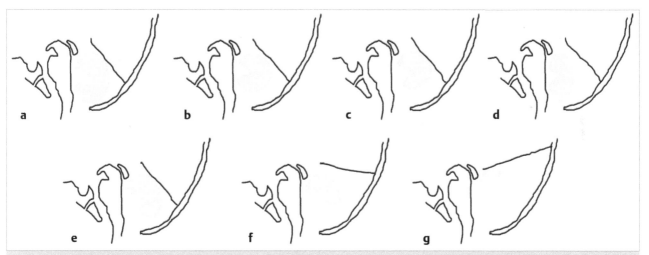

Fig. 4.9 Variety of appearances of the vermis (yellow) in (a) the normal setting, (b) infravermian arachnoid cyst/mega cisterna magna, (c) normal vermis with a prominent infravermian CSF space communicating with the fourth ventricle through a wide foramen of Magendie related to a persistent Blake's pouch cyst, (d) normal vermis with a retrovermian arachnoid cyst, (e) mild inferior vermian hypoplasia representing a mild malformation within the Dandy–Walker spectrum, (f) inferior vermian hypoplasia representing a malformation of moderate severity within the Dandy–Walker spectrum, and (g) an uplifted hypoplastic vermis with a cystically enlarged posterior fossa in a classic Dandy–Walker malformation.

morphologically similar cystic malformations of the posterior fossa, improving the understanding of the disease processes that lead to these malformations but perhaps adding further confusion to daily practice in their management. Therefore, for clinical purposes, mega cisterna magna and retrovermian arachnoid cysts should not be considered to represent abnormalities within the Dandy–Walker spectrum and are unlikely to have clinical or genetic implications (▶ Fig. 4.9)

4.5 Joubert Syndrome

Vermian hypoplasia is not unique to the Dandy–Walker spectrum of malformations of the posterior fossa. Vermian hypoplasia with thickened parallel superior cerebellar peduncles is characteristic of Joubert syndrome (as well as of more rare Joubert-related disorders) (▶ Fig. 4.10).[1] The condition is marked by an abnormal appearance of the fourth ventricle.

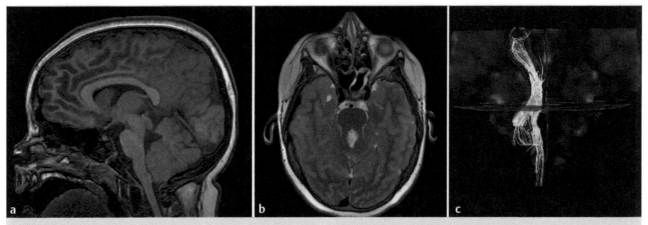

Fig. 4.10 Joubert syndrome. (a) Sagittal T1 W image shows a hypoplastic cerebellar vermis. Because there is no splaying of the cerebellar hemispheres as in a Dandy–Walker malformation, the cerebellar hemisphere can be seen below the hypoplastic vermis on this midline image. (b) Axial T2 W image shows a parallel orientation of the superior cerebellar peduncles, producing a molar tooth appearance. (c) Diffusion tensor fiber tracking shows no evidence of decussation of the fibers of the superior cerebellar peduncle or those of the corticospinal tract.

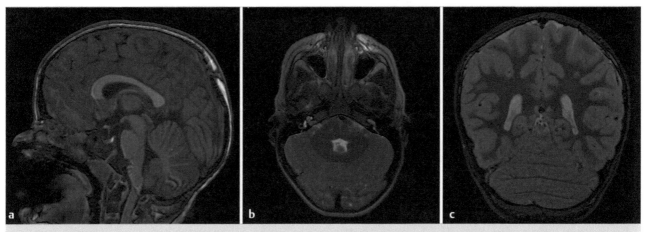

Fig. 4.11 Rhombencephalosynapsis. (a) Sagittal T1 W image shows an atypical fastigial angle of the fourth ventricle, with the foliation pattern of the midline structure more closely resembling that of a cerebellar hemisphere than of the vermis. (b) Axial T2 W image shows no cerebellar interhemispheric fissure or falx cerebelli, and other than a small nodulus, no vermis is identified. (c) Coronal STIR image shows midline continuitity of the folia across both cerebellar hemispheres, confirming a diagnosis of rhombencephalosynapsis.

The thickened parallel superior cerebellar peduncles give an appearance on axial imaging that has been likened to that of a molar tooth. The abnormality in development that causes this appearance is absence of the mesencephalic decussation of the fibers of the superior cerebellar peduncle; there is also absence of the pyramidal decussation of the corticospinal tracts.

4.6 Rhombencephalosynapsis

In the posterior fossa, the analog of holoprosencephaly is rhombencephalosynapsis, in which there is absence of cleavage of the cerebellar hemispheres and a resultant absence of vermian development (▶ Fig. 4.11).[2,3] Axial and coronal images are most commonly used to demonstrate this abnormality, but abnormalities can also be seen on midsagittal images, including an atypical morphology of the fourth ventricle and a folia pattern that looks more like cerebellar hemisphere parenchyma than

like vermis. Rhombencephalosynapsis is often associated with a medial position of the inferior colliculi, a midbrain developmental abnormality associated with a high incidence of aqueductal stenosis. Therefore, attention to the fourth ventricular and to vermian morphology is important in all cases of aqueductal stenosis. More recent work has shown that there is a spectrum of abnormalities in rhombencephalosynapsis, in which some parts of the vermis (most commonly the nodulus) can be present. Gomez–Lopez–Hernandez syndrome is a condition in which the patient has rhombencephalosynapsis, alopecia, and anesthesia in the distribution of the trigeminal nerve.[4,5]

4.7 Pontocerebellar Hypoplasia

Pontocerebellar hypoplasia is an abnormality whose name describes the findings on its imaging, in that there is hypoplasia

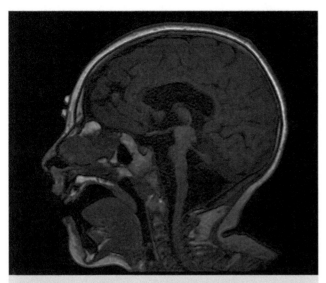

Fig. 4.12 Pontocerebellar hypoplasia. Sagittal T1 W image of the brain of a 4-year-old female with multiple chromosomal abnormalities and seizures shows a small pons and hypoplastic cerebellum, representing a subtype of pontocerebellar hypoplasia.

of the pons and cerebellum (▶ Fig. 4.12).[6,7] Pontocerebellar hypoplasia is a genetic condition with different phenotypes of different subtypes. The primary differential consideration for pontocerebellar hypoplasia is usually one of prior acquired injury, such as perinatal cerebellar hemorrhage or infarction.

4.8 Congenital Muscular Dystrophies

Congenital muscular dystrophies often have cerebellar and brainstem developmental abnormalities.[8] Fukuyama's congenital muscular dystrophy has cerebellar polymicrogyria, cerebellar cystic changes, and brainstem hypoplasia (▶ Fig. 4.13). Walker–Warburg syndrome typically has a kink within a hypoplastic brainstem, and supratentorially has a cobblestone-like lissencephalic cortex. Muscle–eye–brain disease will have pontine hypoplasia, may have cerebellar polymicrogyria, and may also include vermian hypogenesis. Merosin-deficient congenital muscular dystrophy may have mild pontine hypoplasia, but the posterior fossa is otherwise normal .[8]

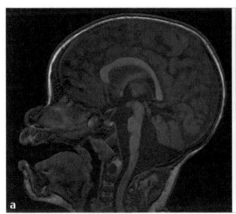
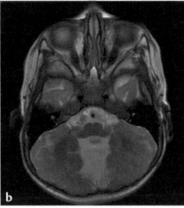

Fig. 4.13 Fukuyama congenital muscular dystrophy. (a) Sagittal T1 W image shows pontine hypoplasia and an abnormal appearance of the vermis. (b) Axial T2 W image of the cerebellum demonstrates polymicrogyria of both cerebellar hemispheres. This finding is rare in the posterior fossa, and in this patient is related to Fukuyama's congenital muscular dystrophy.

4.9 Further Reading

[1] Bosemani T, Orman G, Boltshauser E, Tekes A, Huisman TAGM, Poretti A. Congenital abnormalities of the posterior fossa. Radiographics 2015; 35(1): 200–220

[2] Shekdar K. Posterior fossa malformations. Semin Ultrasound CT MR 2011; 32 (3):228–241

References

[1] Poretti A, Huisman TAGM, Scheer I, Boltshauser E. Joubert syndrome and related disorders: spectrum of neuroimaging findings in 75 patients. AJNR Am J Neuroradiol 2011; 32(8):1459–1463

[2] Ishak GE, Dempsey JC, Shaw DWW et al. Rhombencephalosynapsis: a hindbrain malformation associated with incomplete separation of midbrain and forebrain, hydrocephalus and a broad spectrum of severity. Brain 2012; 135 (Pt 5):1370–1386

[3] Whitehead MT, Choudhri AF, Grimm J, Nelson MD. Rhombencephalosynapsis as a cause of aqueductal stenosis: an under-recognized association in hydrocephalic children. Pediatr Radiol 2014; 44(7):849–856

[4] Choudhri AF, Patel RM, Wilroy RS, Pivnick EK, Whitehead MT. Trigeminal nerve agenesis with absence of foramina rotunda in Gómez-López-Hernández syndrome. Am J Med Genet 2014; 167(1):238-242, doi 10.1002/ajmg.a.36830

[5] Whetsell W, Saigal G, Godinho S. Gomez-Lopez-Hernandez syndrome. Pediatr Radiol 2006; 36(6):552–554

[6] Poretti A, Boltshauser E, Doherty D. Cerebellar hypoplasia: Differential diagnosis and diagnostic approach. Mirzaa GM, Paciorkowski AR, editors. Am J Med Genet C Semin Med Genet 2014;166(2):211–226

[7] Burglen L, Chantot-Bastaraud S, Garel C et al. Spectrum of pontocerebellar hypoplasia in 13 girls and boys with CASK mutations: confirmation of a recognizable phenotype and first description of a male mosaic patient. Orphanet J Rare Dis 2012; 7(1):18

[8] Barkovich AJ. Neuroimaging manifestations and classification of congenital muscular dystrophies. AJNR Am J Neuroradiol 1998; 19(8):1389–1396

5 Perinatal Imaging

5.1 Introduction

Perinatal imaging includes both fetal and neonatal imaging for both congenital defects and acquired abnormalities. Perinatal imaging utilizes ultrasonography to a greater extent than do other applications of neuroradiology, taking advantage of the thin skull and sonographic windows (in particular the anterior fontanelle) of fetuses and neonates, the absence of ionizing radiation in ultrasonography, and the ability to perform the study without sedation and at the patient's bedside if needed. Because clinical examinations in this age group can be challenging, the appropriate interpretation of imaging studies can significantly aid in the care of these young patients.

5.2 Fetal Imaging

Fetal evaluation of abnormalities of the central nervous system (CNS) is most commonly done to evaluate areas of uncertainty on screening examinations done with ultrasonography at various stages of pregnancy. After an abnormality is identified or suspected on a screening examination, a more detailed fetal sonographic evaluation can be performed to characterize the abnormality. When there is need for further clarification of a suspected finding and/or associated abnormalities, fetal magnetic resonance imaging (MRI) can be performed. Fetal MRI is typically performed at 1.5 teslas or a lower field strength.

Recent investigations have begun to use a field strength of 3 teslas for fetal MRI, but the safety and benefits of this have not yet been established.

One of the most common indications for more detailed fetal ultrasonography is for ventriculomegaly, which can be associated with a variety of congenital and acquired abnormalities. Fetal ventriculomegaly is typically defined as a transverse dimension of the atrium of the lateral ventricle that exceeds 10 mm. A finding of ventriculomegaly should prompt a detailed survey of the entire CNS[1]; however, it is occasionally an isolated finding. When ventriculomegaly is present, a follow-up examination should be done to evaluate for its progression, which may result in the need for postnatal shunting (see Chapter 11).

Hydrocephalus can be seen in the setting of germinal matrix hemorrhage (GMH) in utero, which is typically the result of severe maternal stressors, such as an automobile accident or exposure to cocaine (▶ Fig. 5.1). Ventriculomegaly can be related to malformations of the posterior fossa, including a Chiari type II malformation (▶ Fig. 5.2) or a malformation within the Dandy–Walker spectrum (▶ Fig. 5.3), or to supratentorial abnormalities, including agenesis of the corpus callosum (▶ Fig. 5.4). Congenital malformations of the CNS are further discussed in Chapters 3 and 4.

A Chiari type II malformation is nearly always associated with a lumbosacral myelomeningocele (▶ Fig. 5.2), although this can be difficult to see if the back of the fetus is abutting the placenta

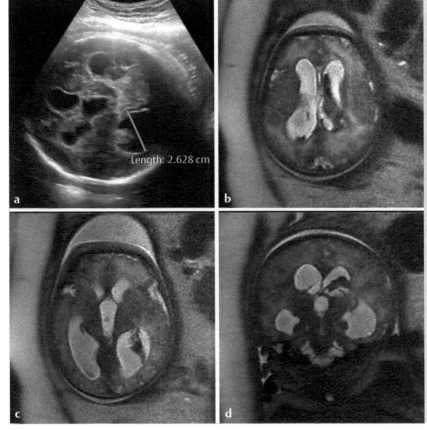

Fig. 5.1 Fetal germinal matrix hemorrhage (GMH). (a) A fetal abdominal ultrasonographic examination performed at approximately 36 weeks, gestational age shows ventriculomegaly of both lateral ventricles and the third ventricle, with echogenic material in the atria of the lateral ventricles. (b,c) Axial single-shot T2 W images and (d) coronal T2 W image show hypointense material in the body of the left lateral ventricle (b,d), extending into the atrium of the left lateral ventricle (c).

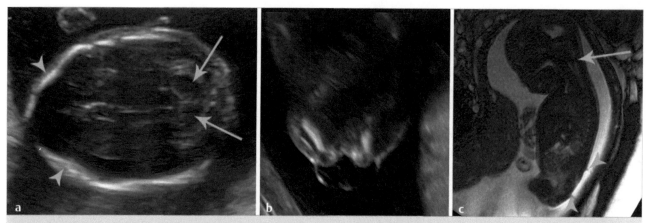

Fig. 5.2 Fetal Chiari type II malformation with myelomeningocele. (a) Ultrasonographic examination of the fetal head in the axial plane obtained at approximately 19 weeks of gestation shows inward bowing of the frontal calvaria (*green arrowheads*), resulting in an appearance described as resembling that of a lemon. There is also an arclike configuration of the cerebellum, described as resembling a banana (*green arrows*). (b) Fetal ultrasonographic examination of the lower lumbar region in the axial plane demonstrates splaying of the posterior elements, with a cystic posterior protrusion representing a myelomeningocele. Neural elements are seen extending to a posterior echogenic structure, the neural placode. (c) Fetal sagittal MRI scan with fast imaging employing steady-state acquisition (FIESTA) shows crowding of the posterior fossa with absence of a cisterna magna (*green arrow*), as well as a cystic-appearing myelomeningocele (*green arrowheads*).

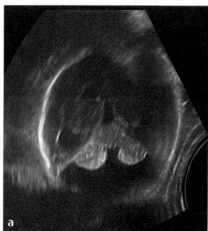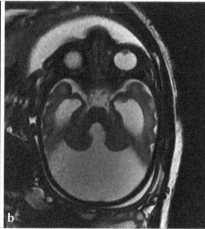

Fig. 5.3 Fetal Dandy–Walker malformation. (a) Axial–oblique fetal ultrasonographic examination shows splaying of the cerebellar hemispheres with communication between the fourth ventricle and cystically dilated posterior fossa without intervening vermis. (b) Axial single-shot T2W image from a fetal MRI scan confirms the Dandy–Walker malformation and ventriculomegaly.

or the amniotic sac/uterus. A Chiari type II malformation is associated with effacement of the cisterna magna on an axial view of the posterior cranial fossa, resulting in a finding referred to as a "banana sign." Owing to the low intracranial pressures in fetuses with a Chiari type II malformation, there is slight inward bowing of the frontolateral aspect of the calvarium, resulting in a finding referred to as a "lemon sign." Cerebellar ectopia through an enlarged foramen magnum cannot always be seen with ultrasonography; it may be better revealed by magnetic resonance imaging (MRI).

Although a Chiari type malformation is marked by a small posterior fossa, the Dandy–Walker spectrum of malformations results in cystic enlargement of the posterior cranial fossa. The extent of vermian hypoplasia in such a malformation can be difficult to determine with ultrasonography, and MRI performs better for this purpose.

Ventriculomegaly can also be seen with congenital supratentorial malformations, and particularly with agenesis of the corpus callosum (ACC), in which there is preferential enlargement of the atria and occipital horns of the lateral ventricles secondary to a loss of parieto-occipital white matter volume (▶ Fig. 5.4), a condition known as colpocephaly. In ACC, a midsagittal view can show absence of the corpus callosum and a radiating gyral pattern, and a coronal view can show a typical high-riding third ventricle. Agenesis of the corpus callosum is commonly associated with an interhemispheric cyst ("cystic meningeal dysplasia").[2] When accompanied by a cyst in a female fetus, ACC raises the possibility of Aicardi syndrome, in which there are also abnormalities of the eye.[3]

An additional indication for more detailed fetal CNS imaging arises from failure to visualize the septi pellucidi in a screening examination. During development there is typically a cavum septum pellucidum. Absence of the septi pellucidi can be seen in the constellation of findings known as septo-optic dysplasia (SOD), in which the optic nerves are hypoplastic. Both endocrine abnormalities and pituitary malformation, in particular ectopic neurohypophysis, and possibly a schizencephalic cleft, may occur in SOD. Hypoplasia of the optic nerve and an ectopic neurohypophysis can be difficult to confirm on prenatal imaging, and postnatal ophthalmic examination and endocrine

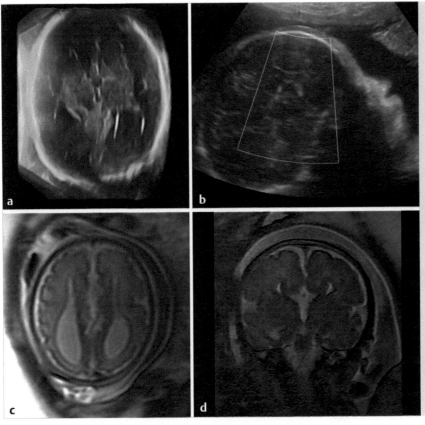

Fig. 5.4 Fetal agenesis of the corpus callosum. (a) Axial fetal ultrasonographic image of the head shows enlargement of the atria of both lateral ventricles. (b) Sagittal Doppler ultrasonographic image shows a low position of the distal branches of the anterior cerebral artery.(c) Axial single-shot T2 W magnetic resonance image of the brain shows parallel lateral ventricles and preferential enlargement of the atria (colpocephaly). (d) Coronal single-shot T2 W magnetic resonance image shows a vertically oriented third ventricle in communication with the interhemispheric fissure without intervening corpus callosum, and a "longhorn" appearance of the third ventricle and lateral ventricles.

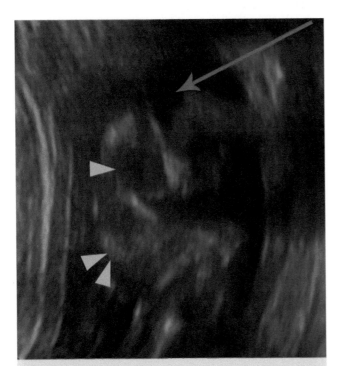

Fig. 5.5 Fetal anencephaly. Sagittal ultrasonographic image of the fetal head shows the eyes (*green arrowhead*) and chin/face (*double green arrowheads*). There is absence of a cranial vault above the level of the eyes (*red arrow*).

testing may be indicated for their detection, as may also be postnatal MRI. At times, absence of the septum pellucidum can be an isolated finding without presumable pathologic consequences, but this must be considered a diagnosis of exclusion.

Septo-optic dysplasia is considered to possibly represent the mildest form of a disorder within the holoprosencephaly spectrum. Although the absence of a septum pellucidum can occasionally be an isolated finding, it should prompt an investigation for other features of disorders within this spectrum of holoprosencephalic disorders

The identification of a more profound parenchymal abnormality makes it important to fully characterize the other (extracranial) findings in the affected fetus, which have prognostic implications for the fetus and possibly genetic implications for any future children. The more severe disorders in the holoprosencephaly spectrum can have an appearance that is confusing to one who is not familiar with the abnormality (refer to ▶ Fig. 3.13, ▶ Fig. 3.14, ▶ Fig. 3.15, and ▶ Fig. 3.16).[4] The more severe disorders within the spectrum (e.g., alobar holoprosencephaly) tend to have poor postnatal prognoses.

A defect in closure of the rostral neural tube can result in an open cranial vault and exposure of the developing tissue of the patient's central nervous system (CNS) to amniotic fluid, resulting in injury to the tissue and failure of formation of the brain (▶ Fig. 5.5). This condition is known as anencephaly (literally "no brain").

In another condition, known as hydranencephaly (literally "water in place of the brain") there is in utero occlusion of both internal carotid arteries, resulting in necrosis of nearly the entirety of the supratentorial parenchyma, other than the

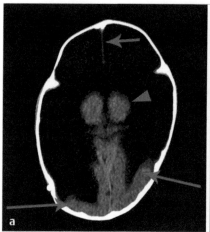
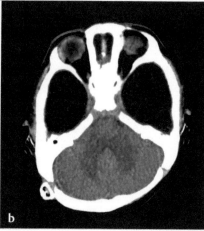

Fig. 5.6 Hydranencephaly. (a) Axial computed tomographic image of the head of a 4-month-old male shows nearly complete absence of the supratentorial parenchyma, except for the thalami (*arrowhead*) and occipital lobes (*long arrows*), both of which areas are supplied by the posterior circulation. The normally separated thalami, as well as the presence of the falx cerebri (*short arrow*), indicate that the patient's disorder does not belong to the holoprosencephaly spectrum. (b) Axial computed tomographic image of the posterior fossa shows a relatively normal appearance of the brainstem and cerebellum, which are supplied by the posterior circulation.

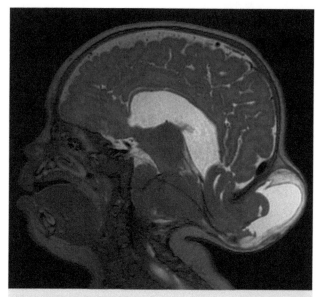

Fig. 5.7 Encephalocele. Sagittal T2W magnetic resonance image of the head of a 7-month-old boy shows brain parenchyma protruding through a defect in the occipital bone, with surrounding meninges and CSF.

thalami and possibly the inferior occipital lobes, which may be supplied by the posterior circulation. The brainstem and cerebellum are typically normal. Because the cerebral hemispheres will have originally formed and cleaved, there will be a normal falx cerebri (▸ Fig. 5.6); however, the postnatal prognosis is poor. The presence of the falx cerebri can differentiate hydranencephaly from alobar holoprosencephaly.

A defect in the calvarium can result in protrusion of the meninges and CSF (meningocele) or brain parenchyma (encephalocele) (▸ Fig. 5.7). An encephalocele can be associated with a phenotype resembling a Chiari type II malformation, known as a Chiari type III malformation. An occipital encephalocele in the setting of renal anomalies and polydactyly can be seen in Meckel–Gruber syndrome.

A large central CSF space without a finding of significant parenchyma can be seen in the setting of severe hydrocephalus, which is important to differentiate from other causes because it has the potential for nearly complete normalization after shunting. The thin rim of peripheralized parenchyma may be difficult to see on ultrasound, which is why fetal MRI can help differentiate devastating conditions like alobar holoprosencephaly and hydranencephaly from a potentially treatable severe hydrocephaly.

It is important to note that the normal sulcation pattern of the brain occurs predominantly in the second half of gestation, and it can be very easy to incorrectly diagnose lissencephaly prior to term gestation. This is important to remember for prenatal imaging, as well as for postnatal imaging in very premature infants.

5.3 Neonatal Imaging

The neonatal brain is easily evaluated with ultrasonography, as the anterior fontanelle is open (in particular in premature infants). This can allow both coronal and sagittal views of the brain, with excellent evaluation of the ventricular system but limited detail of the posterior fossa. In premature infants, it is also possible to have ultrasonographic views through the mastoid fontenelle (▸ Fig. 5.8).

5.4 Germinal Matrix Hemorrhage

Premature infants are at increased risk for germinal matrix hemorrhage (GMH). The germinal matrix is the site of the neuronal proliferation that creates the cortex and is located predominantly along the lateral margins of the bodies of the lateral ventricles. Because of the metabolic demands of neuronal proliferation, the germinal matrix is highly vascular. In the premature infant, the autonomic nervous system is not fully developed and autoregulation is therefore impaired. Any fetal stressor that results in fluctuations in heart rate and/or blood pressure raises the possibility of a hemorrhage in the fragile blood vessels of the germinal matrix. The mildest form of such hemorrhage is a small focus that remains in the subependymal zone, known as a grade I GMH (▸ Fig. 5.9).

When a GMH extends into the ventricle, it is referred to as a grade II GMH (▸ Fig. 5.10). When an intraventricular hemorrhage is of a large volume that distends the ventricular system, it is referred to as a grade III GMH (▸ Fig. 5.11).

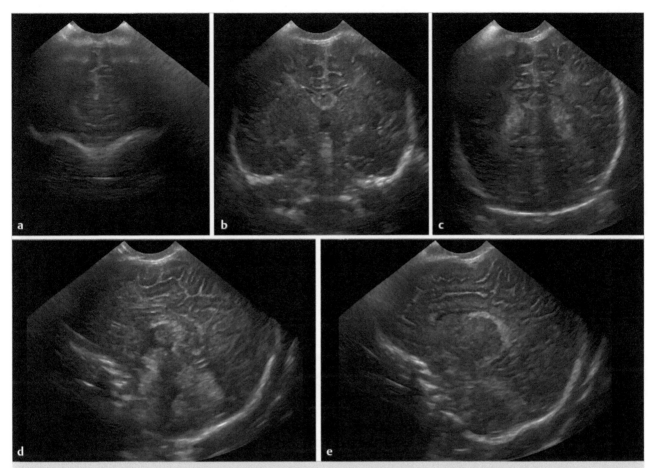

Fig. 5.8 Ultrasonographic image of the anatomy of the head. Three ultrasonographic images are shown, in the coronal plane and extending through the anterior fontanelle from anterior to posterior. (a) The anterior-most image shows the floor of the anterior cranial fossa (orbital roofs). (b) The second image shows the bodies of both lateral ventricles. (c) The posterior-most image, a coronal–oblique image, shows the choroid plexus within the atria of both lateral ventricles. (d) A midsagittal image shows the corpus callosum, the brainstem, and the echogenic vermis posterior to the fourth ventricle. (e) A parasagittal image shows the choroid plexus in the posterior body of the lateral ventricle, but not extending anteriorly to the level of the caudothalamic groove.

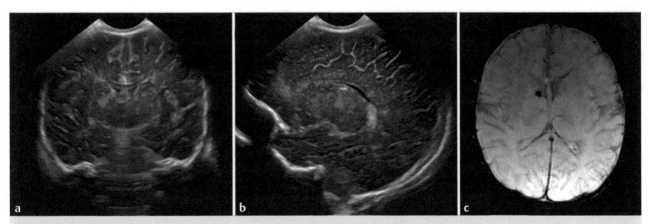

Fig. 5.9 Grade I germinal matrix hemorrhage (GMH). (a) Coronal ultrasonographic image through the anterior fontanelle obtained at 14 days of age shows a focal asymmetry in the subependymal region along the lateral margin of the body of the right lateral ventricle (*red arrowhead*). (b) A sagittal ultrasonographic image shows the asymmetry to be centered at the caudothalamic groove (*red arrowhead*). (c) An axial susceptibility-weighted image from an MRI scan shows hypointensity in the location shown in (b), confirming that the abnormality in this patient's brain represents a focal grade I GMH.

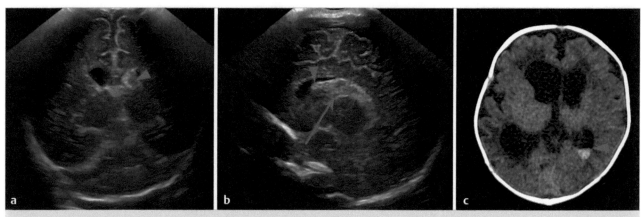

Fig. 5.10 Grade II germinal matrix hemorrhage (GMH). (a) Coronal ultrasonographic image in an 11-day-old premature infant shows echogenic material in the body of the left lateral ventricle (*red arrowhead*). (b) A sagittal image shows that the echogenic material (*red arrowhead*) extends anterior to the expected location of the caudothalamic groove (*red arrow*), which (together with the asymmetry in the subependymal region) confirms that this represents a grade II GMH and not echogenic choroid plexus. (c) Axial computed tomographic image recorded 3 weeks later shows development of ventriculomegaly with layering of blood products in the occipital horn of the left lateral ventricle (*red arrowhead*). Because the ventriculomegaly in this patient is probably related to impaired passage of CSF through the sylvian aqueduct, and not to distention from a blood clot, the diagnosis remains a grade II GMH.

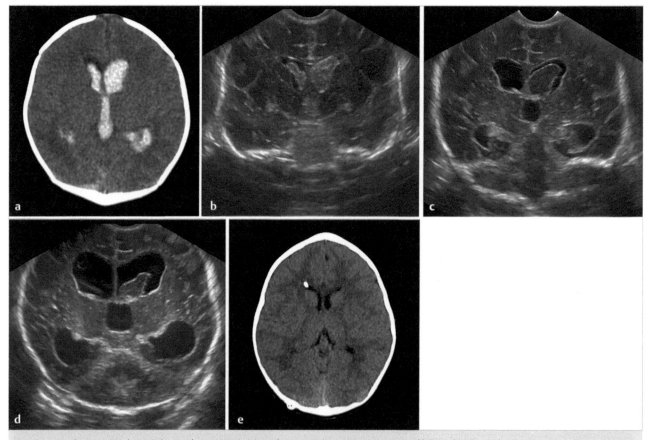

Fig. 5.11 Grade III germinal matrix hemorrhage (GMH). (a) Axial computed tomographic image of bilateral GMH made at an outside institution shows casting of the ventricular system with blood clot, resulting in dilation of the left lateral ventricle and third ventricle, and to a lesser extent of the right lateral ventricle, consistent with grade III GMH. Note that in contrast to the case with intracranial hemorrhage later in life, computed tomography is rarely indicated for the primary evaluation of a GMH, but can aid in surgical planning and evaluation of the posterior fossa. (b) Coronal ultrasonographic image through the anterior fontanelle at 5 days shows echogenic clot in the bodies of both lateral ventricles. (c) Coronal ultrasonographic image made at 13 days shows early retraction of the clots in the ventricles, with less echogenicity. (d) A coronal ultrasonographic image at 20 days shows continued retraction of the clots but development of hydrocephalus. (e) Axial computed tomographic image made at 3 years of age shows a nondilated appearance of the ventricles after shunting, without appreciable parenchymal abnormality.

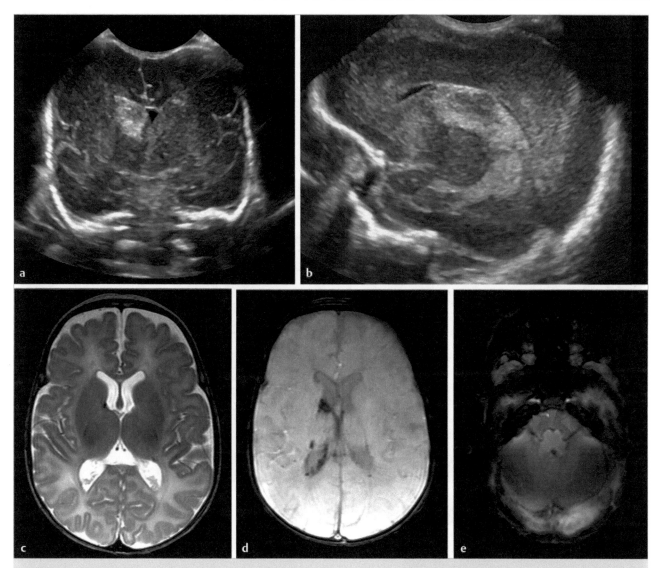

Fig. 5.12 Grade IV germinal matrix hemorrhage (GMH). (a) Coronal and (b) sagittal ultrasonographic images made at made at 6 days of age in a female born prematurely at 24 weeks, gestational age demonstrates an expansile area of intra-axial echogenicity in the region of the right caudate body, representing a hemorrhagic venous infarction (i.e., grade IV GMH). (c) Axial T2 W magnetic resonance image at 4 months of age shows a relatively normal structural appearance of the brain, with a focus of T2 hypointensity along the right caudothalamic groove. (d) An axial susceptibility-weighted magnetic resonance image shows multifocal areas of hypointensity, consistent with hemosiderin deposition that was underestimated on conventional sequences. (e) An axial susceptibility-weighted magnetic resonance image at the level of the medulla shows a hypointense "India-ink" margin to the brainstem, as well as the cisternal segments of several cranial nerves, representing superficial siderosis (*red arrowheads*).

Note that obstruction of the sylvian aqueduct by blood products from a grade II GMH, with resulting hydrocephalus, does not constitute a grade III GMH, but remains a hemorrhage of grade II. Normal choroid plexus within the lateral ventricles can be echogenic, but is typically symmetric and should not extend anteriorly to the level of the caudothalamic groove. When there is uncertainty in differentiating choroid plexus from a GMH, short-term follow-up studies can help. Computed tomography is not a technique for routine characterization of GMH.

Hemorrhage within the parenchyma itself is referred to as a grade IV GMH (▶ Fig. 5.12). However, recent work has strongly suggested that this entity is actually a hemorrhagic venous infarction. Therefore, although there is a progression of severity of GMH from grade I to grade II and grade III, a grade IV GMH is a separate entity, and the application to it of the term "germinal matrix hemorrhage" is somewhat of a misnomer.

It is possible, and in fact common, to have hemorrhage of different grades between the right and left lateral ventricles. It is important to note that grade I GMH is often difficult to detect with CT, and that although CT is typically the mainstay modality for evaluating hemorrhage in other age groups, it is reserved for problem solving in the neonatal period. When possible, cross-sectional evaluation for problem solving and surgical planning should be done with MRI because susceptibility-weighted imaging can show the extent of deposition of blood products and hemosiderin (▶ Fig. 5.12 e).

Germinal matrix hemorrhage is rare in a term infant, and intracranial hemorrhage in a term infant raises the possibility

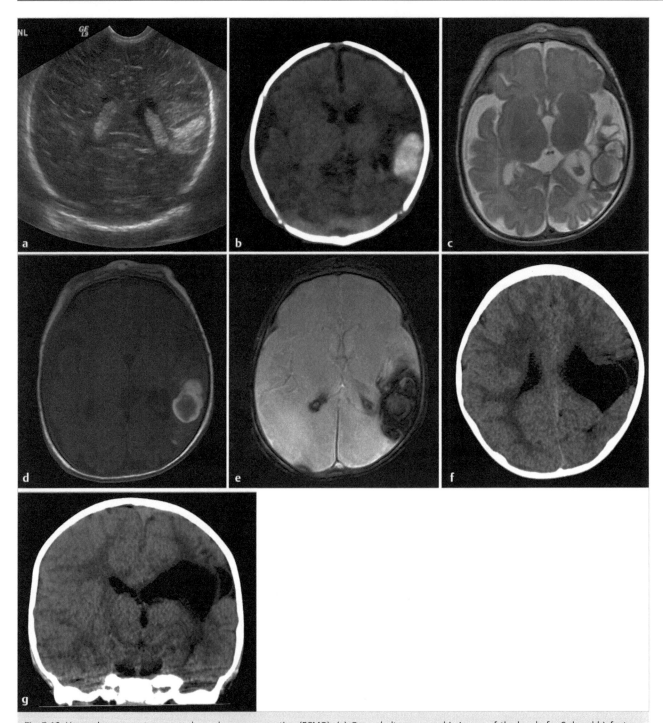

Fig. 5.13 Hemorrhage on extracorporeal membrane oxygenation (ECMO). (a) Coronal ultrasonographic image of the head of a 6-day-old infant on ECMO demonstrates an echogenic, slightly expansile area on the left posterior temporal lobe. (b) A computed tomographic examination at 19 days of life shows a parenchymal hematoma. (c) Magnetic resonance imaging at 24 days of life shows a thin peripheral rim of T2 W hypointense signal with (d) heterogeneous internal signal characteristics on T2 W and T1 W (d) images, susceptibility hypointensity, consistent with blood products in mixed stages of evolution. (f) Axial and (g) coronal computed tomographic images made at 5 years of age show left posterior temporal and inferior parietal encephalomalacia with ex vacuo enlargement of the left lateral ventricle.

of other abnormalities, such as trauma, a coagulopathy, or a vascular malformation.

Because of hemodynamic variations in an anticoagulated patient, daily ultrasonographic studies of the head are often done on children receiving extracorporeal membrane oxygenation (ECMO). The development of an intracranial hemorrhage may result in cessation of ECMO therapy, but the risks and benefits of doing this must be considered on a patient-by-patient basis. Hemorrhages in anticoagulated ECMO patients will not be isolated to the germinal matrix, and a more extensive sonographic survey of the entire brain in such children may therefore be required (▶ Fig. 5.13).

In the setting of GMH, patients often develop hydrocephalus. Serial ultrasonographic examinations can indicate whether the hydrocephalus progresses and may require shunting. For patients who have hydrocephalus, some centers advocate using resistive indices in the pericallosal artery to determine the need for shunting, with high resistive indices (e.g., > 0.8) favoring shunting; however, exact numerical cutoff values of such indices have not been reliably established.[5,6] Another technique used at some centers, without definitive validation, is evaluation of variations in the resistive index in the pericallosal artery during compression of the anterior fontanelle.[7] The management of posthemorrhagic hydrocephalus is complicated, and it is not based on a single value, and shunting is not the only management technique for it, with other techniques for this including ETV and serial lumbar puncture, with variable rates of success.[8,9]

5.5 Hypoxic-Ischemic Encephalopathy

Ischemic injury to the CNS can result from peripartum hypoxia incurred, for example, by in utero stress or by postnatal abnormalities related to cardiac and/or respiratory compromise. Pre-existing cardiac or pulmonary disease increases the risk for ischemic injury to the CNS, also known as hypoxic-ischemic encephalopathy (HIE). Ultrasonography remains a valuable first-line investigational tool for HIE, although MRI demonstrates greater sensitivity and specificity.

Parenchymal edema manifests as increased echogenicity in an ultrasonographic examination (▸ Fig. 5.14); however, this can often be very subtle, especially if there is a bilateral symmetric injury. Diffusion-weighted imaging (DWI) may show

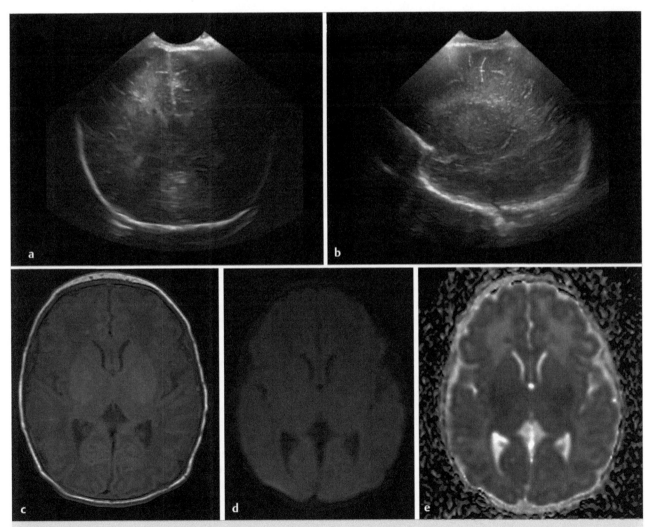

Fig. 5.14 Hypoxic-ischemic encephalopathy demonstrated on ultrasound and MRI. (a) Coronal and (b) right parasagittal ultrasonographic images of the head of a 1-day-old infant male with suspected HIE demonstrates a diffuse homogeneous echogenicity of the cerebral white matter, consistent with edema. (N.B.: It is important to be familiar with the normal echogenicity of white matter as shown with the imaging equipment at a given institution.) (c) Axial T1 W MRI obtained at 5 days of life shows a greater hyperintensity in the globi palladi than within the posterior limb of the internal capsule, consistent with sequelae of HIE. (d) Axial DWI with (e) apparent diffusion coefficient (ADC) mapping shows signs of reduced water diffusion in the posterior lentiform nucleus and in the ventral posterolateral nucleus of the thalami, corresponding with the areas that are actively myelinating at this age.

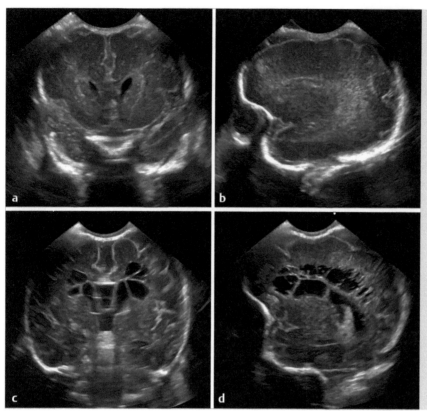

Fig. 5.15 Periventricular leukomalacia. (a) Coronal and (b) parasagittal ultrasonographic images in a 1-week-old premature infant born at approximately 26 weeks of gestational age demonstrates an echogenic appearance to the periventricular white matter, as well as an immature sulcation pattern. (c) Follow-up coronal and (d) parasagittal ultrasonographic images made at 1 month show development of multiple areas of cystic necrosis (also referred to as periventricular leukomalacia) coursing along the margins of the bodies of both lateral ventricles.

these findings more clearly, allowing confident identification of the cause for neurologic symptoms, such as seizure or hypotonia (▶ Fig. 5.15).[10,11,12,13] Hypoxic-ischemic encephalopathy is typically symmetric, and accordingly can be difficult to identify on diffusion-weighted imaging if there is a diffuse abnormality. Because the cerebellum is more resistant to hypoxic injury than the cerebrum, coronal DWI can be helpful for detecting diffuse supratentorial injury. Although MRI is more sensitive and specific, ultrasonography remains an important tool in the rapid evaluation of an unstable infant, or for follow-up.

In many cases, it may not be possible to conduct MRI in the first 7 to 10 days after an injury, and DWI performed after this point may therefore not show an abnormality. Other signs of parenchymal injury may remain, such as a hyperintense signal on T1 W imaging in the globi palladi (▶ Fig. 5.14c), probably related to dystrophic micromineralization. T1 shortening in the globus pallidus in the absence of risk factors for HIE should prompt evaluation of bilirubin levels, since this resembles what is seen in kernicterus.

Ischemic injury can result in cystic necrosis of the periventricular white matter, a process often referred to as periventricular leukomalacia (PVL) (▶ Fig. 5.15). Focal areas of parenchymal injury can create dominant cystic areas known as porencephalic cysts (▶ Fig. 5.16), which may develop communication with the ventricular system. Porencephalic cysts may have susceptibility hypointensity along the margins related to hemosiderin deposition. Collectively, white-matter necrosis/PVL and porencephalic cysts can be referred to as white matter disease of prematurity.

Late-term sequelae of severe white-matter disease of prematurity can result in crowding of gyri, known as ulegyria; this can have an appearance similar to that of polymicrogyria, but has a different pathophysiology and clinical significance (▶ Fig. 5.16 d). In patients with more mild disease that is not prospectively clinically evident, there may be a late presentation with either developmental delay or possibly hemiparesis, if the injury to white matter affects the corticospinal tracts (▶ Fig. 5.17).

Linear areas of subtle echogenicity may be seen in the deep gray nuclei on sonography (▶ Fig. 5.18), a process known as mineralizing vasculopathy. Originally this was seen only in the setting of HIE, other metabolic derangements, and genetic abnormalities, such as trisomies, but increased sensitivity of the transducers used in ultrasonography has led to occasions on which mineralizing vasculopathy can be seen in the absence of other abnormalities and is therefore of uncertain significance.

Evaluation of the newborn with seizures or abnormal movements warrants detailed evaluation for signs of leukodystrophies and/or inborn errors of metabolism, possibly including MRI with MR spectroscopy. Clinical evaluation for dysmorphic features that may be associated with genetic disorders may be helpful, and if there are dysmorphic features, a radiographic skeletal survey should be considered.

Additionally, it is important to be aware that neonatal encephalitis caused by herpes simplex virus (HSV) does not necessarily arise through direct spread from the gasserian ganglion to the medial temporal lobes, and may disseminate through the CSF and/or hematogenously, and can have a somewhat random distribution and possibly spare the temporal lobes (▶ Fig. 5.19).

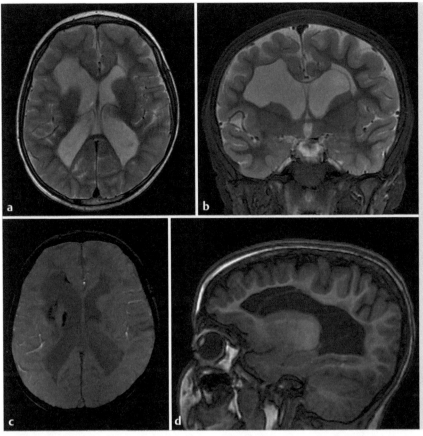

Fig. 5.16 Porencephaly. (a) Axial T2 W magnetic resonance image and (b) coronal short tau inversion recovery image show a right frontal porencephalic cyst that is in communication with the right lateral ventricle, and a left frontal cyst that is not in visible communication with the left lateral ventricle. There is corresponding loss of white-matter volume. (c) Axial susceptibility-weighted image shows multifocal areas of hemosiderin deposition along the margins of the lateral ventricles and the porencephalic cyst, from prior intraventricular hemorrhage. (d) Sagittal T1 W magnetic resonance image shows an area of left frontal subcortical white-matter thinning. The resultant crowding of the overlying gyri from a decreased white-matter volume is known as ulegyria, and should not be confused with polymicrogyria.

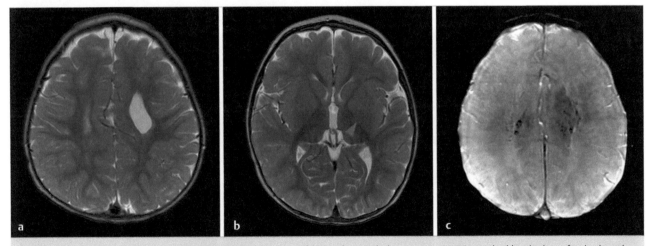

Fig. 5.17 Hemiparesis. (a) Axial T2 W magnetic resonance image made to evaluate right hemiparesis in a 16-month-old male shows focal volume loss at the superior margin of the body of the left lateral ventricle. (b) Axial T2 W image at the level of the deep gray nuclei shows a focal abnormality in the midportion of the left posterior limb of the internal capsule (*red arrowhead*), probably related to Wallerian degeneration in the corticospinal tract. (c) Axial susceptibility-weighted image shows that the volume loss seen in (a) is related to prior germinal matrix hemorrhage.

The T1 W and T2 W signal abnormalities that occur in HSV infection can be difficult to identify in the hypomyelinated neonate, and there may not be any appreciable postcontrast enhancement. Therefore, unexplained areas of diffusion restriction in a neonate with seizures should raise suspicion of HSV encephalitis, and treatment with acyclovir should be started immediately (without waiting for confirmation by polymerase chain reaction on a specimen of CSF). Eventually, there may be areas of hypointense signal on susceptibility-weighted imaging related to hemorrhagic changes common in HSV encephalitis.

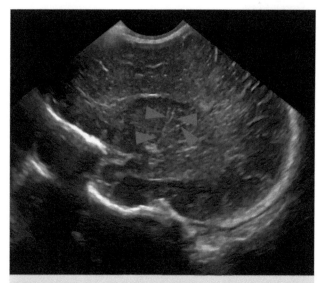

Fig. 5.18 Mineralizing vasculopathy. Sagittal ultrasonographic image of the head of an 11-day-old boy shows branching echogenic structures (*red arrowheads*) within the lentiform nucleus, representing mineralizing vasculopathy.

5.6 Normal Perinatal Findings

Several findings on MRI are commonly encountered in the neonate but not in other age groups. Trace amounts of subdural blood products can be present after parturition, particularly in the posterior fossa and overlying the occipital lobes (▶ Fig. 5.20), and are typically of no clinical significance. It can be challenging to determine the appropriate level of concern for these findings because it is always necessary to be alert for signs of nonaccidental trauma.

A cephalohematoma is an extracranial subperiosteal hematoma that can occur with childbirth, possibly in relation to the location of vacuum extraction (▶ Fig. 5.21). Because a cephalohematoma is a subperiosteal collection (analogous to an epidural hematoma), it will typically be bound by sutures. Although it typically resolves spontaneously, it may calcify (▶ Fig. 5.22).

Caput succedaneum is an extracranial hematoma that is not subperiosteal (and therefore can cross sutures and the midline), and typically resolves spontaneously without complication. In the first days after vaginal birth, the cranial configuration in caput succedaneum is elongated, an effect known as cranial molding (▶ Fig. 5.23), which is a normal process.

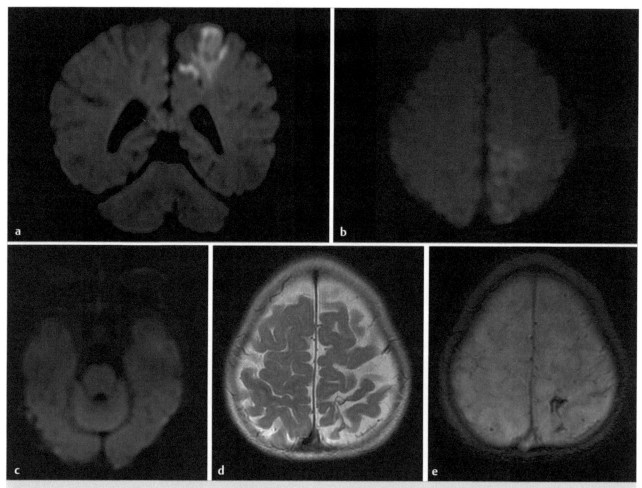

Fig. 5.19 Perinatal herpes simplex virus (HSV) encephalitis. (a) Coronal and (b) axial diffusion-weighted images (DWI) show reduced water diffusion in the left superior parietal lobule in a 3-week-old female with seizures of new onset, which were proven to be related to neonatal HSV encephalitis. (c) Axial DWI through the temporal lobes shows no abnormality, in contrast to what is seen in non-neonatal HSV encephalitis. (d) Axial T2 W image obtained at 10 months of age shows encephalomalacia in the area of involvement, and (e) susceptibility-weighted imaging shows signs of prior hemorrhage.

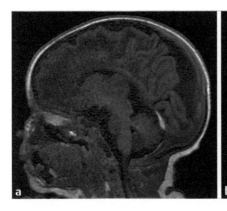
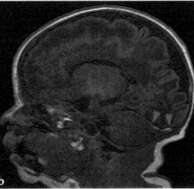

Fig. 5.20 Parturition-related subdural hematoma (SDH). Sagittal T1 W magnetic resonance images of the head of a 7-day-old female infant who underwent magnetic resonance imaging (MRI) as a part of a genetic screen show areas of subdural T1 shortening overlying (a) the cerebellum and (b) occipital poles, which is in a pattern that can be seen with trace quantities of parturition-related blood products (*red arrowheads*).

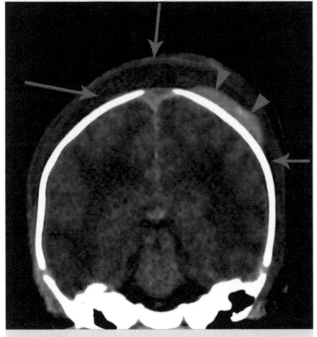

Fig. 5.21 Cephalohematoma. Coronal computed tomographic image of the head of a 1-day-old infant male with scalp swelling after childbirth demonstrates a focal area of subperiosteal blood products overlying the left parietal bone near the vertex, consistent with a cephalohematoma (*red arrowheads*). There is also generalized scalp swelling crossing the midline without being bound by sutures, which is consistent with caput succedaneum (*three red arrows*).

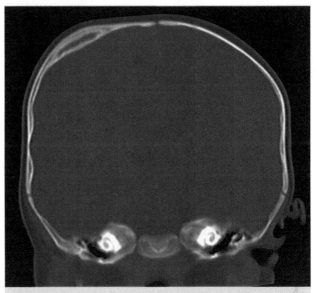

Fig. 5.22 Calcified cephalohematoma. Coronal bone-algorithm computed tomographic scan performed on a 4-month-old child with a palpable area of swelling on the head that became firm over time shows focal thickening of the calvarium without an overlying periosteal reaction, consistent with a calcified cephalohematoma.

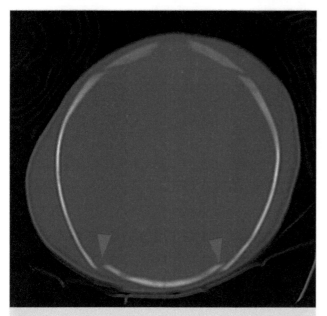

Fig. 5.23 Axial bone-algorithm computed tomographic image of the head of a 1-day-old infant made to evaluate scalp swelling after prolonged childbirth. No fracture is identified, but the occipital bone underlies the posterior margin of the parietal bones (*red arrowheads*), a condition known as calvarial molding, which is a normal and transient postparturition process. Also seen is scalp swelling related to caput succedaneum.

5.7 Further Reading

[1] Yoon HJ, Kim JH, Jeon TY, Yoo S-Y, Eo H. Devastating metabolic brain disorders of newborns and young infants. Radiographics 2014; 34(5):1257–1272

References

[1] Griffiths PD, Reeves MJ, Morris JE et al. A prospective study of fetuses with isolated ventriculomegaly investigated by antenatal sonography and in utero MR imaging. AJNR Am J Neuroradiol 2010; 31(1):106–111

[2] Raybaud C. The corpus callosum, the other great forebrain commissures, and the septum pellucidum: anatomy, development, and malformation. Neuro-radiology 2010; 52(6):447–477

[3] Aicardi J. Aicardi syndrome. Brain Dev 2005; 27(3):164–171

[4] Winter TC, Kennedy AM, Woodward PJ. Holoprosencephaly: a survey of the entity, with embryology and fetal imaging. Radiographics 2015; 35(1):275–290

[5] Goh D, Minns RA, Hendry GM, Thambyayah M, Steers AJ. Cerebrovascular resistive index assessed by duplex Doppler sonography and its relationship to intracranial pressure in infantile hydrocephalus. Pediatr Radiol 1992; 22(4):246–250

[6] Hill A, Volpe JJ. Decrease in pulsatile flow in the anterior cerebral arteries in infantile hydrocephalus. Pediatrics 1982; 69(1):4–7

[7] Taylor GA, Madsen JR. Neonatal hydrocephalus: hemodynamic response to fontanelle compression—correlation with intracranial pressure and need for shunt placement. Radiology 1996; 201(3):685–689

[8] Mazzola CA, Choudhri AF, Auguste KI et al. Pediatric hydrocephalus: systematic literature review and evidence-based guidelines. Part 2: Management of posthemorrhagic hydrocephalus in premature infants. J Neurosurg Pediatr 2014; 14(14) Suppl 1:8–23

[9] Nikas DC, Post AF, Choudhri AF, Mazzola CA, Mitchell L, Flannery AM. Pediatric hydrocephalus: systematic literature review and evidence-based guidelines. Part 10: Change in ventricle size as a measurement of effective treatment of hydrocephalus. J Neurosurg Pediatr 2014; 14(14) Suppl 1:77–81

[10] Ghei SK, Zan E, Nathan JE et al. MR imaging of hypoxic-ischemic injury in term neonates: pearls and pitfalls. Radiographics 2014; 34(4):1047–1061

[11] Shroff MM, Soares-Fernandes JP, Whyte H, Raybaud C. MR imaging for diagnostic evaluation of encephalopathy in the newborn. Radiographics 2010; 30 (3):763–780

[12] Chao CP, Zaleski CG, Patton AC. Neonatal hypoxic ischemic encephalopathy: multimodality imaging findings. Radiographics 2006; 26:S159–S172

[13] Huang BY, Castillo M. Hypoxic-ischemic brain injury: imaging findings from birth to adulthood. Radiographics 2008; 28(2):417–439, quiz 617

6 Trauma and Hemorrhage

6.1 Introduction

Traumatic head injuries are a common occurrence, with an incidence of up to 1.7 million per year in the United States as of 2014.[1,2] Trauma results in costs for early, follow-up, and possibly long-term care, and also has implications with regard to neural development. Head trauma comes in many forms and has many causes, including accidents and sports injuries. Another type of traumatic injury is purposeful trauma, also known as nonaccidental trauma (NAT) or child abuse. The appearance of the developing skull makes it common for unfused sutures to be mistaken for fractures in young children, and conversely, fractures can be mistaken for normal sutures. Radiologic evaluation plays a critical role in the diagnosis and characterization of traumatic head injury, and research has suggested an even larger role for it in the future with advanced imaging techniques.[3,4,5] A correct understanding of normal developmental anatomy throughout childhood, as well as of the various types of intracranial injuries in pediatric trauma, can allow the appropriate identification of injuries, aiding in their treatment and prognosis.

6.2 Hemorrhage

6.2.1 Appearance of Blood on Computed Tomography

Acutely clotted blood has a density on computed tomography (CT) that is higher than that of brain parenchyma, typically up to 60 to 80 HU. The density is related to the concentrated proteins and heme (which contains iron) in the clot. Unclotted blood will not have this high density, and a hyperacute hemorrhage may not have a uniformly high density, as is the case with the "swirl-sign" of active bleeding into an epidural hematoma (▶ Fig. 6.1). Over time, a hematoma will evolve and decrease in size, and the protein and heme in it are resorbed, resulting in the density of the collected blood decreasing at approximate 1 HU per day. A collection of intermediate density (perhaps 30 HU) is commonly said to be a chronic collection, but may represent an acute collection in a patient with severe anemia.

6.2.2 Dating Hemorrhage on Magnetic Resonance Imaging

The appearance on magnetic resonance imaging (MRI) of evolving blood products relates to both the chemical species of heme in an image and the integrity of the erythrocyte. The evolution of hemoglobin from oxyhemoglobin to deoxyhemoglobin to methemoglobin and then to hemosiderin occurs in a sequential manner but with a highly variable time frame (▶ Table 6.1). Additionally, there is cell lysis, typically during the methemoglobin stage of the evolution. The timing with which the entities in the evolution appear depends upon factors like the presence of continuing bleeding, temperature, pH, and oxygen tension, among others. It is therefore strongly recommended that exact dating of blood products not be attempted with MRI, and even an approximate time window should be suggested with caution in the absence of a full understanding of all of the factors that influence the evolution of blood. Mnemonics exist to assist in remembering the appearance of blood at various stages in T1 W and T2 W images; however, using a mnemonic for this reflects a lack of understanding the process in which blood products evolve, and no attempt should be made to date the blood products if using a mnemonic approach. We will focus on T1 W and T2 W imaging, and later deal with susceptibility-weighted imaging (SWI).

Oxyhemoglobin is present in the first few hours after bleeding. Within a few hours, the oxyhemoglobin degrades to deoxyhemoglobin, which has a hyperintense signal on T1 W MRI. This evolution takes longer in environments with higher pO_2 values. After 1 to 5 days, deoxyhemoglobin metabolizes to methemoglobin. Because of proton–electron dipole–dipole interaction (PEDDI), methemoglobin is bright on T1 W imaging. Its hyperintense signal on T1 W imaging is due to PEDDI, but with intact erythrocytes, methemoglobin has hypointense T2 W imaging because of proton relaxation enhancement (PRE). When the erythrocytes lyse, PRE is no longer a factor in the T2 W signal, which then becomes hyperintense. The shortening of the T1 W signal caused by PEDDI is related to the methemoglobin itself and is unaffected by cell lysis. Eventually, the methemoglobin evolves into hemosiderin, which is hypointense on T1 W and T2 W imaging as well as on SWI. Not only is the exact timing of this evolution highly variable, but the evolution of different portions of a hematoma may vary because all of the chemical species in it do not evolve simultaneously.

6.2.3 Subdural Hematoma

A subdural hematoma (SDH) is a collection of blood between the inner and outer dural layers, most commonly related to the traumatic injury of bridging veins. The blood collection that produces an SDH is most commonly located directly subjacent to the site of injury, but with the development of communication of the subdural space, the blood collection in an SDH can redistribute. Subdural hematomas are typically characterized by their location, thickness, and resulting mass effect. These collections are typically of low pressure, filled from venous bleeding, and have a crescentic shape. Because the blood collections in SDH are of low pressure and often do not grow, they are typically followed clinically in the absence of a marked mass effect or neurologic symptoms. However, an SDH can be evacuated neurosurgically if there is concern for its enlargement, a significant mass effect, or a neurologic deficit.

The margins of the falx cerebri and tentorium cerebelli are covered with dural layers, and subdural collections of blood can commonly be seen along these structures (▶ Fig. 6.2). Because the subdural space courses along the surface of these structures, a collection that extends across the falx cerebri or tentorium cerebelli without extension overlying the surface is within the epidural space (▶ Fig. 6.3). Trace subdural blood products overlying the occipital poles and cerebellum can be seen in the early postnatal period in relation to parturition (see Chapter 5), but there will typically be no parenchymal abnormality or resulting mass effect in such cases.

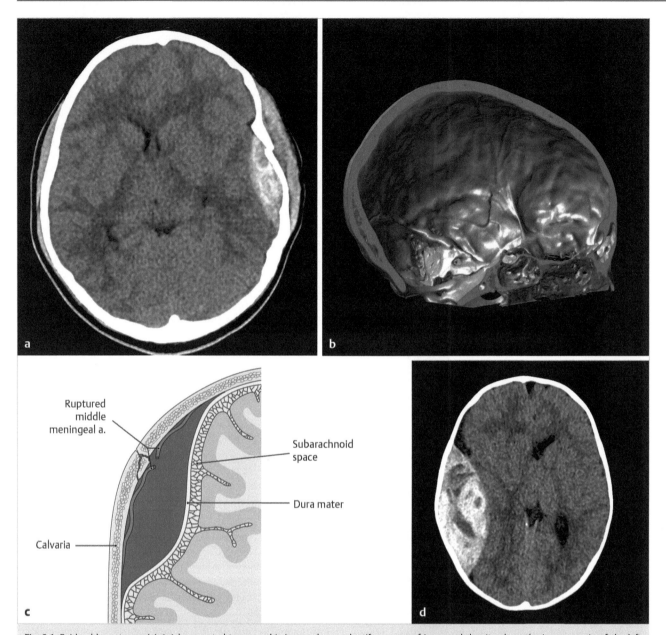

Fig. 6.1 Epidural hematoma. (a) Axial computed tomographic image shows a lentiform area of increased density along the inner margin of the left squamous temporal bone, with an overlying minimally depressed fracture. (b) Three-dimensional reformatting to display the inner table of the skull shows that the fracture crosses vascular grooves of branches of the middle meningeal artery. (c) Diagram showing the relationship of the disruption in the middle meningeal artery caused by the fracture in an extradural location. (d) Axial computed tomographic image in a 1-year-old male after a head injury, showing a large, lentiform epidural hematoma with a heterogeneous internal appearance that may be indicative of active bleeding, with the areas of low density representing blood products that have not yet clotted. "c" From Atlas of Anatomy, © Thieme 2012, Illustration by Markus Voll.

Table 6.1 Appearance of evolving blood products on magnetic resonance imaging

	Blood product	T1-weighted imaging	T2-weighted imaging	Approximate time frame
Hyperacute	Oxyhemoglobin	Isointense	Hyperintense (with a possible hypointense rim)	4–6 h
Acute	Deoxyhemoglobin	Isointense	Hypointense	6 h–3 days
Early subacute	Intracellular methemoglobin	Hyperintense	Hypointense	3–7 days
Late subacute	Extracellular methemoglobin	Hyperintense	Hyperintense	1–6 weeks
Chronic	Hemosiderin	Hypointense	Hypointense	Months to forever

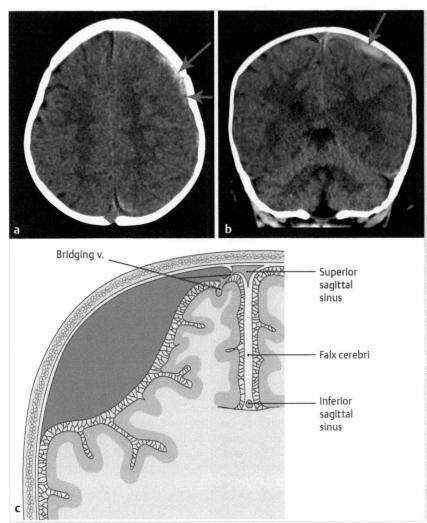

Fig. 6.2 Subdural hematoma. (a) Axial and (b) coronal computed tomographic images in a 7-month-old female following a traumatic injury shows a subdural collection overlying the left frontal lobe (*arrows*), with extension overlying the falx cerebri (*arrowheads*). There is local sulcal effacement but no resulting midline shift. (c) Diagram showing the relationship of the hematoma relative to the arachnoid and dura. Note that the "sub" part of "subdural" is relative to the skin surface and not relative to the brain. "c" From Atlas of Anatomy, © Thieme 2012, Illustration by Markus Voll.

An entity that occurs in young children but rarely in adults is a subdural hematoma with a focal tear in the dural membrane that allows cerebrospinal fluid (CSF) to extend into the subdural space. This is known as a hematohygroma; it can be of lower density on CT than typically expected in an acute collection, and may even be associated with the layering of blood products. An entity with an intermediate-density appearance on CT should not automatically be interpreted as a subacute/chronic hematoma, and the layering of blood products does not automatically indicate an acute-on-chronic hematoma. These concepts are very different from conventional teachings in adult neuroradiology, and awareness of them is exceedingly important (► Fig. 6.4). An elderly patient with underlying brain-parenchymal atrophy may have an asymptomatic chronic hematoma. When there is bleeding into this chronic collection, there will be layering of blood products, which are felt to be acute-on-chronic blood products, and in adults this latter belief is usually correct. In children, however, the assumption might be that a volume of low-density material is a chronic hematoma that was previously present but asymptomatic. Given the relative paucity of extra space in the pediatric skull, however, this is not possible; a low-density portion of a collection would be symptomatic. Awareness of this is important because this finding is sometimes described as a mixed-age subdural hematoma

suggestive of a hematoma related to NAT. Although the findings in such cases could be related to NAT, they are always likely to be acute. Similarly, patients may have a hematohygroma of intermediate density over one hemisphere and a hematoma overlying the other hemisphere; both of these collections could be acute collections, and should therefore be described as mixed-density subdural collections but not as mixed-age subdural collections.

Layering of blood products can also occur within an acute collection in a patient with impaired coagulation as the result of either an intrinsic coagulopathy or pharmacologic therapy. A subdural collection of low density in an anemic patient, such as a child with leukemia, may be an acute, life-threatening emergency. Even the presence of layering blood products may be due to impaired clotting in these patients, who may have thrombocytopenia. Therefore, especially in a patient with anemia or a coagulopathy, such as a leukemia patient, a collection should not be designated as chronic unless a prior study shows that the collection was previously present.

6.2.4 Epidural Hematoma

An epidural hematoma is a collection of blood that occurs between the skull and outer layer of the dura, which is also the

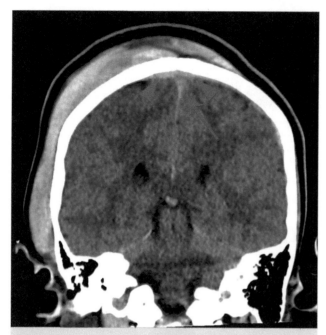

Fig. 6.3 Epidural hemorrhage crossing the falx cerebri. Coronal computed tomographic image in a 14-year-old male with history of head trauma shows an extra-axial hematoma (*arrowheads*). Because this extends between the superior sagittal sinus (*arrow*) and the calvarium and does not extend along the falx cerebri, it represents an epidural hematoma. Note that the hemorrhage crosses the sagittal suture.

shearing of a branch of the middle meningeal artery (▶ Fig. 6.1 b). Because the resulting hematoma is a subperiosteal collection, it will not cross intact sutures; however, because there is usually a fracture that may disrupt the dural insertion at the suture, this is not an inviolable rule. An extra-axial collection between the superior sagittal sinus and the calvarium, and which does not extend along the falx cerebri, is an epidural collection, often related to a venous injury.

Because epidural hematomas usually arise from arterial injury, they are more likely than subdural hematomas to expand and exert a mass effect on the brain parenchyma. Therefore, epidural hematomas require acute neurosurgical evaluation. Historically, this has also mandated acute neurosurgical evacuation of the hematoma and, if possible, cauterization of the injured vessel. Currently, small epidural hematomas in patients with normal mental status and without neurologic symptoms are sometimes observed closely, and a follow-up computed tomographic study of the head is done within 12 to 24 hours to see whether such a hematoma has progressed in size. Some stable hematomas in patients without neurologic symptoms are simply followed with clinical observation; however, the decision to follow such an epidural hematoma is based on the results of a neurosurgeon's clinical evaluation.

periosteum. Consequently, an epidural hematoma could also be referred to as a subperiosteal hematoma. Epidural hematomas are nearly always the result of arterial bleeding caused by vascular injury from a fracture and have a lentiform shape (▶ Fig. 6.1). Therefore, if an extra-axial collection of blood is seen next to a fracture, it should be suspected of having an epidural origin. If it is not possible to differentiate whether a collection is subdural or epidural, "extra-axial" is an appropriate superset of collections into which to categorize the collection.

The most common cause of an epidural hematoma is a fracture of the parietal bone or squamosal temporal bone with

6.2.5 Subarachnoid Hemorrhage

The subarachoid space is located between the brain parenchyma and the overlying dura. In adults the most common cause of subarachnoid hemorrhage (SAH) is a ruptured aneurysm, but this is less common in children, in whom SAH is most often seen in the setting of traumatic injury. Traumatic SAH is usually seen in conjunction with other types of hemorrhage (▶ Fig. 6.5). Subarachnoid hemorrhage can result in chronic staining by hemosiderin of the brain parenchyma, in particular the brainstem, which can be seen on susceptibility-weighted imaging and is known as superficial siderosis (refer to ▶ Fig. 5.12). Superficial siderosis can also be seen as a sequela of hemorrhage from other sources, such as significant germinal matrix hemorrhage (GMH). Chronic coating by hemosiderin deposits of the cisternal segments of cranial nerves may result in symptoms like tinnitus.

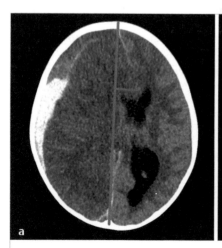
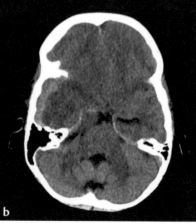

Fig. 6.4 Layering of blood in subdural hematoma. (a) Axial computed tomographic image in a 4-year-old with a recent traumatic injury shows layering of high-density blood products, with the non-dependent portion of the collection having an intermediate density. This results in approximately 19 mm of right-to-left midline shift, and (b) on an axial computed tomographic image at a lower level there is herniation of the uncus of the temporal lobe (*red arrowhead*) with mass effect on the brainstem. The patient was normal before experiencing the injury, and the injury represents an acute subdural collection of mixed density (as opposed to an acute-on-chronic collection). There is additionally diminished gray–white-matter differentiation throughout the right cerebral hemisphere, probably related to a mass effect and vascular compromise.

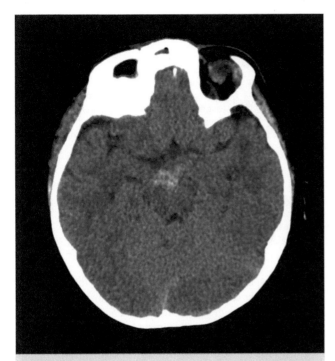

Fig. 6.5 Subarachnoid hemorrhage. Axial computed tomographic image of the head of a 6-year-old after a motor-vehicle accident shows high-density material in the interpeduncular fossa and suprasellar cistern, representing posttraumatic subarachnoid hemorrhage.

6.2.6 Parenchymal Hemorrhage

Parenchymal hemorrhages can occur from contusion, either directly subjacent to the site of impact and/or a fracture, or in relation to impact against a bone, such as the skull base (▶ Fig. 6.6). Parenchymal hemorrhages tend to be associated with the subsequent development of encephalomalacia

(▶ Fig. 6.6 c) and neurologic deficits that relate to the location and volume of parenchyma involved.

6.2.7 Diffuse Axonal Injury/Shear Injury

In addition to causing macroscopic parenchymal hemorrhages, it is now known that traumatic brain injury may result in petechial (microscopic) hemorrhages related to the shearing of white-matter fibers (▶ Fig. 6.7). This shearing injury is postulated to be related to the differing angular momentum of gray and white matter during rapid acceleration–deceleration injuries, particularly when they have a rotational component. The areas of microscopic injury can occur without signs of macroscopic hemorrhage or edema, and despite the brain's having a normal appearance on CT, can be associated with significant neurologic deficits. For this reason, unexplained neurologic deficits in a patient with head trauma warrant an MRI study with SWI. Susceptibility-weighted imaging will show the petechial hemorrhages, which are often at the interface of gray and white matter as well as in the corpus callosum. The abnormalities in shear injury may also show up on diffusion-weighted imaging (DWI) (▶ Fig. 6.7). Multifocal involvement by a shear injury is also known as diffuse axonal injury.

6.3 Pneumocephalus

Intracranial air, known as pneumocephalus, is important to identify on examinations for trauma. This is often best seen on bone-window CT images (▶ Fig. 6.8). Pneumocephalus indicates that there has been a fracture, typically into the paranasal sinuses (such as a fracture through the cribriform plate) or mastoid air cells (such as in a temporal-bone fracture), or an open fracture possibly related to a penetrating injury. Accordingly, the presence of pneumocephalus reflects a high risk for the subsequent development of infection, and its presence therefore prompts the initiation of antibiotic therapy.

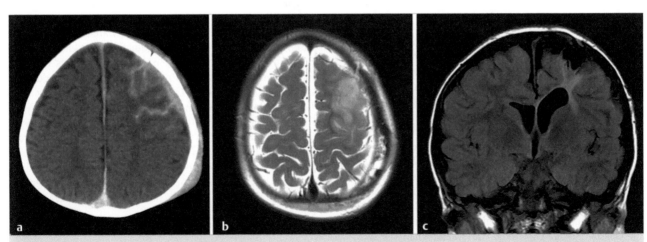

Fig. 6.6 Parenchymal contusion. (a) Axial computed tomographic image in a 14-month-old status post head trauma showing a left frontal fracture and subarachnoid and subdural blood products, with low density of the parenchyma. (b) Axial T2-weighted magnetic resonance image shows a hyperintense signal within the parenchyma, consistent with a contusion. (c) Coronal fluid attenuation inversion recovery (FLAIR) image 6 years after the injury in (a) shows focal volume loss and hyperintense signal (gliosis) within this area of encephalomalacia, with ex vacuo dilation of the left lateral ventricle.

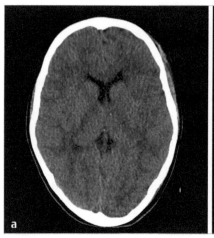
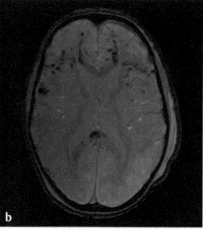

Fig. 6.7 Diffuse axonal injury. (a) Axial computed tomographic image in an 8-year-old child after head injury shows no definite abnormality. The patient remained comatose, with (b) a magnetic resonance imaging (MRI) study showing multifocal areas of hypointensity on susceptibility-weighted imaging thoughout both frontal lobes, as well as within the splenium of the corpus callosum, consistent with petechial hemorrhages in the setting of diffuse axonal injury (shear injury).

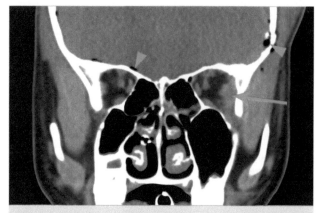

Fig. 6.8 Coronal computed tomographic image showing a hematoma in the lateral extraconal space (*blue arrow*), and multiple foci of pneumocephalus (*blue arrowheads*).

6.4 Mass Effect

A mass effect on subjacent brain parenchyma can produce damage ranging from mild sulcal effacement and flattening to distortion of the ipsilateral lateral ventricle without midline shift, midline shift without uncal herniation, and more severe forms of herniation. Measuring the degree of midline shift is important, and is typically accomplished by drawing a line between the anterior and posterior aspects of the superior sagittal sinus and measuring the distance of deviation from this line of a midline structure, such as the septum pellucidum or third ventricle (▶ Fig. 6.4 a). Apparent midline shift of 1 or 2 mm is typically insignificant and may be artifactual, but changes in midline shift between studies are important to recognize. It is also critical to recognize that bilateral extra-axial collections may not result in a midline shift, for which reason close attention to the perimesencephalic cisterns is warranted. When the uncus of the temporal lobe is pushed medially, effacing the crural cistern and exerting a mass effect on the cerebral peduncle, the result is referred to as uncal herniation. However, herniation is not an all-or-none phenomenon, and therefore effacement of the crural cistern without a mass effect represents an early stage of uncal herniation, whereas more severe forms of herniation result in mass effect on the midbrain and caudal displacement

of the uncus. Because the cisternal segment of the oculomotor nerve normally courses adjacent to the medial margin of the uncus, mass effect on the third nerve and a resulting third-nerve palsy (an inferolaterally directed eye with a dilated pupil, or "down, out, and dilated") is a sign of uncal herniation (▶ Fig. 6.4 b).

After sulcal and ventricular effacement and uncal herniation, there is effacement of the remainder of the perimesencephalic cisterns, and eventually of the prepontine cisterns and cisterna magna. Caudual displacement of the cerebellar tonsils through the foramen magnum as the result of mass effect is known as tonsillar herniation. Tonsillar herniation can be thought of as an "acquired Chiari type I malformation," but this significantly underestimates its potentially ominous implications.

6.5 Sports Injuries

The traumatic injuries discussed thus far are related to single injurious events. Events in high-impact sports, such as in football, from falls off bicycles, or in gymnastics, can cause the same types of injuries, particularly if protective head equipment is not used. However, there is increasing awareness of the implications of repetitive subclinical traumatic injury, known as mild traumatic brain injury (mTBI), particularly in sports like football, hockey, or boxing. Mild traumatic brain injury produces no abnormalities visible on CT or conventional MRI, but mild hemosiderin deposition may be seen on SWI. Studies with diffusion tensor imaging (DTI) have begun to show subtle microstructural alterations in the brain, as manifested by reduced fractional anisotropy in the deep white matter. Although important in population-based studies, these findings have not been reliably applied to the individual patient, and therefore remain findings in research that do not yet have a clear clinical role.

6.6 Fractures

Head trauma may result in fractures of the skull, which, as mentioned above, predispose to arterial injury and the development of epidural hematoma. High-impact injuries are required to fracture a mature skull, but the thin skull of very young children is more susceptible to fracture. In particular, the skull

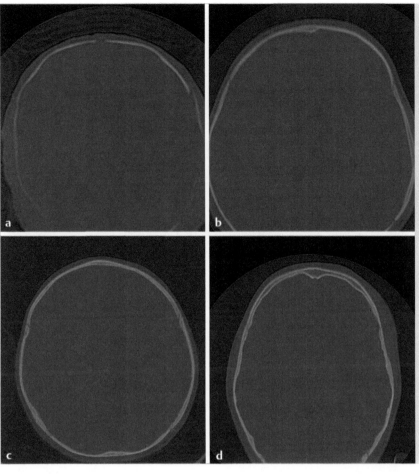

Fig. 6.9 Diploic space comparison. Axial bone algorithm computed tomographic images of the frontal bone of four different patients at (a) 1 day, (b) 9 months, (c) 18 months, and (d) 8 years of age. At 1 day of age (a), the metopic suture is patent and only cortex is visible between the inner and outer table. At 9 months (b), there is focal marrow within the diploic space in the location of the now-closed metopic suture, but the bone is otherwise largely without a diploic space. At 18 months (c), a thin diploic space is visible between separate cortical layers of the inner and outer tables. At 8 years of age (d), a discrete diploic space is identified, with distinct inner- and outer-table cortex.

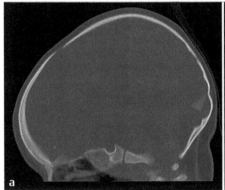
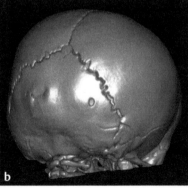

Fig. 6.10 (a) Sagittal bone algorithm computed tomographic image of the head of a 9-month-old girl who fell, showing a focal area of indentation of the skull, further confirmed on (b) three-dimensional images and representing a ping-pong fracture.

within the first year of life has no diploic space, which puts it at higher risk for fracture. The matrix of trabeculations in the diploic space of the mature skull provides support between the inner and outer tables of the skull, resembling the support provided by the vertical strut within an I-beam used in construction, or the central support in corrugated cardboard (▶ Fig. 6.9). The single-layer cortex in young children is prone to greenstick-like depressions, sometimes known as "ping-pong" fractures (▶ Fig. 6.10).

Computed tomography is the mainstay imaging modality for the diagnosis of skull fractures. Skull radiographs may miss more than 25% of calvarial fractures, but the missed fractures are typically small and nondisplaced, and radiography of the skull can therefore be considered in young children who show no neurologic deficits. Fractures directly in the axial plane may be missed on axial computed tomographic images, and sagittal and coronal reformatting can improve the ability to detect these fractures. Dedicated bone algorithm images produced from the scanner are better at depicting fractures than are the bone-window evaluation of soft tissue algorithm data. Extracranial soft tissue swelling can provide a clue as to where to look for a fracture, and close attention to the skull subjacent to areas of extracranial hematomas will improve the diagnostic yield of studies done with CT, but this should not be the only area scrutinized for fractures. Three-dimensional reconstructions of the skull are very helpful in detecting fractures, providing

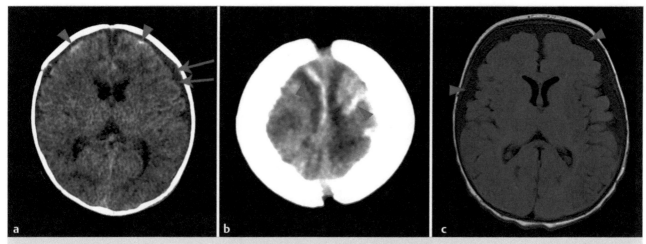

Fig. 6.11 Nonaccidental trauma and cortical vein thrombosis. (a) Axial computed tomographic image of the head of a 1-month-old child shows foci of extra-axial blood products (*arrowheads*) and prominence of the extra-axial space, which has a density higher than that of the CSF within the ventricles (*arrows*). (b) Axial computed tomographic image near the vertex shows linear areas of high density (*red arrowheads*), possibly representing thrombosed cortical veins. (c) Axial fluid attenuation inversion recovery image shows bilateral subdural collections (*red arrowheads*) that have incomplete suppression (as compared with the ventricular system), consistent with proteinaceous fluid and probably indicative of hematohygromas, resulting from a tear in the dura that allows cerebrospinal fluid into a hematoma.

improvements in both sensitivity and specificity. In young children, three-dimensional (3D) reconstructions can help prevent misdiagnosing a suture as a fracture and conversely, mistakenly identifying a fracture as a suture. Three-dimensional reconstructions are especially helpful for identifying the contour irregularity of ping-pong fractures at locations where there may not be a cortical break.

6.7 Nonaccidental Trauma

Nonaccidental trauma is a condition for which one would hope to have nearly perfect imaging sensitivity and specificity, to avoid missing the diagnosis and at the same time avoiding hesitancy in ruling out NAT in cases without abuse. Nonaccidental trauma is most commonly seen in children under 2 years of age, but can be seen at any age (including adulthood and advanced age). Considering this diagnosis and communicating with caregivers are the most important considerations for identifying it.

Being alert to the possibility of NAT is important even when there is no reported history of trauma. An abused child may come to clinical attention for nontraumatic reasons, such as seizure or lethargy. For this reason, seeking possible fractures is important even if there are no signs of trauma, particularly in children under 2 years of age.

Unexplained skull fractures or the intracranial finding of blood products must bring attention to the possibility of NAT and prompt a search for other findings, such as other skeletal injuries, cutaneous injuries, or signs of malnourishment.[6,7,8] Subdural hematomas of mixed age are especially concerning for possible NAT, although it is critical to recognize that mixed-density collections are not always of mixed age and can be related to acute hematohygromas from the simultaneous tearing of bridging veins, resulting in the hematomatous component of such lesions, and a laceration of the arachnoid, resulting in its hygromatous component.[9] The presence of cortical-vein thrombosis is also more common in NAT than in other forms of

trauma (▶ Fig. 6.11).[10] Ultimately, a multidisciplinary approach to evaluating all information about the patient, the traumatic injury, and the home environment may be needed to help clarify the findings in a particular case of possible NAT. Yet despite one's best efforts, it may often be impossible to identify the cause of a child's injuries or the circumstances surrounding them.

References

[1] Marin JR, Weaver MD, Yealy DM, Mannix RC. Trends in visits for traumatic brain injury to emergency departments in the United States. JAMA 2014; 311 (18):1917–1919

[2] Faul M, Xu L, Wald MM, Coronado VG. Centers for Disease Control and Prevention. Traumatic Brain Injury in the United States: Emergency Department Visits, Hospitalizations and Deaths. 2010;1–74 http://www.cdc.gov/traumaticbraininjury/pdf/blue_book.pdf

[3] Wintermark M, Sanelli PC, Anzai Y, Tsiouris AJ, Whitlow CT, ACR Head Injury Institute. Imaging evidence and recommendations for traumatic brain injury: Conventional neuroimaging techniques. J Am Coll Radiol 2015; 12(2): e1–e14

[4] Wintermark M, Sanelli PC, Anzai Y, Tsiouris AJ, Whitlow CT, American College of Radiology Head Injury Institute. Imaging evidence and recommendations for traumatic brain injury: Advanced neuro- and neurovascular imaging techniques. AJNR Am J Neuroradiol 2015; 36(2):E1–E11

[5] Wintermark M, Coombs L, Druzgal TJ et al. American College of Radiology Head Injury Institute. Traumatic brain injury imaging research roadmap. AJNR Am J Neuroradiol 2015; 36(3):E12–E23

[6] Duhaime AC, Christian CW, Rorke LB, Zimmerman RA. Nonaccidental head injury in infants—The "shaken-baby syndrome." N Engl J Med 1998; 338(25): 1822–1829

[7] Piteau SJ, Ward MGK, Barrowman NJ, Plint AC. Clinical and radiographic characteristics associated with abusive and nonabusive head trauma: A systematic review. Pediatrics 2012; 130(2):315–323

[8] Zuccoli G, Panigrahy A, Haldipur A et al. Susceptibility weighted imaging depicts retinal hemorrhages in abusive head trauma. Neuroradiology 2013; 55(7):889–893

[9] Wittschieber D, Karger B, Niederstadt T, Pfeiffer H, Hahnemann ML. Subdural hygromas in abusive head trauma: Pathogenesis, diagnosis, and forensic implications. AJNR Am J Neuroradiol 2015; 36(3):432–439

[10] Adamsbaum C, Rambaud C. Abusive head trauma: Don't overlook bridging vein thrombosis. Pediatr Radiol 2012; 42(11):1298–1300

7 Neurocutaneous Syndromes

7.1 Introduction

A variety of heterogeneous syndromes and syndromic associations produce findings in the central nervous system and the skin, and often elsewhere in the body. These entities are known as neurocutaneous syndromes, or phakomatoses. Some of these syndromes are commonly encountered in a pediatric neuroradiology setting (▶ Table 7.1), while others are more rare (▶ Table 7.2). The genetics of some phakomatoses are well described and understood, while others have no specific genetic foundation that has yet been described (e.g., the posterior fossa malformations–hemangiomas–arterial anomalies–cardiac defects–eye abnormalities–sternal cleft and supraumbilical raphe [PHACES] syndrome). Notwithstanding this, familiarity with the phakomatoses, in particular the more commonly encountered entities among this group of syndromes, can aid in their recognition and appropriate treatment. Accurately recognizing a phakomatosis can prevent its misdiagnosis and can help determine when family genetic evaluation and counseling may be beneficial. Although the genetic causes of many neurocutaneous syndromes have been identified, the family history for such a disorder will often be negative and cases of the syndrome will be the result of new sporadic mutations.

7.2 Tuberous Sclerosis Complex

Tuberous sclerosis complex (TSC), or Bourneville disease, is a neurocutaneous syndrome with characteristic manifestations in the brain, eyes, and skin, as well as the heart, lung, and kidneys.[1] The most common presenting symptom is seizures, present in approximately 80% of patients with TSC. Defects in two genes, *TSC-1* and *TSC-2*, which encode the proteins tuberin and hamartin, respectively, are responsible for TSC. Tuberin and hamartin form the TSC dimer, which inhibits the mammalian target of rapamycin (mTOR) pathway. Defects in either *TSC-1* or *TSC-2* result in dysfunction of the dimer and unregulated (or underregulated) mTOR activity. The findings characteristic of this in the central nervous system (CNS) include eponymous cortical tubers, which the neurologist Désiré-Magloire Bournville, after whom the disease was named, thought resembled potato spuds. Given the firmness of the tubers, the name "tuberous sclerosis" emerged (literally, "hard potato"). The tubers in tuberous sclerosis complex are areas of cortical thickening and gyral expansion, producing abnormal subcortical T2/fluid-attenuated inversion recovery (FLAIR) signals (▶ Fig. 7.1). The signal abnormality of the lesions tapers as they extend inward to the lateral margin of the lateral ventricles, which was the embryologic location of the germinal matrix. Historically, the cortical abnormalities in TSC have been referred to as "tubers" in the radiology literature, and the subcortical linear extensions of these abnormalities toward the location of the germinal matrix have been described as radial migration lines. In fact, the tubers and the radial migration lines are not two separate entities, and the histologic pattern is that of cortical dysplasia (in particular, focal cortical dysplasia [FCD] type IIb) (▶ Fig. 7.1). The areas of dysplasia can at times have calcifications, and there can occasionally be cystic changes. It is worth

noting that in the newborn, these areas of dysplasia are best depicted on T1 W imaging (▶ Fig. 7.2), and are typically difficult to identify on T2 W and FLAIR imaging because of the high water content of the surrounding unmyelinated brain. From approximately 3 to 24 months of patient age, the areas of dysplasia can be difficult to see on either T1 W or T2 W/FLAIR imaging because of ongoing myelination.

Another characteristic feature of TSC is subependymal hamartomatous nodules along the margins of the lateral ventricles (▶ Fig. 7.1). These nodules frequently calcify, which can be best depicted on computed tomographic scans; however, magnetic resonance imaging (MRI) (and particularly susceptibility-weighted imaging [SWI]) can often give clues about their calcification. The subependymal nodules will often enhance after the injection of gadolinium because there is no intact blood–brain barrier. Large (>10 mm) or enlarging nodules are low-grade neoplasms known as subependymal giant-cell astrocytomas (SEGAs), but even small nodules probably fall within this pathophysiologic spectrum. The most common place for SEGAs is along the lateral margin of the lateral ventricles at the level of the foramina of Monro (▶ Fig. 7.1). It is important to note that subependymal nodules and SEGAs are not "tubers."

Although traditionally treated with surgical resection, SEGAs have now been shown to involute on therapy with mTOR inhibitors, such as rapamycin or everolimus. These inhibitors reduce the size of SEGAs to a point at which they have decreased mass effect, which can facilitate their elective surgical resection or allow their observation without surgery.[2]

Cerebellar findings are less common than cerebral findings in TSC, but they do occur. Attention to the globes, especially on computed tomographic scans and in SWI, can show signs of retinal hamartomas (▶ Fig. 7.3). Although the latter is an important observation, dilated funduscopic examination is more sensitive, and a majority of retinal hamartomas are not visible on imaging.

There are no associated spinal findings in TSC, but if spinal imaging is done, attention to the imaged portions of the kidneys is warranted to look for signs of angiomyolipomas. The characteristic skin lesions in TSC include facial angiofibromas (adenoma sebaceum), ash-leaf spots, and shagreen patches. Adolescent and young adult females with tuberous sclerosis are at increased risk for developing a lymphangioleiomyomatosis-like interstitial lung disease with thin-walled cystic changes. Infants with TSC may have cardiac rhabdomyomas, which may even be detected in utero, but these tend to spontaneously regress.

7.3 Sturge–Weber Syndrome

Sturge–Weber syndrome (SWS), or encephalotrigeminal angiomatosis, is a neurocutaneous syndrome that is typically sporadic and has a characteristic cutaneous manifestation of a unilateral port-wine stain (nevus flammeus) conforming to the dermatome of a branch of the trigeminal nerve.[3,4] The vascular dysplasia responsible for this is marked by regional maldevelopment/absence of cortical veins overlying a portion of a cerebral hemisphere (ipsilateral to the port-wine stain). Absence of

Table 7.1 Summary of the common phakomatoses

	Other name	Cutaneous findings	Central nervous system neoplasms	Optic findings	Inheritance	Chromosome	Visceral/other
Tuberous sclerosis	Bourneville disease	Ash-leaf spots, facial angiofibroma (adenoma sebaceum), shagreen patch	SEGA	Retinal hamartomas	Autosomal dominant	*TSC-1* gene: chromosome 9 *TSC-2* gene: chromosome 16	Cardiac rhabdomyomas, lymphangioleiomyomatosis-like lung disease, renal angiomyolipomas
Neurofibromatosis type 1	von Recklinghausen disease	Café au lait spots, subcutaneous neurofibromas	Optic pathway gliomas, pilocytic astrocytomas, neurofibromas	Optic pathway gliomas, Lisch nodules	Autosomal dominant	Chromosome 17	Moyamoya, scoliosis, plexiform neurofibromas, lateral thoracic meningocele
Neurofibromatosis type 2	MISME syndrome		Schwannomas (esp. vestibular), meningiomas, ependymomas	Juvenile subcapsular cataract	Autosomal dominant	Chromosome 22	
Sturge–Weber syndrome	Encephalotrigeminal angiomatosis	Port-wine stain		Choroidal hemangioma, nevus of Ota	Sporadic	Chromosome 3	
von Hippel–Lindau disease	Retinocerebellar angiomatosis		Hemangioblastomas (cerebellar, spinal cord), endolymphatic sac tumors	Retinal hemangioblastomas	Autosomal dominant	Chromosome 3	Renal cell carcinoma, pancreatic neuroendocrine tumors, pheochromocytoma, epididymal cysts

MISME = multiple inherited schwannomas, meningiomas, and ependymomas; SEGA = subependymal giant-cell astrocytoma.

Table 7.2 Key features of less common neurocutaneous syndromes

Syndrome	Comment
Cowden	Lhermitte–Duclos disease, thyroid and breast cancers
Posterior fossa malformations–hemangiomas–arterial anomalies–cardiac defects–eye abnormalities–sternal cleft and supraumbilical raphe syndrome (PHACES)	Hemangiomas, posterior fossa abnormalities
Hereditary hemorrhagic telangiectasia	Arteriovenous malformations, and may present with brain abscess due to pulmonary shunt
Neurocutaneous melanosis	Leptomeningeal melanin deposits (T1 shortening)
McCune–Albright syndrome	Café au lait spots, precocious puberty, polyostotic fibrous dysplasia

the cortical veins impairs the venous drainage of the cortex in this territory, and there is a resultant leptomeningeal angiomatous prominence (▶ Fig. 7.4) that manifests as leptomeningeal enhancement; additionally, there may be prominence of medullary veins draining to the deep venous system (▶ Fig. 7.4). There will often be ipsilateral prominence of the choroid plexus in the atrium of the lateral ventricles (▶ Fig. 7.4). The venous stasis resulting from impaired cortical drainage results in chronic venous congestion in the affected regions of the cortex, causing cell death, volume loss, and calcification. The cortical calcifications are sometimes said to have a tram-track appearance.

Close attention to the orbit on postcontrast imaging in patients with SWS may show retinal enhancement from a choroidal angioma of the eye. This puts patients with SWS at increased risk for glaucoma (▶ Fig. 7.5). Unlike most of the more common neurocutaneous syndromes, Sturge–Weber syndrome does not have a characteristic neoplastic association.

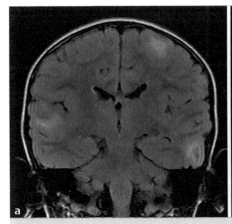
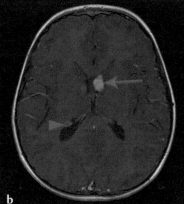
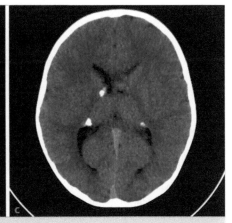

Fig. 7.1 Tuberous sclerosis complex (TSC). (a) Coronal fluid-attenuated inversion recovery (FLAIR) image of the head of a 5-year-old boy with TSC shows areas of subcortical hyperintense signal in the left superior frontal gyrus, left inferior temporal gyrus, and right superior and middle temporal gyri, representing areas of dysplasia ("tubers"). (b) Axial T1 W image plus contrast shows several enhancing subependymal nodules along the lateral margins of the bodies of the lateral ventricles (*arrowhead*). A larger lesion is seen along the lateral margin of the anterior body of the left lateral ventricle, just anterior to the foramen of Monro, representing a SEGA (*red arrow*). (c) Axial computed tomographic image shows calcification within three subependymal nodules, but no significant calcifications are seen within this SEGA (although SEGAs can have calcification).

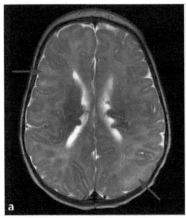
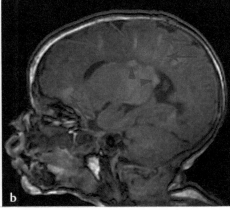

Fig. 7.2 Tuberous sclerosis (TSC) in a newborn. (a) Axial T2 W image of a 3-month-old with TSC shows contour irregularity of the lateral ventricles related to intermediate T2 hypointense subependymal nodules (*arrowheads*). Close attention reveals areas of dysplasia (*red arrows*) in the left parietal lobe and right frontal lobe, which are difficult to see because of the unmyelinated background. (b) Sagittal T1 W image shows multiple linear areas of T1 shortening extending to the cortex (*red arrows*), representing areas of dysplasia better seen on T1 with an unmyelinated background. Subependymal nodules are also seen in T1 W images (*arrowheads*).

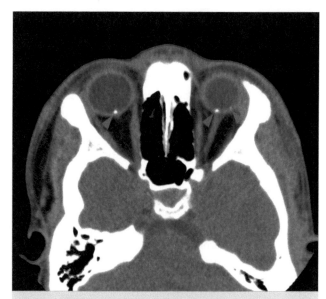

Fig. 7.3 Astrocytic hamartomas. Axial computed tomographic image in a 16-year-old with tuberous sclerosis (TSC) shows areas of focal calcification along the retinas of the globes of both eyes (*arrowheads*). Although the posterior-most lesions could be mistaken for drusen, the more peripheral one on the left is not associated with the head of the optic nerve and therefore is not related to drusen. This patient's age of 16 years is older than would be expected for retinoblastoma, but an examination of the dilated pupil by an ophthalmologist is warranted to further evaluate this finding even in the setting of known TSC.

7.4 Neurofibromatosis Type 1

Neurofibromatosis type 1 (NF1) is the most common neurocutaneous syndrome, with an incidence of approximately 1 in 4,000 individuals, and is related to a genetic abnormality on chromosome 17. Neurofibromatosis type 1 is typically suspected if there is a family history of it or if there are cutaneous stigmata, particularly café au lait spots and/or axillary freckling. Magnetic resonance imaging is the optimum technique for evaluation of the brain in patients with NF1 and will commonly show patchy areas of T2/FLAIR hyperintense signal in the globi palladi, dentate nuclei, deep cerebellar white matter, thalami, and brainstem (▶ Fig. 7.6). These findings were previously referred to as hamartomas but have more recently been recognized to represent myelin vacuolization.[5] The brainstem lesions in NF1 can be expansile, and if they do expand, close follow-up is warranted to exclude a nonenhancing glial neoplasm. Parenchymal tumors are not uncommon in NF1 and are typically of low grade, such as pilocytic astrocytomas.

Tumors of the optic pathway are also a common feature in NF1, and like the parenchymal tumors in the disease are often also pilocytic astrocytomas. Close attention to the optic nerves, chiasm, and tract is required in all studies of patients with NF1 because gliomas can range from subtle, nonenhancing fusiform enlargements (▶ Fig. 7.7a) to focal, exophytic enhancing lesions.

Vascular dysplasias can be associated with NF1, and in the CNS these can include moyamoya (▶ Fig. 7.7b).[6] Signs of moyamoya on conventional MRI can be subtle, including asymmetric flow voids in the middle cerebral artery (MCA) and possibly leptomeningeal enhancement; any suspicious features warrant follow-up with magnetic resonance angiography, and may warrant confirmatory cerebral angiography. It is relevant to note that the gene for familial moyamoya syndrome, like the NF1 gene, is on chromosome 17.[7]

Neurofibromatosis type 1 can be associated with dysplasia of the sphenoid bone, resulting in asymmetry in the anterior margin of the middle cranial fossa (▶ Fig. 7.8).[8] Nerve-sheath tumors are a common feature in NF1, and can be seen in the scalp, orbit, or along cranial nerves (▶ Fig. 7.9), but are most commonly seen in the spine and are further discussed in Chapter 27. Cranial nerve involvement in NF1 typically occurs

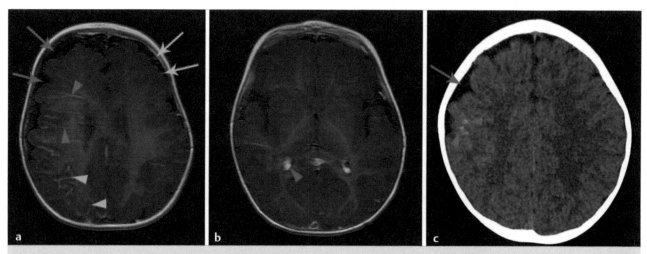

Fig. 7.4 Sturge–Weber syndrome (SWS). (a) Axial T1 plus contrast in a 9-month-old with SWS shows loss of right frontal brain volume, with absence of cortical veins overlying the right frontal lobe (*red arrows*, as compared with *green arrows* on the left). Transmantle collateral vessels provide venous drainage for the right frontal cortex to the deep venous system (*red arrowheads*). Pial collaterals (*green arrowheads*) provide venous drainage for the right parietal and occipital lobes. (b) Axial T1 plus contrast image at a lower level shows ipsilateral hypertrophy of the choroid plexus (*red arrowhead*). (c) Axial computed tomographic image obtained at 3 years of age shows volume loss (*red arrow*) and areas of cortical calcification (*red arrowheads*); note that the dense calcifications sometimes shown as characteristic of SWS are usually not present until later in the disease process.

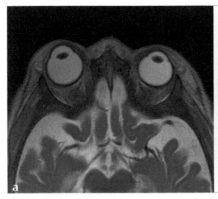
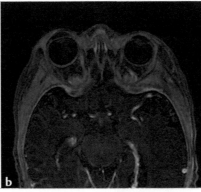

Fig. 7.5 Glaucoma in Sturge–Weber syndrome (SWS). (a) Axial T2 W image in a 5-month-old boy with SWS shows an increased depth of the anterior chamber of the right eye, corresponding with clinical signs of glaucoma. (b) Axial T1 plus contrast image shows asymmetric enhancement of the retina of the right eye, related to a retinal angioma. There is also partial visualization of right posterior temporal and occipital leptomeningeal enhancement.

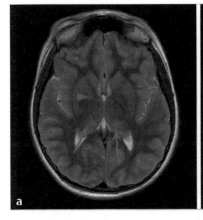
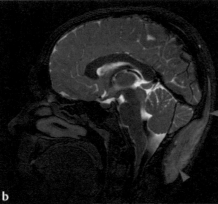

Fig. 7.6 Myelin vacuolization. (a) Axial T2 W image in a 14-year-old girl with neurofibromatosis type 1 (NF1) shows areas of hyperintense signal in the right globus pallidus (*arrowhead*) and bilateral thalami (*arrows*), consistent with areas of myelin vacuolization. (b) Sagittal T2 W–fat suppression (FS) image shows an extracranial soft tissue mass in the occipital region (*red arrowheads*), consistent with en-plaque plexiform neurofibromas.

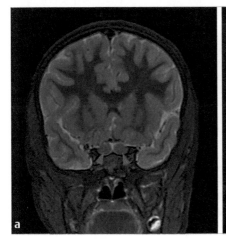
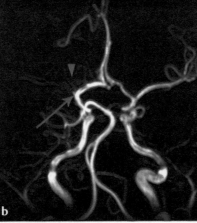

Fig. 7.7 Optic glioma/moyamoya. (a) Coronal short tau inversion recovery (STIR) image in a 5-year-old girl with neurofibromatosis type 1 (NF1) shows thickening of the canalicular segments of both optic nerves (*arrowheads*). (b) Maximum intensity projection (MIP) image from a magnetic resonance angiogram shows nonvisualization of the right middle cerebral artery from the carotid terminus (*arrow*), with prominent serpentine lenticulostriate moyamoya collateral vessels (*arrowhead*).

in extraforaminal segments of the nerves, in contrast to the cisternal segment involvement in NF2.

Neurofibromatosis type 1 can be associated with buphthalmos. Hamartomas of the iris known as Lisch nodules are common in NF1, but cannot be seen by imaging.

7.5 Neurofibromatosis Type 2

Neurofibromatosis type 2 (NF2) is a tumor-prone neurocutaneous syndrome with an origin on chromosome 22,[9] with patients developing multiple inherited meningiomas, schwannomas, and ependymomas (the origin of the term "MISME syndrome").

Patients with NF2 typically do not present until young adulthood, although they sometimes present in childhood or adolescence. The most commonly known association of NF2 is with bilateral vestibular schwannomas (▶ Fig. 7.10a), although schwannomas in patients with NF2 can occur throughout any of the true cranial nerves. The optic nerve (cranial nerve II [CN II]) is formally a tract of the CNS, and has no Schwann cells. The olfactory nerve (CN I) is also a tract of the CNS, but Schwann cells are present in the distal branches of this nerve that extend through the cribriform plate, making possible the occurrence of CN I schwannomas (typically at or below the level of the cribriform plate). The presence of a unilateral vestibular

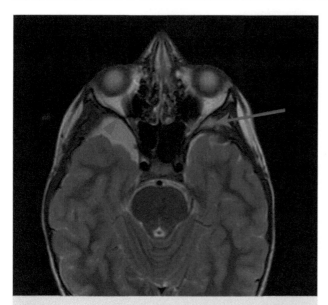

Fig. 7.8 Sphenoid dysplasia. Axial T2 W image in a 9-year-old boy shows prominence of the cerebrospinal fluid (CSF) space at the anterior aspect of the right middle cranial fossa, with a hypoplastic sphenoid bone (*arrowhead*). In contrast, the greater wing of the left sphenoid bone (*arrow*) is normal.

schwannoma, any meningioma, or multicentric ependymoma (or a combination of these) in a child should prompt evaluation for NF2 (▶ Fig. 7.10b).

7.6 von Hippel–Lindau Syndrome

von Hippel–Lindau (vHL) syndrome is a tumor-associated condition in which the most common finding in the CNS is multifocal hemangioblastomas in the cerebellum and spinal cord (▶ Fig. 7.11). The incidence of vHL syndrome is approximately 1 in 40,000, and it more commonly presents in young adulthood than in childhood or adolescence.[10] The cerebellar hemangioblastomas in the syndrome have an appearance that overlaps that of pilocytic astrocytomas. Hemangioblastomas can also be present in the retina of patients with vHL syndrome, and patients with the syndrome are also at risk for papillary cystadenoma of the endolymphatic sac ("endolymphatic sac tumor").

Visceral findings in vHL syndrome include renal cell carcinoma (which can be multicentric), pancreatic neuroendocrine tumors, pheochromocytomas, and cysts of the epididymis (males) and broad ligament (females).[11]

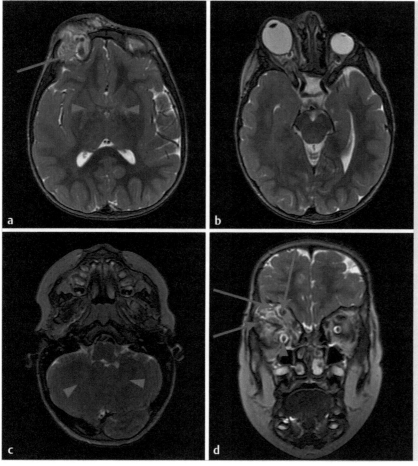

Fig. 7.9 Orbital neurofibroma–buphthalmos. (a) Axial T2 W image in a 5-year-old girl with neurofibromatosis type 1 (NF1) shows areas of myelin vacuolization in both globi palladi (*arrowheads*) and partial visualization of right orbital plexiform neurofibromas (*arrow*). (b) Axial T2 W image at the level of the orbits shows an elongated right globe (increased axial length), representing buphthalmos. (c) Axial T2 W image at the level of the cerebellum shows areas of myelin vacuolization in the deep cerebellar white matter and in the region of the dentate nuclei. (d) Coronal T2 W image at the level of the posterior orbits shows multiple plexiform neurofibromas in the superior intraconal and extraconal space of the right orbit (*arrows*), and a relatively normal-appearing right optic nerve (*arrowhead*), indicating these findings do not represent an optic nerve glioma.

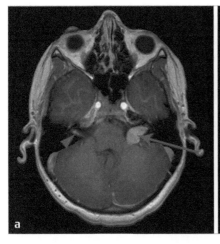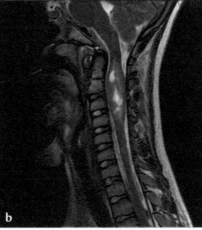

Fig. 7.10 Neurofibromatosis type 2 (NF2) vestibular schwannoma/spinal ependymoma. (a) Axial T1 plus contrast image of the internal auditory canals (IACs) in an 11-year-old boy shows a mass filling and expanding the left IAC (*arrow*), extending through the porus acusticus and effacing the cerebellopontine angle cistern. A smaller enhancing lesion is seen in the right IAC (*arrowhead*), representing bilateral vestibular scwannomas in the setting of NF2. (b) Sagittal T2 W image of the cervical spine shows an expansile intramedullary lesion extending from C1 through C4, which in the setting of NF2 probably represents an ependymoma.

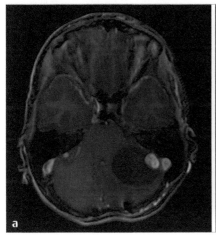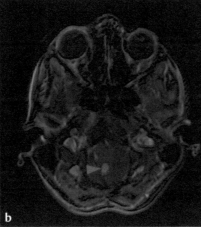

Fig. 7.11 Hemangioblastoma. (a) Axial T1 plus contrast image in a 15-year-old girl shows a cystic lesion with an enhancing mural nodule in the left cerebellar hemisphere. (b) Axial T1 plus contrast image at the level of the foramen magnum demonstrates an enhancing lesion in the region of the obex (*red arrowhead*). These represent multifocal hemangioblastomas in the setting of von Hippel–Lindau syndrome.

7.7 Other Neurocutaneous Syndromes

7.7.1 Posterior Fossa Malformations, Hemangiomas, Arterial Anomalies, Cardiac Defects, Eye Abnormalities, and Sternal or Ventral Defects Syndrome

Posterior fossa malformations, hemangiomas, arterial anomalies, cardiac defects, eye abnormalities, and sternal or ventral defects (PHACES) syndrome is an association of abnormalities that has only recently been recognized, and which falls under the spectrum of neurocutaneous syndromes.[12,13] The name of the syndrome describes the findings that a neuroradiologist may characteristically encounter in patients in whom it occurs. Accordingly, the imaging of any hemangioma of the head and neck should include close attention to the posterior fossa for malformations that raise the possibility of PHACES. Likewise, an abnormality of the posterior fossa (such as a Dandy–Walker malformation) should prompt a search for signs of a soft tissue hemangioma.

7.7.2 Neurocutaneous Melanosis

The diagnosis of neurocutaneous melanosis is commonly based on dermatologic criteria.[14,15] When patients with this condition present for imaging of the CNS, the primary concern is the presence, severity, and distribution of leptomeningeal deposits of melanin. These deposits can be seen as areas of T1 shortening.[15,16] Melanin may also be present in the amygdala and/or hippocampus, in which case its presence can be associated with seizures.

7.7.3 Hypomelanosis of Ito

Hypomelanosis of Ito is a neurocutaneous syndrome with hypopigmented skin lesions. Among a variety of associated findings are hemimegalencephaly in some patients. If a patient with hypomelanosis of Ito has seizures, high-resolution imaging is warranted to ensure the absence of a subhemispheric megalencephaly, which may involve only portions of a cerebral hemisphere and can be missed without appropriate attention.

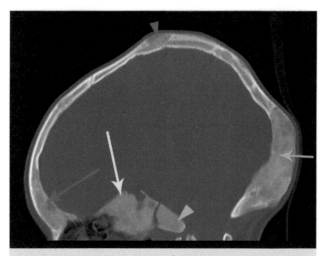

Fig. 7.12 Polyostotic fibrous dysplasia in McCune-Albright syndrome. Sagittal bone algorithm computed tomographic image shows multifocal areas of expansile osseous lesions with a "ground-glass" internal matrix and without aggressive periosteal reaction. Areas involved include the frontal bone (*red arrow*), parietal bone (*red arrowhead*), occipital squama (*green arrow*), basiocciput (*green arrowhead*), and basisphenoid (*white arrow*). This represents polyostototic fibrous dysplasia, which can be seen in McCune–Albright syndrome. When an isolated finding, fibrous dysplasia of the skull is most commonly seen within the basisphenoid bone.

7.7.4 McCune–Albright Syndrome

McCune–Albright syndrome is a neurocutaneous disorder marked by unilateral café au lait spots that have irregular borders and have been described as resembling the coast of Maine (in contrast to the café au lait spots in NF1, which have smoother borders, sometimes leading to their being described as looking like the "coast of California"). Patients with McCune–Albright syndrome will present with endocrine abnormalities, including precocious puberty. Another characteristic feature of the syndrome is polyostotic fibrous dysplasia (▶ Fig. 7.12).[17]

7.7.5 Hereditary Hemorrhagic Telangiectasia

Hereditary hemorrhagic telangiectasia (HHT), also known as Osler–Weber–Rendu syndrome, is a neurocutaneous disorder with associated vascular dysplasias.[18] Direct involvement of the CNS can be seen, with pial arteriovenous malformations, possibly presenting with very subtle leptomeningeal enhancement. As a result of pulmonary arteriovenous malformations and the resultant right-to-left shunting in HHT, patients with this condition can present with paradoxical emboli, whose consequences can include strokes and brain abscesses.[19]

7.7.6 Cowden Syndrome

Cowden syndrome is a hamartomatous overgrowth syndrome related to a mutation in the phosphatase and tensin homolog (PTEN) gene, in which there may be a dysplastic gangliocytoma

of the cerebellum (Lhermitte–Duclos disease). Other findings include an increased risk of breast and thyroid cancer and testicular lipomatosis. Cowden syndrome can also be referred to as PTEN hamartoma tumor syndrome (PHTS).[20]

7.8 Final Comments

A multitude of other neurocutaneous syndromes exist, but their description is beyond the scope of this chapter or book.[21]

References

[1] Northrup H, Krueger DA, International Tuberous Sclerosis Complex Consensus Group. Tuberous sclerosis complex diagnostic criteria update: Recommendations of the 2012 International Tuberous Sclerosis Complex Consensus Conference. In: Vol 49. 2013:243–54 http://dx.doi.org/10.1016/j.pediatrneurol.2013.08.001

[2] Wheless JW, Klimo P Jr. Subependymal giant cell astrocytomas in patients with tuberous sclerosis complex: Considerations for surgical or pharmacotherapeutic intervention. J Child Neurol 2014; 29(11):1562–1571

[3] Sudarsanam A, Ardern-Holmes SL. Sturge-Weber syndrome: From the past to the present. Eur J Paediatr Neurol 2014; 18(3):257–266

[4] Comi AM. Presentation, diagnosis, pathophysiology, and treatment of the neurological features of Sturge-Weber syndrome. Neurologist 2011; 17(4):179–184

[5] Karlsgodt KH, Rosser T, Lutkenhoff ES, Cannon TD, Silva A, Bearden CE. Alterations in white matter microstructure in neurofibromatosis-1. PLoS ONE 2012; 7(10):e47854

[6] Kaas B, Huisman TA, Tekes A, Bergner A, Blakeley JO, Jordan LC. Spectrum and prevalence of vasculopathy in pediatric neurofibromatosis type 1. J Child Neurol 2013; 28(5):561–569

[7] Mineharu Y, Liu W, Inoue K et al. Autosomal dominant moyamoya disease maps to chromosome 17q25.3. Neurology 2008; 70(24 Pt 2):2357–2363

[8] Jacquemin C, Bosley TM, Svedberg H. Orbit deformities in craniofacial neurofibromatosis type 1. AJNR Am J Neuroradiol 2003; 24(8):1678–1682

[9] Asthagiri AR, Parry DM, Butman JA et al. Neurofibromatosis type 2. Lancet 2009; 373(9679):1974–1986

[10] Kaelin WG Jr. Molecular basis of the VHL hereditary cancer syndrome. Nat Rev Cancer 2002; 2(9):673–682

[11] Leung RS, Biswas SV, Duncan M, Rankin S. Imaging features of von Hippel-Lindau disease. Radiographics 2008; 28(1):65–79, quiz 323

[12] Metry D, Heyer G, Hess C et al. PHACE Syndrome Research Conference. Consensus Statement on diagnostic criteria for PHACE syndrome. Pediatrics 2009; 124(5):1447–1456

[13] Nozaki T, Nosaka S, Miyazaki O et al. Syndromes associated with vascular tumors and malformations: A pictorial review. Radiographics 2013; 33(1):175–195

[14] Peretti-Viton P, Gorincour G, Feuillet L et al. Neurocutaneous melanosis: Radiological-pathological correlation. Eur Radiol 2002; 12(6):1349–1353

[15] Ginat DT, Meyers SP. Intracranial lesions with high signal intensity on T1-weighted MR images: Differential diagnosis. Radiographics 2012; 32(2):499–516

[16] Smith AB, Rushing EJ, Smirniotopoulos JG. Pigmented lesions of the central nervous system: radiologic-pathologic correlation. Radiographics 2009; 29(5):1503–1524

[17] Bousson V, Rey-Jouvin C, Laredo J-D et al. Fibrous dysplasia and McCune–Albright syndrome: Imaging for positive and differential diagnoses, prognosis, and follow-up guidelines. Eur J Radiol 2014; 83(10):1828–1842

[18] Shovlin CL. Hereditary haemorrhagic telangiectasia: Pathophysiology, diagnosis and treatment. Blood Rev 2010; 24(6):203–219

[19] Mathis S, Dupuis-Girod S, Plauchu H et al. Cerebral abscesses in hereditary haemorrhagic telangiectasia: A clinical and microbiological evaluation. Clin Neurol Neurosurg 2012; 114(3):235–240

[20] Pilarski R, Burt R, Kohlman W, Pho L, Shannon KM, Swisher E. Cowden syndrome and the PTEN hamartoma tumor syndrome: Systematic review and revised diagnostic criteria. J Natl Cancer Inst 2013; 105(21):1607–1616

[21] Edelstein S, Naidich TP, Newton TH. The rare phakomatoses. Neuroimaging Clin N Am 2004; 14(2):185–217.

8 Neoplasms

8.1 Introduction

Neoplasms of the central nervous system (CNS) are the most common solid neoplasms in children and come in a variety of forms. The most common location for pediatric tumors of the CNS is in the posterior fossa, in contrast to those in adults. Adult primary brain tumors are most commonly in the supratentorial brain; however, tumors in children can arise and spread throughout the brain as well as the spine. Many of the most common pediatric primary neoplasms of the CNS can spread via leptomeningeal seeding; therefore, upon detecting them it is imperative to perform contrast-enhanced magnetic resonance imaging (MRI) of the entire neural axis (brain and total spine) to look for disease. Imaging of the spine must extend into the sacrum to include the end of the thecal sac. Although some tumors, such as pilocytic astrocytoma, are not typically metastatic to the leptomeninges, the exact histologic characterization of these tumors depends on their surgical biopsy/resection, and the author therefore believes that all tumors should have an appropriate preoperative workup.

8.2 Tumors Commonly (But Not Exclusively) Found in the Posterior Fossa

8.2.1 Pilocytic Astrocytoma

Among the most common pediatric tumors of the brain is pilocytic astrocytoma, often referred to as juvenile pilocytic astrocytoma (JPA). Juvenile pilocytic astrocytomas are World Health Organization (WHO) grade I tumors that are typically managed surgically, and if their gross–total resection is achieved, adjuvant therapy is often not given unless there are suspicious changes on follow-up by imaging. The classic description on

imaging of a JPA of the posterior fossa is that of a cystic lesion with an enhancing nodule (▶ Fig. 8.1). The presence of enhancement should not be a dissuasion from recognizing this lesion as a low-grade tumor. The apparent diffusion coefficient (ADC) values of JPAs tend to be high, in the range of 1500×10^{-6} mm^2/sec. Although JPAs are intra-axial tumors, they can have exophytic components. And although the cyst-with-nodule appearance of a JPA is very common in the cerebellum, it is less characteristic of pilocytic astrocytomas found elsewhere. Brainstem pilocytic astrocytomas can present as solid enhancing lesions and a discrete brainstem or deep gray-matter lesion without surrounding edema and without low ADC values is nearly always a pilocytic astrocytoma (▶ Fig. 8.2). Gliomas of the optic pathway, most commonly seen in the setting of neurofibromatosis type 1, are also classified histologically as pilocytic astrocytomas, and may represent fusiform thickenings of the orbital segment of the optic nerve or focal exophytic chiasmatic lesions. Most pediatric intramedullary neoplasms of the spinal cord are pilocytic astrocytomas (further discussed in Chapter 27). Pilocytic astrocytomas have a very low (although not zero) potential for metastatic spread and malignant degeneration. They rarely calcify, and apart from those that occur in the spinal cord, they rarely exhibit internal hemorrhage.

8.2.2 Ependymoma

Ependymomas are tumors arising from the ependymal lining of the brain, and in children occur most commonly in the posterior fossa (▶ Fig. 8.3). Ependymomas are usually low-grade (WHO grade II) tumors, with ADC values between those of a JPA and a medulloblastoma.[1] The WHO grade III variant of ependymoma, known as anaplastic ependymoma, is a more aggressive form of ependymoma. Ependymomas of the posterior fossa are most often extra-axial, and can fill the fourth ventricle and extend through one (or both) foramina of Luschka. Once it

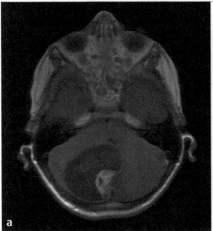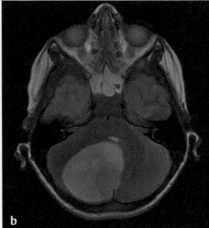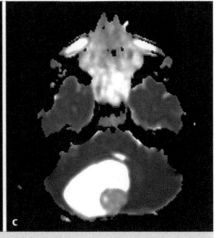

Fig. 8.1 Juvenile pilocytic astrocytoma. (a) Postcontrast axial T1 W image of the posterior fossa shows a cystic lesion in the medial aspect of the right cerebellar hemisphere, resulting in effacement of the fourth ventricle. There is an enhancing mural nodule, as well as thin enhancement along an internal septation. (b) Axial T2 W image shows a relatively hyperintense appearance of the nodule, corresponding to a high internal water content. (c) Axial ADC map shows a hyperintense signal (diffusion of 1750×10^{-6} mm^2/sec), indicating facilitated diffusion in this pilocytic astrocytoma (WHO grade I).

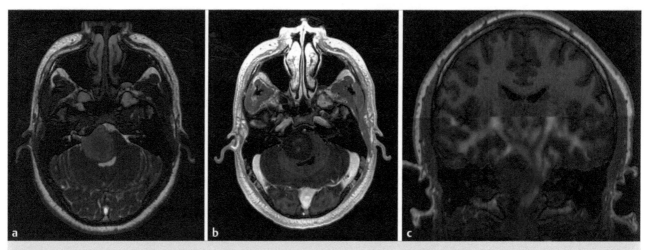

Fig. 8.2 Juvenile pilocytic astrocytoma of the brainstem. (a) Axial fast imaging employing steady-state acquisition image shows a circumscribed intra-axial mass in the right aspect of the pons The mass is focally exophytic and extends into the right porus acusticus. (b) Axial T1 plus contrast image shows heterogeneous internal enhancement. (c) Coronal T1 W image with an overlay of a directionally encoded fractional anisotropy map shows that the mass effect results in deviation of the fibers of the corticospinal tract as opposed to infiltration (which is seen in diffuse intrinsic pontine gliomas). This lesion is a pilocytic astrocytoma.

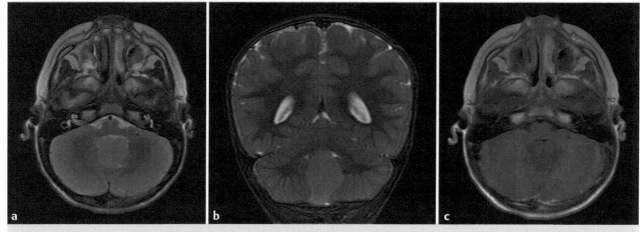

Fig. 8.3 Ependymoma. (a) Axial T2 W image shows a mass of intermediate intensity within the fourth ventricle. (b) Coronal short tau inversion recovery image shows that the mass extends caudally through the foramen of Magendie. (c) Axial T1 plus contrast image shows that the lesion does not demonstrate significant enhancement. This lesion was an ependymoma.

extends through a foramen of Luschka, an ependymoma can insinuate itself into the lateral medullary cistern and extend superiorly into the cerebellopontine-angle cistern and caudally to (and through) the foramen magnum. The tendency of ependymomas to spread through crevices has been described as "toothpaste-like" spread, and can result in mass effect on, or the encasement of, cranial nerves. Optimal survival after the resection of an ependymoma comes from maximal tumor removal at the time of initial surgery, suggesting that careful attention to the extent of such a tumor (and particularly if it has spread through the basal cisterns) is highly important in helping to guide the neurosurgeon. Adjuvant radiation therapy is used after the removal of an ependymoma. Chemotherapy has not yet proven effective against ependymoma.

Because ependymomas sometimes demonstrate only minimal enhancement, the evaluation of all imaging sequences of these tumors, as with all tumors, and as opposed simply to

postcontrast T1 W images, is important. Supratentorial ependymomas are often intra-axial lesions (▶ Fig. 8.4).

8.2.3 Medulloblastoma

Medulloblastoma (MB) is a high-grade tumor of the posterior fossa, and has more recently been categorized as belonging to a subset of primitive neuroectodermal tumor (PNET), for which reason it is sometimes referred to as PNET–MB. Medulloblastoma can result in obstructive hydrocephalus when it occurs in the fourth ventricle, and it is prone to dissemination through the cerebrospinal fluid. Spinal metastatic deposits of these tumors are also possible, and as pediatric neoplasms of the CNS, their workup should involve a contrast-enhanced magnetic resonance imaging (MRI) study of the brain and entire spine (▶ Fig. 8.5). Although medulloblastoma most commonly occurs within the fourth ventricle, a cerebellar hemispheric variant,

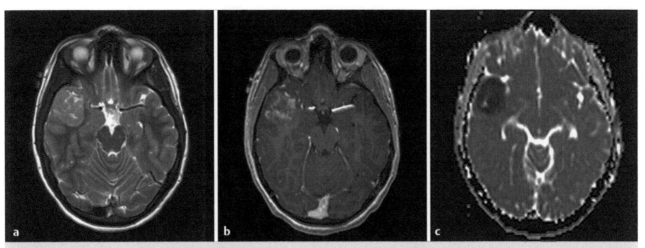

Fig. 8.4 Supratentorial ependymoma. (a) Axial T2 W image demonstrates a relatively circumscribed mass in the right temporal pole, with small internal cystic areas. (b) Axial T1 plus contrast image shows heterogeneous enhancement within the lesion, which was confirmed to be an anaplastic ependymoma. (c) Axial ADC map shows a hypointense appearance of the lesion (diffusion of 500×10^{-6} mm^2/sec), corresponding with the high degree of cellularity of an anaplastic ependymoma.

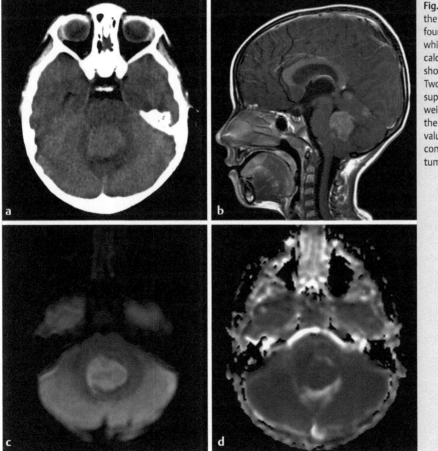

Fig. 8.5 Medulloblastoma. (a) Axial CT image of the posterior fossa shows a mass within the fourth ventricle that is hyperdense relative to white matter and shows no macroscopic calcification. (b) Sagittal T1 plus contrast image shows the mass nearly filling the fourth ventricle. Two metastatic deposits are seen along the superior margin of the vermis. (c) Axial diffusion-weighted image shows a hyperintense signal for the lesion, and (d) an axial ADC map shows low values (diffusion of 675×10^{-6} mm^2/sec), confirming the highly cellular nature of the tumor.

known as a desmoplastic nodular medulloblastoma, can occur, and is the most common type of this neoplasm found in older adolescents and young adults. More recent work has classified medulloblastomas on the basis of their genetic profiles in terms of the *WNT* and *Hedgehog* genes.

Previously, the presence of calcification had been suggested as a means of differentiating ependymoma from medulloblastoma, but this occurred before the advanced characterization of these tumors with MRI and is of little practical use in the clinical setting, since both tumors may or may not have calcification.

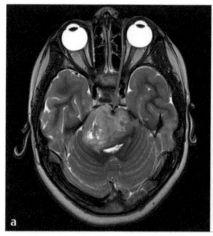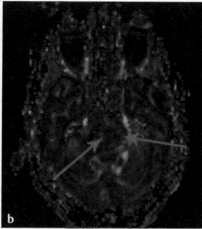

Fig. 8.6 Diffuse intrinsic pontine glioma (DIPG). (a) Axial T2 W image of the head of a 6-year-old girl shows an expansile lesion within the pons that results in partial effacement of the fourth ventricle as well as nearly 270° of coverage of the basilar artery (*arrow*). The fiber bundle of the left corticospinal tract is seen (*arrowhead*) surrounded by tumor, confirming the tumor as an infiltrating lesion. (b) Axial directionally encoded fractional anisotropy map from diffusion tensor imaging shows the descending fibers of the left corticospinal tract (*red arrows*), corresponding to the area seen in the T2 W image in (a); however, the fibers of the right corticospinal tract are attenuated and involved by tumor. This represents a DIPG.

Apparent diffusion coefficient values have proven more effective for attempting to differentiate ependymoma from medulloblastoma than the presence of calcifications, but this alone is not foolproof because anaplastic ependymoma (WHO grade III) can have low ADC values, and atypical teratoid rhabdoid tumor (AT/RT) can have similarly low ADC values. Regardless of histologic characteristics, the ADC values of ependymoma correlate well with tumor grade and cellularity. The high nuclear to cytoplasmic ratio results in both medulloblastoma and AT/RT tumor having appearances of higher density than that of ependymoma on computed tomography, even in the absence of macroscopic calcification.

There are primitive neuroectodermal tumors that are not MB, yet which present as aggressive tumors with low ADC values and a propensity for leptomeningeal spread. Supratentorial PNETs are usually variants of tumors other than medulloblastoma.

8.2.4 Atypical Teratoid Rhabdoid Tumor

Atypical teratoid rhabdoid tumor (AT/RT) is a highly cellular and aggressive tumor that is most commonly seen in the first few years of life. On imaging, and clinically, AT/RT can be difficult to differentiate from medulloblastoma, and both types of tumor have a propensity for causing leptomeningeal metastatic disease. Atypical teratoid/rhabdoid tumor can be a mass in the fourth ventricle, like medulloblastoma and ependymoma, or an intra-axial lesion.

8.2.5 Diffuse Intrinsic Pontine Glioma

Diffuse intrinsic pontine glioma (DIPG) is an intra-axial tumor that has characteristic features on imaging, including diffuse enlargement of the pons/brainstem with a T2 hyperintense appearance. Because of brainstem enlargement with this tumor, there is "encasement" of the basilar artery (▶ Fig. 8.6), a feature strongly suggestive of DIPG. Diffuse intrinsic pontine glioma is not a surgically curable disease, and the treatment for it is radiation therapy. It is most often a low-grade tumor, but can have areas of malignant degeneration. Adjunctive techniques including ADC values, perfusion imaging, and multivoxel MR-spectroscopy can aid in determining more aggressive/cellular components of a DIPG. Atypical or aggressive features in a suspected DIPG warrant biopsy.

8.3 Tumors That Tend to Present in the Supratentorial Compartment

8.3.1 Tumors in the Sellar Region

A cystic mass arising in the suprasellar region may very well be a craniopharyngioma, particularly if there are signs of calcification and proteinaceous fluid within some of the cystic components. Craniopharyngiomas can present as the result of a mass effect on the optic pathway, obstructive hydrocephalus, and/or endocrine alterations. When large, craniopharyngiomas can extend superiorly into the third ventricle. Although craniophyaryngiomas were originally treated surgically, their management has more recently shifted toward radiation therapy (▶ Fig. 8.7).

A leading differential consideration with suprasellar lesions is a glioma of the optic pathway. Histologically, such gliomas are often pilocytic astrocytomas, and they rarely calcify without prior radiation treatment. A glioma of the optic pathway can present as a fusiform enlargement of the optic nerve, chiasm, and/or tract, typically with an associated T2-hyperintense signal and variable enhancement pattern, or a focal exophytic lesion that tends to have mixed solid and cystic components with heterogeneous enhancement (▶ Fig. 8.8). Gliomas of the optic pathway may present as the result of visual disturbance or a mass effect, or can be found in the asymptomatic stage in patients undergoing surveillance scans for entities like neurofibromatosis type 1.

Germinomas are suprasellar lesions that tend to present as irregularly shaped, enhancing lesions along the pituitary stalk. Their presentation may be endocrinologic or related to a mass effect. Germinomas can also occur in the pineal region. If a germinoma is suspected, sampling of cerebrospinal fluid (CSF) with analysis for germ-cell markers is warranted in the workup. Noninfectious granulomatous processes, and particularly Langerhans' cell histiocytosis, are the primary considerations in the differential diagnosis of germinomas. Sarcoidosis can have an appearance overlapping that of germinomas, but it is rare in children.

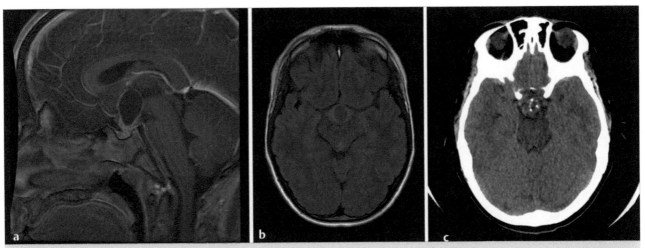

Fig. 8.7 Craniopharyngioma. (a) Sagittal T1 plus contrast image of the head of a 16-year-old boy with delayed puberty shows a cystic suprasellar lesion with a peripheral rim of enhancement. The lesion is distinct from the pituitary gland. (b) Axial fluid attenuation inversion recovery image showing the central contents of the cyst demonstrates incomplete suppression. (c) Axial computed tomographic image shows areas of calcification within the suprasellar lesion, which was confirmed to be a craniopharyngioma.

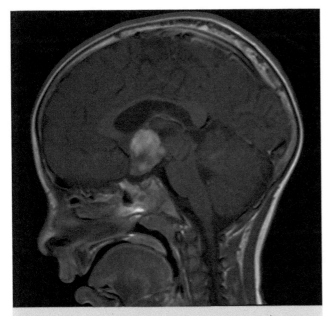

Fig. 8.8 Chiasmic glioma. Sagittal T1 plus contrast image shows a predominantly solid, slightly heterogeneous suprasellar enhancing mass that fills the anterior recesses and body of the third ventricle. This represents a chiasmatic glioma, which histologically is a pilocytic astrocytoma.

A non-neoplastic entity that warrants awareness and that can mimic a suprasellar mass is an ectopic neurohypophysis. An ectopic neurohypophysis can appear as a globular mass in the region of the infundibular recess of the third ventricle. The most important clue to recognizing this entity is the absence of an orthotopic neurohypophysis. An ectopic neurohypophysis can show contrast enhancement and will also have intrinsic T1 shortening (see Chapter 13).

Pituitary adenomas are rare in children, but when present will resemble those in adults. Small lesions (microadenomas) typically present as the result of endocrine signs related to hormone secretion. Larger lesions (macroadenomas) tend to be nonsecreting and therefore to grow without detection until they exert a mass effect on adjacent structures, such as the optic chiasm.

8.4 Syndrome-associated Tumors

Contrast-enhancing masses along the margins of the lateral ventricles in the setting of tuberous sclerosis (TSC) can represent a subependymal giant-cell astrocytoma (SEGA). Differentiation of a SEGA from a routine subependymal nodule of TSC can be difficult, but SEGAs most commonly occur at the level of the foramina of Monro (see Chapter 7). Subependymal giant-cell astrocytoma should be strongly suspected if a lesion exceeds 10 mm in maximum dimension or is enlarging. The size of subependymal lesions can be difficult to measure without the use of intravenous contrast material, and for this reason gadolinium-enhanced MRI is warranted for the evaluation of TSC. Subependymal giant-cell astrocytomas can cause obstructive hydrocephalus and have traditionally been managed with surgical resection. They have been shown to involute after the administration of inhibitors of mammalian target of rapamycin (mTOR).

Gliomas of the optic pathway are seen with increased frequency in neurofibromatosis type 1 (NF1), can occur anywhere along the optic pathway, may or may not show contrast enhancement, and may or may not have cystic components. Accordingly, careful attention to the optic pathway is warranted in patients with NF1, as gliomatous lesions may be very subtle at first presentation, providing the opportunity for their close follow-up and, according to need, their early treatment to minimize visual compromise. Approximately half of gliomas of the optic pathway occur in patients without additional features of NF1.

Hemangioblastomas have a cyst with an appearance like that of a contrast-enhancing nodule, resembling that of pilocytic

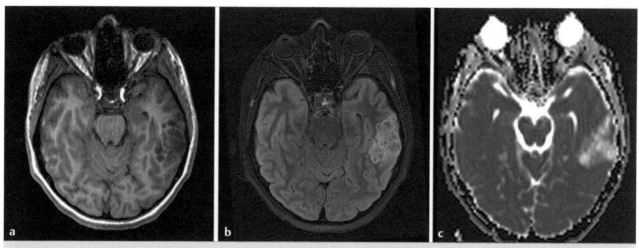

Fig. 8.9 Dysembryoplastic neuroepithelial tumor (DNET). (a) Axial T1 W image through the level of the midbrain and temporal lobes shows a multilobulated lesion in the left temporal lobe with circumscribed hypointense areas. (b) Axial fluid-attenuated inversion recovery image shows a hyperintense signal associated with the wall and septations of the multicystic lesion. (c) Axial apparent diffusion coefficient map shows a hyperintense signal within the lesion, confirming facilitated diffusion (diffusion of 2060×10^{-6} mm^2/sec) in this lesion, which was shown to be a DNET, a World Health Organization grade I lesion.

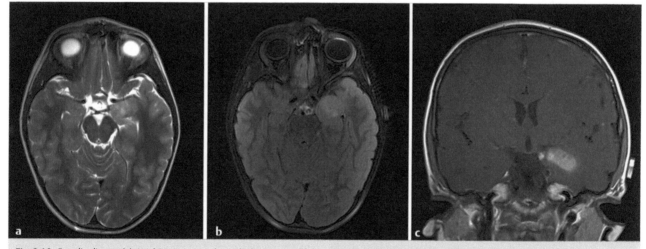

Fig. 8.10 Ganglioglioma. (a) Axial T2 W image through the temporal lobes shows a slightly expansile hyperintense lesion with internal microcystic changes in the region of the left amygdala. (b) Axial fluid-attenuated inversion recovery image shows the lesion to be hyperintense and without a discrete margin. (c) Coronal T1 plus contrast image shows enhancement within the lesion. This represented a ganglioglioma.

astrocytoma, but are extremely rare in children who do not have von Hippel–Lindau disease.

Meningiomas can occur in children, but are much less common than in adults. A meningioma in a child should raise the consideration of NF2.

8.5 Seizure-associated Tumors

Several low-grade tumors tend to present with seizures, most commonly dysembryoplastic neuroepithelial tumor (DNET) (▶ Fig. 8.9) and ganglioglioma (▶ Fig. 8.10). Both have mixed cystic and solid components, involve cortex and juxtacortical white matter, and because they are low-grade lesions, have higher ADC values ($> 1000 \times 10^{-6}$ mm^2/sec). Although the appearances on imaging of DNET and ganglioglioma overlap,

ganglioglioma commonly shows contrast enhancement, whereas DNET rarely does. Both tumors may have calcifications, but this is more common with ganglioglioma. Both DNET and ganglioglioma have a propensity for involving the temporal lobes, and particularly the region of the amygdala and hippocampus, but both of these tumors can occur anywhere in the brain. Close attention to fluid-attenuated inversion recovery (FLAIR) images is warranted to evaluate the extent of the lesions of DNET and ganglioglioma. Cystic components of these tumors tend to have incomplete suppression on FLAIR because of proteinaceous components.

Another supratentorial cystic tumor with a nodular area of soft tissue and that can present with seizures is a pleomorphic xanthoastrocytoma (PXA) (▶ Fig. 8.11). The solid portion of a PXA is often at the periphery of the tumor, will typically

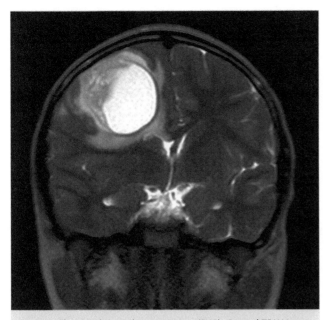

Fig. 8.11 Pleomorphic xanthoastrocytoma (PXA). Coronal T2 W image of the head of a 9-year-old boy shows a mass in the right posterior frontal lobe, with a peripheral nodular area of soft tissue and a surrounding rim of edema. The mass results in partial effacement of the body of the ventricles and right-to-left midline shift. This represented a PXA.

over several years cannot differentiate an LGG from cortical dysplasia because LGG may remain unchanged for periods exceeding 5 years. Postcontrast enhancement effectively excludes cortical dysplasia from differential diagnostic consideration. If surgical management of an LGG is not pursued, continued surveillance is warranted.

Multiple juxtacortical cystic structures that show no enhancement, no surrounding abnormality in their FLAIR signal, no diffusion abnormality, and the complete suppression of cystic components on FLAIR are most likely prominent Virchow–Robin (perivascular) spaces, which can be mistaken for a DNET if not carefully studied.

8.6 Tumors of the Pineal Region

Lesions of the pineal region can be difficult to characterize and manage. Cysts of the pineal gland can raise concern about a neoplastic etiology, but cysts are very common and pineal tumors are not. The normal pineal parenchyma enhances after administration of gadolinium, but a pineal cyst with enhancing pineal tissue can be difficult to comfortably diagnose as a physiologic finding. Features that should raise concern include large size of a cyst (greater than 10 mm), peripherally splayed calcifications, and thick, enhancing cyst walls with nodular enhancement. Pineal parenchymal tumors can be low grade (pineocytoma) or high grade (pineoblastoma). Pineoblastoma is histologically classified as a type of primitive neuroectodermal tumor (PNET). The leading differential consideration for a suspected pineal tumor is that of a germinoma (see the section of this chapter on suprasellar tumors); differentiation can be aided by sampling of CSF as well as diffusion-weighted imaging (DWI), because pineal germinomas usually have high ADC values.[2,3]

Pineal tumors can present as the result of mass effect on the tectal plate and resulting effacement of the sylvian aqueduct and corresponding obstructive triventricular hydrocephalus.

Another mass in the pineal region that can present with obstructive hydrocephalus from effacement of the sylvian aqueduct is a tectal glioma, which is usually a low-grade tectal tumor (▶ Fig. 8.12). Tectal gliomas may not require treatment, and are often managed by endoscopic third ventriculostomy to deal with the issues of CSF transit that these tumors raise, and with imaging surveillance. If a tectal glioma enlarges or

enhance, and may have an apparent dural tail caused by local dural irritation/inflammation. Pleomorphic xanthoastrocytoma is a WHO grade II tumor, but a WHO grade III anaplastic variant exists.

Oligodendroglioma is an additional consideration for a cortical/juxtacortical tumor in the setting of seizures and that has heterogeneous enhancement and some calcification. However, oligodendroglioma is less commonly seen in children than other epilepsy-associated tumors, such as DNET, ganglioglioma, and PXA.

Differentiation of a nonenhancing, low-grade glioma (LGG) from cortical dysplasia can be very difficult for the pathologist, let alone the radiologist. The finding of cystic components favors LGG, but cortical dysplasia can also be cystic. Stability

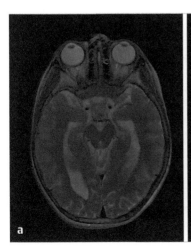
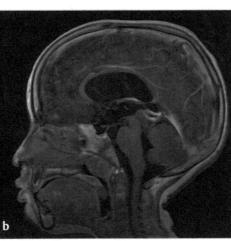

Fig. 8.12 Tectal glioma. (a) Axial T2 W image shows a hyperintense lesion in the tectal plate. (b) Sagittal T1 plus contrast image shows ill-defined expansion of the quadrigeminal (tectal) plate, with effacement of the sylvian aqueduct, without postcontrast enhancement within the tectal glioma.

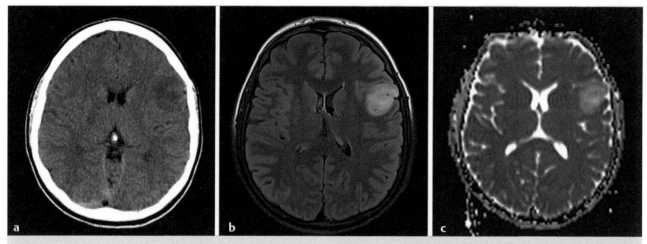

Fig. 8.13 Low-grade glioma. (a) Axial computed tomographic image of the head of a 14-year-old boy with a first-time seizure shows an ill-defined hypointense area in the left inferior frontal gyrus. (b) Axial fluid-attenuated inversion recovery image shows a cortical and subcortical hyperintense signal with focal cortical thickening. (c) Axial attenuated diffusion coefficient map shows facilitated diffusion (diffusion of 1500×10^{-6} mm^2/sec). There was no abnormal postcontrast enhancement. This was a fibrillary astrocytoma, a World Health Organization grade II lesion.

becomes more aggressive, its treatment is more likely to involve radiation therapy than surgical resection, but an atypically appearing lesion may require biopsy to aid in determining its optimal treatment.

A large pineal cyst can be difficult to differentiate from an arachnoid cyst in a cavum vellum interpositum; a feature that can aid in its characterization is the location of the internal cerebral veins. A lesion arising from the vellum interpositum or the splenium of the corpus callosum will inferiorly displace the internal cerebral veins, whereas a pineal-region lesion will superiorly displace the veins.

8.7 Tumors in the First Year of Life

Although pediatric brain tumors most commonly represent the "big three" in the posterior fossa, consisting of MB, JPA, and ependymoma, the situation is different in the first 6 to 12 months postnatally. Tumors in the latter period tend to be supratentorial and include lesions like teratoma, desmoplastic infantile ganglioglioma (DIG), and high-grade gliomas (HGG). Desmoplastic infantile gangliogliomas are larger than regular gangliogliomas and are more likely to present due to mass effect rather than seizures.

8.8 Other Tumors (Mainly Supratentorial)

Although they are less common than in adults, high-grade gliomas (HGG) can occur in children and can include anaplastic astrocytoma and glioblastoma. Low-grade gliomas (LGG) include fibrillary astrocytoma (▶ Fig. 8.13), a WHO grade II tumor that is typically an infiltrating lesion and does not show postcontrast enhancement. Low-grade gliomas, including DIPG, can transform into HGG, including glioblastoma.

Depending on the location of an HGG, its management may involve a combination of biopsy, resection, chemotherapy, and radiation. Advanced imaging is important for determining the most aggressive part of the tumor for appropriate selection of a biopsy site, often through the use of ADC maps and perfusion imaging. Multivoxel spectroscopy can also be helpful in determining biopsy-site selection in a suspected HGG. It is important to know that the highest-grade part of an HGG may not enhance, and correspondingly, that enhancing parts of such a tumor do not necessarily represent the most aggressive parts of the lesion.

Supratentorial intraventricular tumors in children are most commonly of choroid plexus origin (other than in patients with TSC, in whom SEGA is the most common type of tumor).[4] Tumors of the choroid plexus can be low-grade choroid plexus papillomas (CPP) or high-grade choroid plexus carcinomas (CPC) (▶ Fig. 8.14). Choroid plexus tumors in children most commonly occur in the trigone of the lateral ventricles, although they can occur in the third and fourth ventricles. Because of their vascularity, preresection embolization of these lesions is sometimes attempted.

Meningiomas are rare in children without a history of NF2 or prior radiation therapy. Contrast-enhancing masses based in the dura in children may represent hemangiopericytomas.

8.9 Treatment

For most pediatric neoplasms of the CNS, maximal cytoreductive surgery results in the best prognosis. Gross–total surgical resection may be possible for many lesions, including JPA, ependymoma, MB, ganglioglioma, PXA, and others. With a gross–total resection, certain lesions, such as low-grade tumors (JPA, ganglioglioma, and PXA) and mature teratoma of the pineal region, typically do not require adjunct chemotherapy or radiation and are followed with imaging surveillance. For other tumors, adjunct radiation therapy is common. Radiation may be delivered locally to the site of surgery, or to the whole brain, or to the entire brain and spine (craniospinal). The more localized the radiation, the lower the risks of impaired brain

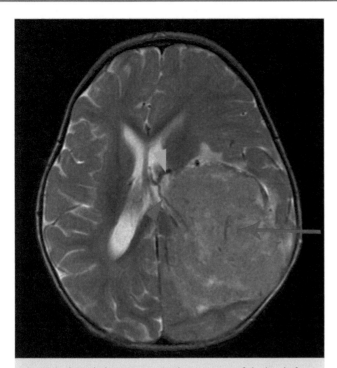

Fig. 8.14 Choroid plexus tumor. Axial T2W image of the head of a 15-month-old girl shows a large supratentorial mass that expands the atrium of the left lateral ventricle (*red arrow*). There is ipsilateral prominence of the thalamostriate vein (*green arrowhead*), and enlargement of what may be a feeding choroidal artery (*red arrowhead*). This was a carcinoma of the choroid plexus.

development; however, if there is documented CSF dissemination of disease, a wider field of radiation coverage is typically needed. Surgery guided by intraoperative MRI has been shown to result in a high rate of gross-total resection, with a 30-day rate of tumor-related return to the operating room of less than 1%.[5] However, certain tumors, such as DIPG, are not amenable to gross-total resection. Treatment strategy for craniopharyngioma is evolving, and in the absence of significant mass effect or hydrocephalus, radiation therapy without surgery has resulted in tumor-related outcomes similar to those with surgery, with a lower rate of endocrine complications.[6]

References

[1] Rumboldt Z, Camacho DLA, Lake D, Welsh CT, Castillo M. Apparent diffusion coefficients for differentiation of cerebellar tumors in children. AJNR Am J Neuroradiol 2006; 27(6):1362–1369

[2] Dumrongpisutikul N, Intrapiromkul J, Yousem DM. Distinguishing between germinomas and pineal cell tumors on MR imaging. AJNR Am J Neuroradiol 2012; 33(3):550–555

[3] Choudhri AF, Whitehead MT, Siddiqui A et al. Diffusion characteristics of pediatric pineal tumors. Neuroradiol J 2015; 28(2):209–216

[4] Smith AB, Smirniotopoulos JG, Horkanyne-Szakaly I. From the radiologic pathology archives: Intraventricular neoplasms: Radiologic-pathologic correlation. Radiographics 2013; 33(1):21–43

[5] Choudhri AF, Klimo P Jr, Auschwitz TS, Whitehead MT, Boop FA. 3 T intraoperative MRI for management of pediatric CNS neoplasms. AJNR Am J Neuroradiol 2014; 35(12):2382–2387

[6] Kiehna EN, Merchant TE. Radiation therapy for pediatric craniopharyngioma. Neurosurg Focus 2010; 28(4):E10

9 Seizures

9.1 Introduction

Seizures are a common neurologic finding in children, with approximately 400,000 children in the United States having epilepsy. In addition to patients with documented seizures of varying types (▶ Table 9.1), it is common for studies to be requested to evaluate seizure like activity, such as staring spells or pseudoseizures. Although uncomplicated febrile seizures do not require imaging of the brain, nearly all other instances of seizures in children will eventually result in imaging. Accordingly, this is a common indication for imaging in pediatric neuroradiology, and an understanding of the disease processes in seizure disorders, and a logical approach to establishing protocols for imaging and to image interpretation, is critical.

9.2 Imaging Modalities

In the emergent setting, computed tomography (CT) may be done on a patient with a seizure so as to rapidly exclude intracranial hemorrhage or other acute abnormalities (particularly posttraumatic seizures). However, magnetic resonance imaging (MRI) is predominantly the mainstay modality for the evaluation of seizures. In the absence of signs of infection or known predisposing factors (e.g., a neurocutaneous disorder), or signs of a tumor (in particular ganglioglioma and dysembryoplastic neuroepithelial tumor), intravenous contrast enhancement is typically not required for the evaluation of seizures through MRI. Vascular imaging, such as computed tomographic angiography (CTA) or magnetic resonance angiography (MRA), may help if there are signs of vascular abnormality or prior stroke.

Certain surgical procedures can aid in the treatment of some patients with epilepsy (▶ Table 9.2). In patients who are considered candidates for epilepsy surgery, advanced imaging modalities, including functional MRI (fMRI), and in nuclear medicine, single-photon emission computed tomography (SPECT) perfusion and positron emission tomography (PET), may be useful;

these are discussed in the surgical planning section of this chapter. Magnetoencephalography is a technique that detects the focal magnetic field that arises from neuronal activation and can aid in the spatial localization of epileptic discharges with greater accuracy than can surface electroencephalography (EEG). However, although magnetoencephalography is a helpful technique, it is not widely available at present.

Understanding the normal hippocampal anatomy is critical for the evaluation of seizures because both developmental and acquired abnormalities of the hippocampus can be associated with seizures (▶ Fig. 9.1). A normal variant in the hippocampal region that warrants awareness is a choroidal-fissure cyst; if the adjacent parenchyma is normal, and the cyst contents follow cerebrospinal fluid (CSF) behavior in all sequences, including suppression on fluid-attenuated inversion recovery (FLAIR) and facilitated diffusion, as well as lack of enhancement with the administration of contrast medium, then what is being seen is a normal hippocampal variant, usually without pathologic consequence (▶ Fig. 9.2).

9.3 Mesial Temporal Sclerosis/Hippocampal Sclerosis

Evaluation of the hippocampi, particularly in the coronal plane, is important in all seizure evaluations. Hippocampal volume loss with a hyperintense signal on T2 W/FLAIR imaging, related to gliosis, is a feature of mesial temporal sclerosis (MTS), also known as hippocampal sclerosis (▶ Fig. 9.3). The entire hippocampus may be involved, although other patterns of involvement, such as of sections CA1 and CA4, or isolated involvement of CA4 (end-fimbrial sclerosis), have been described. It is important to be aware that this process can be bilateral in up to 20% of patients with MTS, which carries two potential diagnostic pitfalls. First, a bilateral symmetric abnormality can be missed unless there is familiarity with the normal hippocampal morphology. Second, a bilateral asymmetric abnormality could

Table 9.1 Types of seizures

Type		Description
Focal		Previously called partial seizures, and previously subdivided into simple partial and complex partial seizures. Seizures that are (on a conceptual basis) believed to originate and remain within a single cerebral hemisphere.
Generalized (seizures that involve both cerebral hemispheres, typically with alteration and/or loss of consciousness)	Absence	Brief loss of consciousness without an appreciable postictal state (formerly classified as petit mal seizures)
	Myoclonic	Brief shock-like muscle jerking
	Tonic	Sudden increased tone of a muscle or group of muscles. Consciousness is usually preserved.
	Clonic	Alternating contraction and relaxation of a muscle or group of muscles
	Tonic–clonic	Increased tone within a muscle or group of muscles, followed by alternating contraction and relaxation (formerly designated grand mal seizures). When prolonged (>10 minutes), this is referred to as status epilepticus, which is a medical emergency.
	Atonic	Sudden loss of muscle tone, often resulting in the patient falling ("drop attack")
Gelastic		Seizures that may manifest as laughing spells, typically associated with a hypothalamic hamartoma

Used with permission from Berg AT, Berkovic SF, Brodie MJ, et al. Revised terminology and concepts for organization of seizures and epilepsies: Report of the ILAE Commission on Classification and Terminology, 2005–2009. Epilepsia. 2010;51(4):676–85.

Table 9.2 Types of surgery for epilepsy

Surgery	Description
Temporal lobectomy	Surgical resection of the temporal lobe. Temporal lobectomy procedures are often characterized by surgeons as the distance from the temporal pole that was resected (e.g., a 3-cm temporal lobectomy vs. a 4-cm temporal lobectomy). This usually involves resection of the temporal pole, uncus, and amygdala, and may or may not involve resection of the head of the hippocampus.
Corpus callosotomy	Transection of the corpus callosum, often to prevent seizure propagation in patients with atonic seizures, so as to prevent drop attacks (i.e., the patient retains control of half of the body and does not fall). The callosotomy may involve the entire corpus callosum, spare the splenium (sometimes called a 90% callosotomy), or spare the splenium and isthmus (sometimes called a 70% callosotomy).
Hemispherectomy (functional)	Resection and/or disconnection of a cerebral hemisphere. This involves a temporal lobectomy, resection of the insula and portions of the frontal and parietal lobes, and a corpus callosotomy to disconnect the remaining parenchyma.
Topectomy	A focal surgical resection of an epileptogenic focus, possibly involving a structural lesion, such as cortical dysplasia or a cavernoma.
Vagal-nerve stimulator	An implanted device with an electrode that wraps around the vagal nerve and intermittently stimulates it.

be mistaken for a unilateral process, which is important because in some cases the less atrophied side of the hippocampus may be the cause of seizures. Therefore, caution is warranted before the structural findings suggestive of MTS are definitively linked with the physiologic implications of the location of origin of a seizure. Determining the true cause of seizures is the reason for more detailed workup, including EEG, possible intraoperative monitoring with grid electrodes or depth electrodes, SPECT perfusion studies, and possibly MEG. An imaging feature supportive of MTS is volume loss in the ipsilateral fornix and mammillary body, related to Wallerian degeneration along the circuit of Papez.

Mesial temporal sclerosis has been shown to be more common in individuals with a childhood history of febrile seizures,

but the exact cause–effect relationship of the two disorders remains unclear. Although MTS is typically a disease of adolescence and adulthood, it can be seen in children as young as 2 years of age who have a mutation of the cellular type 1A voltage-gated sodium channel (SCN1A).

9.4 Congenital Malformations

Seizures can be associated with a variety of congenital malformations. This is particularly true of cortical dysplasia, in which there are abnormal neurons and altered cortical development. There are several subtypes of cortical dysplasia,[1] and it can be generally stated that type I focal cortical dysplasia is most commonly visible on T1-weighted (T1 W) imaging and that type II focal cortical dysplasia is most commonly visible on T2-weighted (T2 W) and FLAIR imaging (refer to ▶ Fig. 3.2). A subtype of type II cortical dysplasia characteristically produces a transmantle signal abnormality that fans outward as it extends from the original location of the germinal matrix toward the peripheral cortex. This is known as focal cortical dysplasia type IIB (FCB IIB), also referred to as Taylor-type cortical dysplasia or focal cortical dysplasia with balloon cells. The dysplastic abnormality described above is pathognomonic for focal cortical dysplasia type IIB and is also identical to the that of the dysplasia ("tubers") seen in tuberous sclerosis complex (further discussed in Chapter 3 and Chapter 7, respectively). Other types of cortical dysplasia can be difficult to differentiate from a low-grade tumor, such as a fibrillary astrocytoma, and follow-up studies to document the stability of a lesion are therefore warranted if its surgical resection is not pursued. Given that low-grade neoplasms may not show appreciable growth over the course of several years, the 2-year stability rule used for many other tumor-mimicking lesions does not apply in this situation. It is important to be aware that cortical dysplasia can be occult even on high-resolution MRI, and it may only be evident upon histopathologic confirmation after resection of a focus of seizure; accordingly, other means of identifying the location of epileptogenic cortex, such as SPECT perfusion and MEG, can play a role in these patients.

An additional malformation of development that can be associated with seizures is gray-matter heterotopia (refer to ▶ Fig. 3.3, ▶ Fig. 3.4, and ▶ Fig. 3.5), with epileptogenic

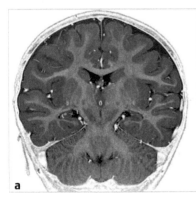
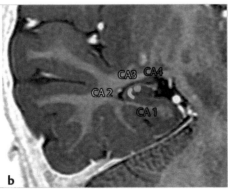

a   b

Fig. 9.1 Hippocampal anatomy. (a) Coronal short tau inversion recovery (STIR) image of the hippocampi with black-and-white inversion shows a normal hippocampal anatomy. (b) A magnified view of the right hippocampus shows the normal morphology of the hippocampal subparts CA1 through CA4.

CA3 CA4
CA2
CA1

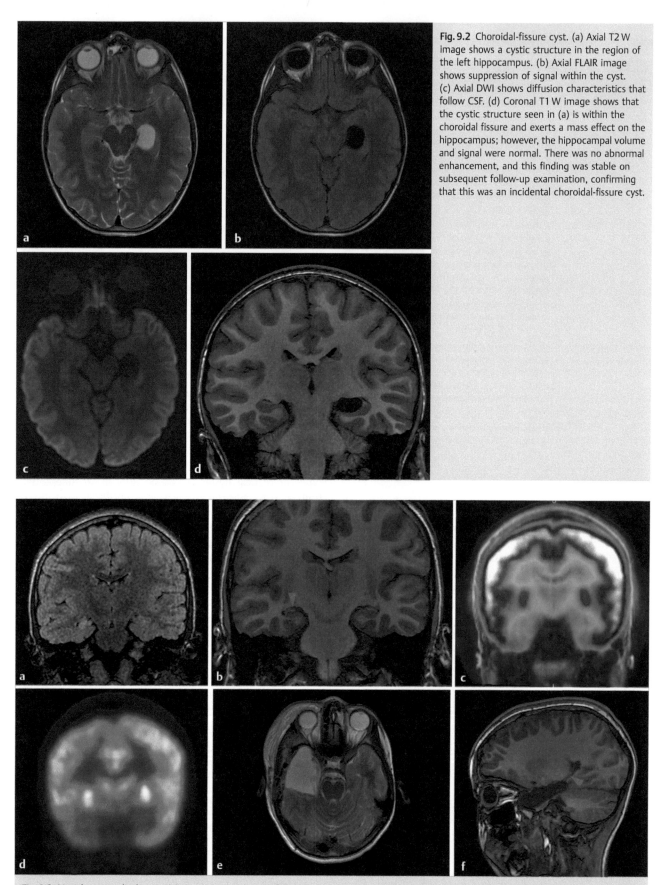

Fig. 9.2 Choroidal-fissure cyst. (a) Axial T2 W image shows a cystic structure in the region of the left hippocampus. (b) Axial FLAIR image shows suppression of signal within the cyst. (c) Axial DWI shows diffusion characteristics that follow CSF. (d) Coronal T1 W image shows that the cystic structure seen in (a) is within the choroidal fissure and exerts a mass effect on the hippocampus; however, the hippocampal volume and signal were normal. There was no abnormal enhancement, and this finding was stable on subsequent follow-up examination, confirming that this was an incidental choroidal-fissure cyst.

Fig. 9.3 Mesial temporal sclerosis. (a) Coronal FLAIR image of the head of an 11-year-old male with seizures shows an asymmetrically hyperintense signal in the right hippocampus (*red arrowhead*). (b) A coronal T1 W image shows an asymmetrically smaller volume of the right (*red arrowhead*) than of the left hippocampus. (c) An interictal coronal HMPAO–SPECT perfusion image fused to a T1 W magnetic resonance image shows subtly decreased perfusion in the right temporal lobe. (d) An interictal coronal 18F-deoxyglucose–positron-emission tomographic image shows diminished metabolism in the right temporal lobe (note the improved spatial resolution and signal-to-noise ratio as compared with those in HMPAO–SPECT imaging). (e) Axial T2 W image after a right temporal lobectomy shows absence of the right temporal pole, uncus, amygdala, and hippocampus. (f) Sagittal T1 W image shows that only the hippocampal tail remains (*red arrowhead*). The patient's condition was confirmed to be right-sided hippocampal sclerosis (mesial temporal sclerosis).

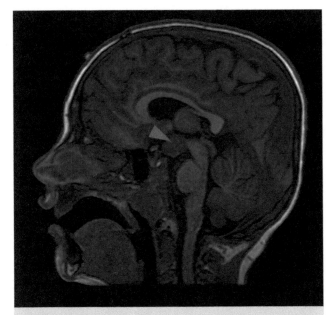

Fig. 9.4 Hypothalamic hamartoma. Sagittal T1 W image in a 4-year-old boy with gelastic seizures demonstrates a nodular area of thickening (*red arrowhead*) associated with the floor of the third ventricle. This did not demonstrate postcontrast enhancement, and represents a hypothalamic hamartoma (hamartoma of the tuber cinereum).

the third ventricle, which is a portion of the hypothalamus known as the tuber cinereum (▶ Fig. 9.4). Although a hypothalamic hamartoma will demonstrate slight T1 and T2 prolongation in comparison to the adjacent hypothalamus, and will have facilitated diffusion, it should produce no postcontrast enhancement. The presence of postcontrast enhancement should raise suspicion for a neoplasm like pilocytic astrocytoma.

An additional but more severe congenital malformation associated with seizures is hemimegalencephaly (literally, half the brain is too big) (▶ Fig. 9.5). Patients with hemimegalencephaly have hamartomatous/dysplastic overgrowth of one cerebral hemisphere with relative sparing of the other. There can be accelerated myelination in the abnormal hemisphere, and the lateral ventricle is larger in the affected hemisphere. Hemimegalencephaly is typically sporadic, but it can be a part of a rare neurocutaneous disorder known as hypomelanosis of Ito. Because the affected hemisphere has little normal function, seizure control may require a hemispherectomy. Although an anatomic hemispherectomy can be a challenging procedure with a complicated postoperative course, including superficial siderosis and abnormal CSF dynamics, a functional hemispherectomy can have similar seizure control with fewer long-term complications. A functional hemispherectomy involves a temporal lobectomy, resection of the insula, and partial parieto-occipital resection. The frontal and occipital poles remain, but are disconnected from the remainder of the brain by a corpus callosotomy (▶ Fig. 9.5).

discharges possibly arising from the heterotopic gray matter. If the heterotopia is multifocal, it may pose a diagnostic challenge if some sort of ablative procedure or resection is planned.

A hamartoma of the hypothalamus can be the cause of seizures, and particularly of a type of seizures that manifests with laughter, known as gelastic seizures. This lesion can be difficult to identify if the hypothalamus is not scrutinized. It may arise from the main portion of the hypothalamus or from the floor of

9.5 Seizures Associated with Neoplasms

Some pediatric tumors are associated with seizures. Resection of the tumor and any adjacent affected parenchyma can result in significant (or complete) seizure control. The two most

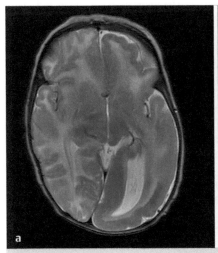
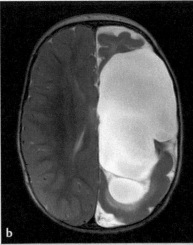
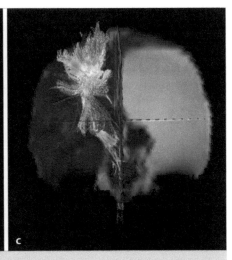

Fig. 9.5 Hemimegalencephaly/hemispherectomy. (a) Axial T2 W image in a 1-month-old female with intractable seizures shows hamartomatous overgrowth of the left cerebral hemisphere, with dysplastic cortex and ipsilateral ventricular enlargement. (b) Axial T2 W image at 20 months of age after the patient underwent a functional hemispherectomy, in which the temporal lobe, insula, and a majority of the frontal and parietal lobes were resected, with the remnant parenchyma of the frontal and occipital poles disconnected through a corpus callosotomy. (c) Fiber tracking on diffusion tensor imaging shows no fibers traversing the midline through the corpus callosum to the remnant left-hemispheric parenchyma, confirming disconnection of the two cerebral hemispheres.

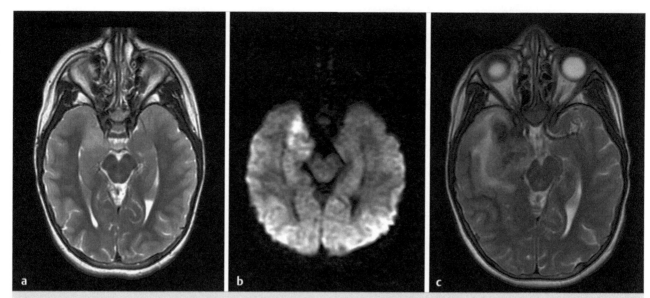

Fig. 9.6 Herpes simplex virus (HSV) encephalitis. (a) Axial T2W image in an 8-year-old female with fevers and a seizure shows an edematous appearance of the uncus of the right temporal lobe. (b) Axial DWI shows a hyperintense signal in this region. (c) Axial T2W image made 1 week after the image in (b) shows extension of the edematous area and development of T2 hypointense areas, consistent with hemorrhage in this patient with HSV encephalitis.

common neoplasms associated with seizures are ganglioglioma and dysembryoplastic neuroepithelial tumor (DNET). Both entities tend to occur within the temporal lobe and have cystic components, and therefore can be difficult to differentiate on imaging. Because both ganglioglioma and DNET are low-grade tumors (World Health Organization [WHO] grade I), their exact preoperative histologic differentiation may not be required. The presence of enhancing components and calcification favors the diagnosis of ganglioglioma (refer to ▶ Fig. 8.10), whereas a predominantly multicystic appearance favors DNET (refer to ▶ Fig. 8.9).

Another tumor that can be associated with seizures is pleomorphic xanthoastrocytoma (PXA), a WHO grade II tumor, which tends to have a larger unilocular cystic component than other supratentorial cystic seizure-associated tumors such as ganglioglioma (refer to ▶ Fig. 8.11). The enhancing nodule in PXA tends to be peripherally located, and may be adherent to the dura. There is a WHO grade II variant of ganglioglioma, and a WHO grade III variant of PXA (anaplastic PXA).

9.6 Neurocutaneous Disorders

Two neurocutaneous syndromes have a high association with the development of seizures: tuberous sclerosis complex (TSC) (refer to ▶ Fig. 7.1 and ▶ Fig. 7.2) and Sturge–Weber syndrome (SWS) (refer to ▶ Fig. 7.4). The imaging features of these entities are further discussed in Chapter 7. Hypomelanosis of Ito is a rare neurocutaneous disorder that is sometimes associated with hemimegalencephaly. Dysplastic/hamartomatous cortex is the origin of the seizures in hypomelanosis of Ito. Cortical dysplasia (tubers) constitute the epileptogenic foci in TSC. Gliosis from chronic venous ischemia is the origin of the seizures in SWS. These topics are further discussed in Chapter 7.

9.7 Seizures Associated with Inflammatory Conditions

A variety of inflammatory conditions can result in seizures, including infectious and noninfectious inflammation. In terms of meriting awareness, the most important infectious cause of seizures is encephalitis caused by herpes simplex virus (HSV). Beyond the neonatal period, HSV encephalitis typically arises from reactivation of the virus within the gasserian (trigeminal) ganglion in the region of Meckel's cave (▶ Fig. 9.6). Therefore, the adjacent portions of the temporal lobe are the first areas involved by the infection. The involved parenchyma will demonstrate reduced water diffusion and a hyperintense T2/fluid-attenuated inversion receevery (FLAIR) signal, and possibly postcontrast enhancement. When any of these features are seen, especially in the setting of a febrile seizure, the diagnosis of HSV encephalitis should be considered and treatment with acyclovir should be initiated until confirmation of the presence of HSV through a polymerase chain reaction (PCR) for HSV done on the patient's CSF. If the PCR for HSV is negative, other differential considerations become more likely, including glioma, trauma, venous congestion, and causes of inflammation other than HSV infection. Although these other entities can be entertained from the time of the initial evaluation, it is still imperative to treat the patient with acyclovir until there is a negative PCR result for HSV.

Patients with seizures of acute onset during or after a febrile illness may develop a condition called febrile infection-related epilepsy syndrome (FIRES). Patients with this syndrome are typically without a pre-existing history of epilepsy, and upon its onset have prolonged status epilepticus, often requiring monitoring in the intensive care unit (ICU). Because of the extensive metabolic demands of prolonged status epilepticus, the patient may have profound parenchymal volume loss.[2]

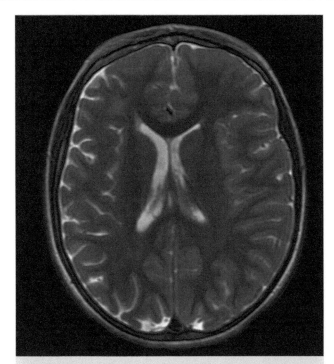

Fig. 9.7 Rasmussen encephalitis. Axial T2 W image in a 6-year-old girl with intractable seizures shows right hemispheric volume loss with prominence of sulci and asymmetric enlargement of the right lateral ventricle, representing sequelae of Rassmussen encephalitis.

A chronic inflammatory process that results in profound seizures arising from a single hemisphere is Rassmussen encephalitis (▶ Fig. 9.7). Over time, this condition results in the ipsilateral loss of volume of one cerebral hemisphere, which may eventually require either corpus callosotomy or hemispherectomy for seizure control.

9.8 Seizures Related to Focal Noninflammatory Processes

Areas of prior parenchymal injury (gliosis) can be epileptogenic. The gliosis may have been caused by prior surgery, an infection or inflammatory process, trauma, or stroke. Additionally, the deposition of hemosiderin from any of these processes is a risk factor for epileptogenic activity. Gliosis and the deposition of hemosiderin cause seizure development late after the resection of a tumor, and if the margins of the resection cavity are proven to be the source of such seizures, the gliotic tissue may be resected.

A cavernoma is a focal dysplastic area of blood vessels prone to microhemorrhage (further discussed in Chapter 12). Hemosiderin surrounding a cavernoma may be the cause of seizures (▶ Fig. 9.8). The diagnosis of a cavernoma is based on the presence of a continuous peripheral rim of hemosiderin around a heterogeneous (often circumscribed) lesion. The presence of an associated developmental venous anomaly (DVA) further

increases the likelihood that a lesion is a cavernoma. Although a cavernoma in a patient with seizures is a possible source of the seizures, a DVA alone, without an associated cavernoma, is probably of no significance in this regard. If a DVA is seen in a patient with seizures, susceptibility-weighted imaging (SWI) is helpful for identifying a possible associated cavernoma.

9.9 Medication-related Effects

Chronic antiepileptic therapy may result in cerebellar volume loss (▶ Fig. 9.9). Myelinic edema, visible on T2 W imaging and possibly on diffusion-weighted imaging (DWI), can be seen in the globi palladi, hypothalamus, and within the central tegmental tracts of the pons (▶ Fig. 9.10) after administration of the antiepileptic agent vigabatrin.[3] Familiarity with this appearance is important for avoiding the mistaken identification of this medication-related effect as a stroke or other form of metabolic injury, and for alerting the patient's neurologist about the possibility of medication toxicity.

9.10 Surgical Planning

For patients with focal epilepsy who are candidates for surgery, advanced diagnostic techniques focus on two separate but related goals. One is localizing and confirming the origin of the seizures, and the other is related to mapping and attempting to preserve normal brain functions. In terms of detecting the onset of seizures, single-photon emission computed tomography (SPECT) can be done with a radiotracer that localizes to brain parenchyma in proportion to blood flow and shows greater activity in gray- than in white-matter structures. When the radiotracer is injected in an interictal state, it is likely to show hypoperfusion around areas of epileptogenic cortex. If the tracer can be injected immediately after the onset of a seizure, during inpatient seizure monitoring, it may reveal the hyperemia that occurs during the seizure, in what is known as an ictal SPECT study. Co-registration of the ictal and interictal SPECT signals allows subtraction imaging for maximizing the likelihood of identification of areas with interictal hypoperfusion and ictal hyperperfusion; the resulting data can be displayed as an overlay on an MRI readout to aid in the spatial localization of a focus of seizure activity (▶ Fig. 9.3 c). To confirm the findings in an ictal SPECT study, subdural grid electrodes can be placed to record electroencephalographic readings with a higher density and better spatial localization than can be done with skin leads.

For surgical planning, fMRI can aid in localizing cortex that controls motor and visual functions (▶ Fig. 9.8 e). Functional MRI can lateralize language (i.e., determine which cerebral hemisphere is dominant for language tasks), and localize receptive and expressive language to specific areas of cortex. There is no reliable noninvasive means of lateralizing memory, and the Wada test remains useful for this purpose. Wada tests, however, are difficult to perform in many adolescents and nearly impossible in younger children. Passive mapping of motor and language function can be performed on sedated patients.[4]

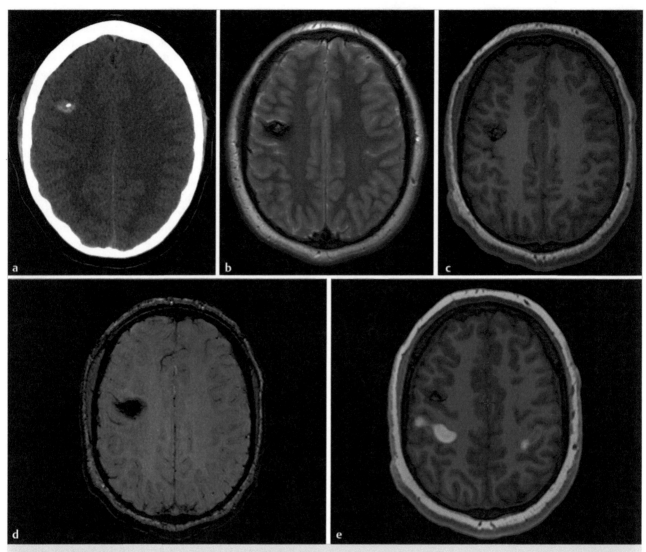

Fig. 9.8 Cavernoma. (a) Axial CT image in a 15-year-old boy with a seizure of new onset shows a right frontal area of increased density with a focal internal area of calcification. (b) Axial T2 W and (c) T1 W images show a peripheral hypointense rim with a heterogeneous central signal. (d) Axial susceptibility-weighted image shows a diffuse hypointense appearance of this lesion, which represents a cavernoma. (e) Functional MRI made during a left-hand motor task (orange) and overlaid on a T1 W image shows that motor activity of the left upper extremity is located posteriorly to the cavernoma, which was subsequently successfully resected.

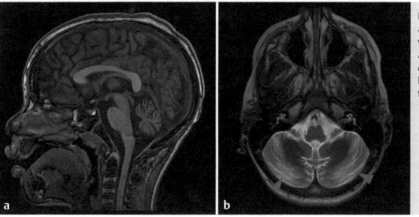

Fig. 9.9 Cerebellar volume loss. (a) Sagittal T1 W and (b) axial T2 W images in a 4-year-old female with seizures show prominence of the CSF space along the folia of the cerebellar hemispheres (*red arrowheads*) and vermis. Mild cerebellar volume loss can be a result of chronic antiepileptic therapy.

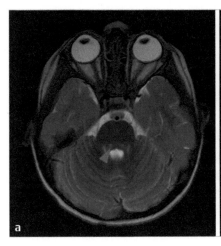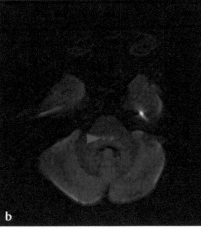

Fig. 9.10 Chronic antiepileptic therapy with vigabatrin (Sabril). (a) Axial T2 W image and (b) axial DWI of the brainstem in a 2-year-old female child with seizures show a hyperintense signal associated with the central tegmental tracts bilaterally (*red arrowheads*). This pattern, as well as abnormalities in the globi palladi, hypothalami, and thalami, can be related to myelinic edema in patients taking the antiepileptic medication vigabatrin. Identification of this finding may be important for guiding dose modification/cessation of this medication and preventing investigative studies for other metabolic abnormalities.

9.11 Further Reading

[1] Berg AT, Berkovic SF, Brodie MJ et al. Revised terminology and concepts for organization of seizures and epilepsies: Report of the ILAE Commission on Classification and Terminology, 2005–2009. Epilepsia 2010; 51(4):676–685

References

[1] Blümcke I, Thom M, Aronica E et al. The clinicopathologic spectrum of focal cortical dysplasias: A consensus classification proposed by an ad hoc Task Force of the ILAE Diagnostic Methods Commission. Epilepsia 2011; 52(1): 158–174

[2] Rivas-Coppola MS, Shah N, Choudhri AF, Morgan R, Wheless JW. Chronological evolution of magnetic resonance imaging findings in children with febrile infection-related epilepsy syndrome. Pediatr Neurol. 2015 Sep 25. pii: S0887-8994(15)00437-3. doi: 10.1016/j.pediatrneurol.2015.09.003. [Epub ahead of print] PMID: 26597039

[3] Pearl PL, Vezina LG, Saneto RP et al. Cerebral MRI abnormalities associated with vigabatrin therapy. Epilepsia 2009; 50(2):184–194

[4] Choudhri AF, Patel RM, Whitehead MT, Siddiqui A, Wheless JW. Cortical activation through passive-motion functional MRI. Am J Neuroradiol 2015 Sep;36(9):1675-1681. doi: 10.3174/ajnr.A4345

10 Infection and Inflammation

10.1 Introduction

Inflammatory conditions of both infectious and noninfectious origin can result in neurologic symptoms and have a variety of appearances on imaging. The appearances on imaging of some of these disorders are characteristic, whereas others can have nonspecific appearance requiring a differential diagnostic approach. In some instances, the ability to narrow the differential diagnosis can by itself aid in determining the appropriate treatment and/or additional diagnostic tests for an inflammatory condition. Familiarity with the laboratory profiles of CSF abnormalities in different infectious and inflammatory processes is important (▶ Table 10.1).

10.2 Infection

10.2.1 Meningitis

The most common infectious condition of the central nervous system (CNS) is meningitis. Meningitis is not a diagnosis based on imaging, and imaging is generally not indicated in this condition unless there are atypical features or focal neurologic deficits. Testing of cerebrospinal fluid (CSF) is the primary means of confirming the diagnosis of meningitis. In patients with known meningitis, there are two primary reasons why imaging may be performed. The first is to seek signs of a source of the infection, such as osseous erosion from the mastoid air cells or paranasal sinuses, and the second is to seek signs of an abscess. Although computed tomography (CT) can reveal signs of osseous dehiscence, an abscess is best seen on contrast-enhanced magnetic resonance imaging (MRI) with diffusion-weighted imaging (DWI).

On MRI, meningitis will appear as leptomeningeal enhancement, usually without any parenchymal signal abnormality. Leptomeningeal enhancement is most commonly evaluated on postcontrast T1 W images, although postcontrast fluid-attenuated inversion recovery (FLAIR) images are especially sensitive to it. Contrast-enhanced CT is rarely indicated in meningitis, because in most situations a high-quality unenhanced CT scan will identify any extra-axial collections or parenchymal edema, and contrast-enhanced MRI is more sensitive than contrast-enhanced CT in identifying inflammation. Computed tomographic examination without and with contrast enhancement will double the radiation dose delivered to the patient while yielding only slightly more information than will unenhanced CT. Performing only a postcontrast CT scan will limit the ability to detect hemorrhage. Therefore, the preferred diagnostic evaluation in suspected meningitis would be an unenhanced CT scan and, if there are abnormalities or further clinical concern, subsequent MRI without and with contrast enhancement. Ultimately, it should be remembered that a lumbar puncture is the most important tool in diagnosing meningitis (▶ Table 10.1).[1]

10.2.2 Abscess

An abscess will typically have a peripheral contiguous rim of enhancement and centrally will demonstrate reduced water diffusion (▶ Fig. 10.1). When the abscess is intra-axial, there will be surrounding edematous changes. An abscess, also known as an empyema, can occur in the subdural or epidural space (▶ Fig. 10.2), in which case it is usually secondary to conditions like sinonasal/mastoid disease or penetrating trauma, or is postoperative.

10.2.3 Encephalitis

Encephalitis is a condition in which there is inflammation of the brain parenchyma itself, of either infectious or noninfectious origin. Because bacterial infection of the brain will usually lead to necrosis/abscess, encephalitis of infectious origin is typically related to a viral infection. A special consideration among viral encephalitides is herpes simplex virus (HSV) encephalitis, which most commonly presents as a febrile seizure. Such encephalitis is most often related to HSV-1 virus involved in an orofacial infection (such as a cold sore), in which there is reactivation of the virus in the trigeminal ganglion (also known as the gasserian ganglion) (refer to ▶ Fig. 9.6). Accordingly, the adjacent portion of the medial temporal lobe will be preferentially involved, as evidenced on imaging through a hyperintense T2/FLAIR signal, reduced water diffusion, and possibly postcontrast enhancement, with the eventual development of hemorrhagic necrosis. If this diagnosis is suspected, treatment with acyclovir should be started immediately (not waiting for confirmation of the diagnosis). Only upon a negative result of polymerase chain reaction (PCR) for HSV on a CSF specimen should acyclovir therapy be discontinued.

In the neonatal period, HSV infection is more commonly related to the HSV-2 virus, may not involve the temporal lobes, and can have a scattered and random distribution (see Chapter 5) from hematogenous and/or CSF dissemination.

Other viral encephalitides tend to cause nonspecific edema predominantly in the gray matter, most often without abnormal enhancement, hemorrhagic changes, or diffusion abnormality.

Table 10.1 Results of lumbar puncture in inflammatory and infectious disorders of the central nervous system

Condition	Results
Normal*	Protein 15 to 60 mg/100 mL of CSF, glucose 50 to 80 mg/100 mL, cell count 0 to 5 white cells, no red blood cells
Bacterial meningitis	Elevated neutrophil count, decreased glucose concentration; protein concentration can be elevated
Viral meningitis	Elevated lymphocyte count, normal to mildly decreased glucose concentration
Noninfectious inflammatory process	Minimally elevated lymphocyte count, normal glucose concentration, mildly elevated protein concentration
Neoplasm with cerebrospinal fluid dissemination	Markedly elevated protein concentration; perform cytology on cerebrospinal fluid sample if concern exists about possible neoplasm

*Note that normal ranges will vary slightly among laboratories.

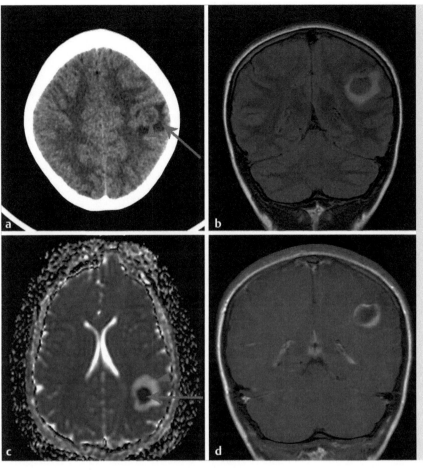

Fig. 10.1 Abscess. (a) Axial computed tomographic image of the head of a 10-year-old girl shows a round lesion (*red arrowhead*) with a surrounding rim of edema (*red arrow*). (b) Coronal fluid-attenuated inversion recovery image shows an ovoid lesion with a rim of hyperintense signal. (c) Axial ADC map shows a hypointense area centrally (*red arrow*) representing restricted diffusion, with a peripheral rim of hyperintense signal (*red arrowhead*) representing facilitated diffusion. (d) Coronal T1 W plus contrast image shows a peripheral rim of enhancement and no central enhancement. This represents an abscess with a peripheral rim of vasogenic edema.

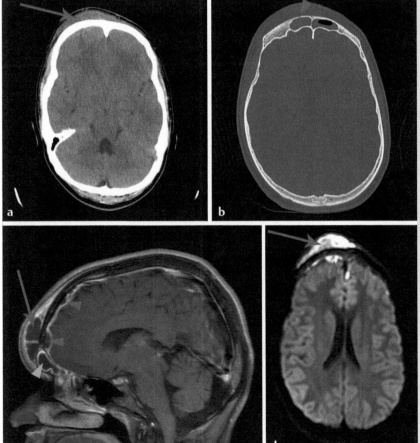

Fig. 10.2 Pott's puffy tumor/frontal empyema. (a) Axial computed tomographic image of the head of a 16-year-old boy with headache, fever, and new forehead swelling shows extracranial soft tissue swelling in the scalp (*red arrow*) and an extra-axial collection overlying the right frontal pole (*red arrowhead*). (b) Bone algorithm image shows a focal area of dehiscence in the outer cortex of the right frontal sinus (*red arrowhead*). (c) Sagittal T1 plus contrast image shows a peripherally enhancing fluid collection overlying the right frontal sinus (*red arrow*), representing an extracranial abscess (Pott's puffy tumor). There is pachymeningeal thickening overlying the right frontal lobe, with focal areas of fluid collection consistent with empyemas (*red arrowheads*). There is also fluid within a peripherally enhancing frontal sinus (*green arrowhead*). (d) Axial diffusion-weighted image shows diffusion restriction within the extracranial fluid (*red arrow*) and intracranial collections (*red arrowheads*), confirming that these findings are empyemas/abscesses. The collection extends along the falx cerebri, indicating that it has a subdural component as well as a presumed epidural component.

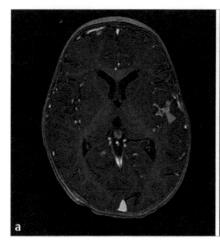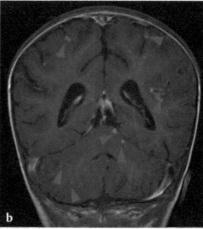

Fig. 10.3 Tuberculous meningitis. (a) Axial T1 plus contrast image of the head of a 1-year-old girl with fevers and altered mental status shows thick leptomeningeal enhancement along the left sylvian fissure (*arrowhead*). (b) Coronal T1 plus contrast image shows multifocal areas of leptomeningeal enhancement (*red arrowheads*), representing tuberculous meningitis.

10.2.4 Atypical Infections

Atypical infectious processes must be considered in specific circumstances in which there are abnormalities on imaging of the pediatric brain. Such circumstances relate to the patient's history of exposure to regionally prominent diseases. Lyme meningitis, related to spirochetal infection by *Borrelia burgdorferi*, can result in enhancement along the cisternal segments of cranial nerves. The enhancement will be smooth and without thickening, and will be rare in patients without a history of being bitten by a tick of the genus *Ixodes* and/or travel to areas in which Lyme disease is endemic.

Two infectious processes that are rare in the United States but are commonly encountered globally and of which it is important to be aware are neurocysticercosis and tuberculosis. Neurocysticercosis is a parasitic infection caused by the pig tapeworm *Taenia solium*. It is transmitted through undercooked pork and results in partly cystic and partly calcified lesions within the brain, and commonly presents with seizures. Seizures can occasionally be an isolated finding. Most patients with cysticercosis have multiple intracranial lesions; however, occasionally a patient will have only a single lesion, which makes imaging diagnosis more challenging. When there is uncertainty, evaluation for the involvement of other organs, including the finding of calcified intramuscular lesions in the extremities, can increase confidence in the diagnosis of cysticercosis.

Mycobacterium tuberculosis is an organism most widely known for causing pulmonary infections, but it can also cause meningitis, with thickened, contrast-enhancing leptomeningeal deposits (▶ Fig. 10.3). The investigation of a patient with this condition is likely to elicit a positive history of exposure, and awareness of the appearance of tuberculous meningitis on imaging is important because the causative bacterium may not show up on gram stain and may not grow in culture for weeks to months, even in special culture medium.

10.3 Inflammatory Processes

Noninfectious inflammatory processes can be among the most confusing disease processes to identify. They are more difficult to confirm than infectious processes and are more commonly encountered than inborn errors of metabolism. A majority of noninfectious inflammatory processes are immune-mediated demyelinating conditions. Contrast-enhanced MRI is the mainstay of evaluation for these conditions.

Multiple sclerosis (MS) is a noninfectious, immune-mediated inflammatory and demyelinating condition (▶ Fig. 10.4). Although much more common in adults, it can occur in adolescents and rarely also in children. As in adults, MS in pediatric patients shows a female predominance and is more common in geographic locations farther away from the Equator (higher latitudes) than closer to it. The most common appearance of a demyelinating plaque of MS is that of an ovoid lesion that is hyperintense on T2 W/FLAIR imaging, with the long axis of the lesion following the course of the medullary veins (perivenular orientation).[2,3] Areas of acute demyelination will show postcontrast enhancement, often with a peripheral discontinuous rim. Although not unique to MS, a discontinuous rim is characteristic of noninfectious inflammatory processes and helpful in differentiating them from an infectious or neoplastic process. Lesions of MS can occur within the corpus callosum, brainstem, cerebellum, and optic nerve ("optic neuritis"), and within the spinal cord (▶ Fig. 10.5). Although FLAIR imaging is helpful for identifying lesions of MS in the supratentorial brain, lesions in the posterior fossa are often easier to identify on conventional T2 W magnetic resonance images.

Acute disseminated encephalomyelitis (ADEM) is a noninfectious, immune-mediated inflammatory process that follows an immune response to an infectious agent, typically a virus, but possibly a bacterial pathogen or attenuated virus/viral antigens in a vaccine (▶ Fig. 10.5).[4] The theory for the development of ADEM is that the immune response cross-reacts with myelin, resulting in inflammation. Acute disseminated encephalomyelitis can take on many patterns, possibly related to the type of immune cross-reactivity that causes it. No specific relationship has yet been elucidated between the immune response that causes a particular phenotype of ADEM and the appearance of the condition on imaging. Acute disseminated encephalomyelitis can involve any area that is myelinated, including the thalamus, which consists predominantly of gray matter but has a large myelinated component because of its numerous afferent and efferent connections.

In ADEM as in all demyelinating processes, careful attention should be paid to the optic nerves, even if only on a brain

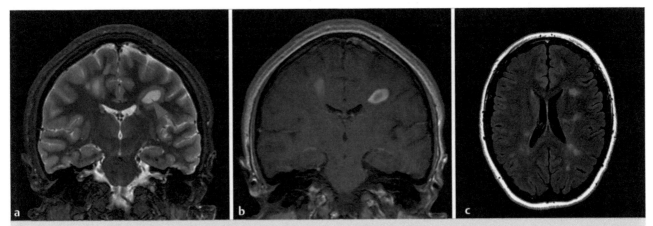

Fig. 10.4 Multiple sclerosis (MS). (a) Coronal short tau inversion recovery image shows an ovoid hyperintense lesion in the left posterior frontal white matter, with its long axis along the trajectory of medullary veins (*red arrowhead*). (b) T1 plus contrast imaging shows enhancement, consistent with an area of active demyelination in the setting of MS. (c) Axial fluid-attenuated inversion recovery image shows multiple additional areas of hyperintense signal in white matter.

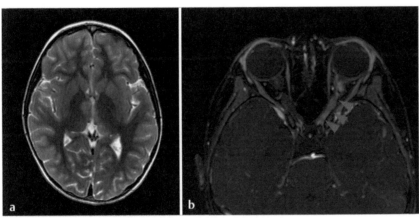

Fig. 10.5 Acute disseminated encephalomyelitis (ADEM). (a) Axial T2 W image of the head of a 7-year-old girl with altered mental status and vision changes shows heterogeneous areas of T2 hyperintense signal in both thalami. (b) Axial T1 plus contrast fat-suppressed image of the orbits shows enhancement of the canalicular and orbital segment of the left optic nerve (*arrowheads*), consistent with optic neuritis in the setting of ADEM. Note that the involvement of deep gray matter is much less common in multiple sclerosis than in ADEM, but both disorders can present with optic neuritis.

protocol study. If the patient has specific visual complaints, dedicated orbital MRI is warranted in addition to MRI of the brain. It is also important to be aware that the middle cerebellar peduncle is a large white-matter tract that is often involved in demyelinating conditions. It is relevant to note that the definition of ADEM based on clinical consensus requires the patient to be encephalopathic, but that encephalopathy is not clearly defined (and may include fatigue or irritability), and that from a pathophysiologic standpoint, the disease process in ADEM (regardless of name or classification given to it) does not require encephalopathy.

Neuromyelitis optica (NMO), also known as Devic's disease, is an immune-mediated condition that characteristically involves the optic nerves and spinal cord (▶ Fig. 10.6).[5] Brain involvement does not exclude the diagnosis of NMO, but will typically not be the predominating feature of this condition. The immune mediator of NMO is known to be an autoantibody to the aquaporin-4 protein. The involvement of the spinal cord in NMO tends to be expansile, long-segment involvement, as compared with the more focal, minimally or nonexpansile involvement by the lesions in MS. Like NMO, ADEM can also cause lesions of the spinal cord, which in both conditions can be mistaken for intramedullary spinal cord tumors.

Another immune-mediated encephalitis meriting awareness in imaging of the pediatric CNS is encephalitis caused by autoimmune antibodies to the N-methyl-D-aspartate (NMDA) receptor.[6] The clinical and imaging features of this encephalitis can be nonspecific, including acute encephalopathy and memory loss with nonenhancing, gray-matter-predominant areas of signal abnormality without signs of infection. This is seen with increased frequency in patients with mature teratomas of the ovaries. Although these teratomas are not malignant lesions, encephalitis caused by antibody to the NMDA receptor in patients with these lesions can be considered a paraneoplastic condition. Although it can be a severe condition, immunomodulatory therapy, including intravenous immunoglobulin, offers the potential for reversing it, as does resection of any identified neoplastic lesion.

Limbic encephalitis is an immune-mediated encephalitis with involvement of the limbic system, particularly the hippocampi and cingulate gyri. Although in adults limbic encephalitis is usually paraneoplastic and warrants a whole-body oncologic screening protocol, it tends to be idiopathic in children. A recently described entity in children with a limbic encephalitis-like presentation and intractable status epilepticus is febrile infection-related epilepsy syndrome (FIRES).[7,8] Little is

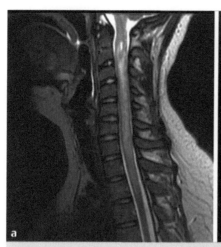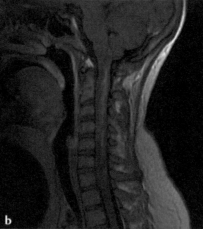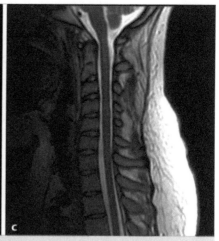

Fig. 10.6 Acute disseminated encephalomyelitis (ADEM)/neuromyelitis optica (NMO)/idiopathic transverse myelitis (ITM) spine. (a) Sagittal T2 W image of the cervical spine of a 17-year-old girl shows a hyperintense signal from a long-segment expansile area of central cord throughout the cervical spinal cord. (b) Sagittal T1 plus contrast image shows heterogeneous enhancement within the lesion, extending superiorly toward the obex. (c) Sagittal T2 W image of the cervical spine at 5 months after treatment shows resolution of the expansile lesion, with mild residual signal abnormality of the spinal cord. This patient had aquaporin-4 autoantibodies detected in her cerebrospinal fluid, representing neuromyelitis optica (Devic's disease). The appearances of ADEM and ITM can be similar.

known about this condition, other than that it can include a rapidly developing encephalomalacia and that the seizures in the condition may respond to a ketogenic diet.

Abnormalities in the signals generated by parenchymal tissue can also result from vascular-mediated processes. Vasculitis refers to a noninfectious inflammatory process involving blood vessels, typically arteries.[9] Its results can include brain-parenchymal abnormalities that appear identical to those in conditions like ADEM, although hemorrhagic changes and gliosis are more common in vasculitides.[10]

As observed in Chapter 12, the diagnosis of vasculitis can be difficult to confirm. When computed tomographic and magnetic resonance arteriography are normal, digital subtraction angiography (DSA) may be needed. Even in the setting of a normal result of DSA, vasculitis cannot be excluded. In theory, a brain biopsy is the gold standard for diagnosing vasculitis, yet even this will often not yield a definitive diagnosis.

Another vasculopathy causing abnormality in white-matter signaling is posterior reversible encephalopathy syndrome (PRES),[11,12] which may be a variant of the disease process known as reversible cerebral vasoconstriction syndrome (RCVS).[13,14] Posterior reversible encephalopathy syndrome is believed to to be a condition in which autonomic dysregulation impairs homeostatic autoregulation and (presumably) leads to an increased interstitial water content from high arteriolar and capillary pressures. The primary risk factors for the occurrence of PRES include severe hypertension, immunosuppressant therapy, and pregnancy. Findings in its radiologic investigation will most commonly be predominantly parieto-occipital (hence the term "posterior" in its name), and upon correction of the factors underlying it (such as normalization of blood pressure or the cessation of immunosuppressant), it will typically resolve (hence the term "reversible" in its name). It is important to note that there is not always posterior involvement in PRES, and that it may not be fully reversible. It can occasionally involve the frontal lobes without parieto-occipital involvement, and it can involve the cerebellum. The syndrome will rarely have a hemor-

rhagic component, and the identification of blood products in an imaging study done for PRES should raise concern about a process like vasculitis.

References

[1] Wright BLC, Lai JTF, Sinclair AJ. Cerebrospinal fluid and lumbar puncture: A practical review. J Neurol 2012; 259(8):1530–1545

[2] Verhey LH, Sled JG. Advanced magnetic resonance imaging in pediatric multiple sclerosis. Neuroimaging Clin N Am 2013; 23(2):337–354

[3] Miller TR, Mohan S, Choudhri AF, Gandhi D, Jindal G. Advances in multiple sclerosis and its variants: Conventional and newer imaging techniques. Radiol Clin North Am 2014; 52(2):321–336

[4] Wender M. Acute disseminated encephalomyelitis (ADEM). J Neuroimmunol 2011; 231(1–2):92–99

[5] Makhani N, Bigi S, Banwell B, Shroff M. Diagnosing neuromyelitis optica. Neuroimaging Clin N Am 2013; 23(2):279–291

[6] Jones KC, Benseler SM, Moharir M. Anti-NMDA receptor encephalitis. Neuroimag Clin N Am 2013; 23(2):309–320

[7] Rivas-Coppola MS, Shah N, Choudhri AF, Morgan R, Wheless JW. Chronological evolution of magnetic resonance imaging findings in children with febrile infection-related epilepsy syndrome. Pediatr Neurol. 2015 Sep 25. pii: S0887-8994(15)00437-3. doi: 10.1016/j.pediatrneurol.2015.09.003. [Epub ahead of print] PMID: 26597039

[8] van Baalen A, Häusler M, Boor R et al. Febrile infection-related epilepsy syndrome (FIRES): A nonencephalitic encephalopathy in childhood. Epilepsia 2010; 51(7):1323–1328

[9] Moharir M, Shroff M, Benseler SM. Childhood central nervous system vasculitis. Neuroimaging Clin N Am 2013; 23(2):293–308

[10] Abdel Razek AAK, Alvarez H, Bagg S, Refaat S, Castillo M. Imaging spectrum of CNS vasculitis. Radiographics 2014; 34(4):873–894

[11] Bartynski WS. Posterior reversible encephalopathy syndrome, Part 1: Fundamental imaging and clinical features. AJNR Am J Neuroradiol 2008; 29(6):1036–1042

[12] Bartynski WS. Posterior reversible encephalopathy syndrome, Part 2: Controversies surrounding pathophysiology of vasogenic edema. AJNR Am J Neuroradiol 2008; 29(6):1043–1049

[13] Miller TR, Shivashankar R, Mossa-Basha M, Gandhi D. Reversible cerebral vasoconstriction syndrome, Part 1: Epidemiology, pathogenesis, and clinical course. AJNR Am J Neuroradiol 2015

[14] Miller TR, Shivashankar R, Mossa-Basha M, Gandhi D. Reversible cerebral vasoconstriction syndrome, Part 2: Diagnostic work-up, imaging evaluation, and differential diagnosis. AJNR Am J Neuroradiol 2015; 36(9):1580–1588

11 Hydrocephalus

11.1 Introduction

Hydrocephalus is the pathologic accumulation of excess cerebrospinal fluid (CSF) within the head, typically within the ventricular system and typically with increased intraventricular pressure. It can be seen both on a congenital and an acquired basis, and it is a condition frequently encountered in pediatric neuroradiology. Although the most basic understanding of hydrocephalus is easy to grasp, the frequency and complexity of this disease process make it helpful to understand more about the pathophysiologic mechanisms responsible for it as well as treatment options for it.

11.2 Basic Model for Hydrocephalus

The most basic model for understanding hydrocephalus, which admittedly is now known to be a gross oversimplification, remains a reasonable starting point in describing the condition. Cerebrospinal fluid (CSF) is predominantly formed by the choroid plexus in the atria of both lateral ventricles of the brain. The CSF then travels through the foramina of Monro into the third ventricle (▶ Fig. 11.1), with the fluid propelled in a pulsatile manner by displacement resulting from arterial expansion during systole. From the third ventricle, CSF traverses the sylvian aqueduct (between the mesencephalic tegmentum and quadrigeminal plate). From the fourth ventricle, outflow of CSF occurs inferiorly into the cisterna magna through the foramen of Magendie, and laterally into the lateral medullary cisterns through the foramina of Luschka. Cerebrospinal fluid is eventually resorbed by the dura and arachnoid granulations, and enters the blood.

It is estimated that in adults, up to 500 mL of CSF is produced per day, but the volume of CSF at any given time is approximately 150 mL, indicating a multifold turnover of the entire volume of CSF every day. Thus, there is a balance between the volume of CSF produced, CSF transit, and the ability to resorb CSF. Alterations in any of these factors can result in hydrocephalus.

The most commonly encountered pattern of hydrocephalus relates to obstruction of the sylvian aqueduct (aqueductal

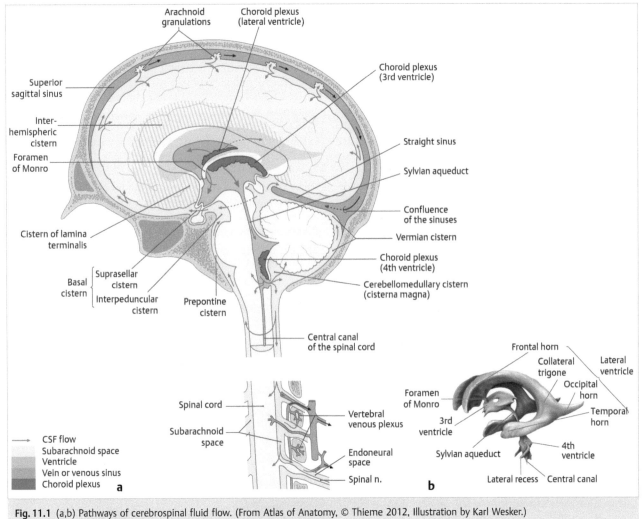

Fig. 11.1 (a,b) Pathways of cerebrospinal fluid flow. (From Atlas of Anatomy, © Thieme 2012, Illustration by Karl Wesker.)

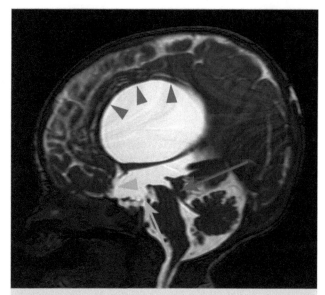

Fig. 11.2 Aqueductal stenosis. Sagittal image made with fast imaging employing steady-state acquisition of the head a 3-day-old boy with hydrocephalus shows effacement of the sylvian aqueduct (*red arrow*), with resulting anterior bowing of the lamina terminalis (*green arrowhead*), inferior bowing of the floor of the third ventricle (*green arrow*), and upward bowing of the corpus callosum (*red arrowheads*). The fourth ventricle is nondilated in this patient with congenital aqueductal stenosis.

stenosis or obstruction) (▶ Fig. 11.2). The sylvian aqueduct can be narrowed or obstructed by blood products after intraventricular hemorrhage or by inflammatory debris in the setting of meningitis, or it can be extrinsically compressed by a mass (such as a pineal tumor or tectal glioma). Aqueductal stenosis can be congenital, with an X-linked form of the disorder. It is also an associated feature in many cases of rhombencephalosynapsis, an abnormality in hindbrain cleavage that results in incomplete lateral migration of the inferior colliculi (mesencephalosynapsis) and resulting underdevelopment of the inferior aspect of the sylvian aqueduct.

Stenosis or obstruction of the sylvian aqueduct will result in excessive accumulation of CSF within the lateral and third ventricles, a pattern known as triventricular hydrocephalus.

At varying degrees of severity of stenosis, there will be fullness of the frontal and temporal horns of the lateral ventricles, anterior bowing of the lamina terminalis, inferior bowing of the floor of the third ventricle, and splaying of the chiasmatic and infundibular recesses of the third ventricle. The fourth ventricle is not dilated in this condition. Historically, stenosis or obstruction of the sylvian aqueduct has been referred to as obstructive hydrocephalus.

If the fourth ventricle is also dilated, in a pattern referred to as tetraventricular hydrocephalus (▶ Fig. 11.3), the assumption is that the sylvian aqueduct is patent. This has historically been ascribed to the overproduction and/or underabsorption of CSF, and it is referred to as communicating hydrocephalus; however, this term is often inaccurately applied and misleading. Many patients with a tetraventricular hydrocephalus actually do have an obstruction, with arachnoid webs or membranes obstructing the outflow of CSF from the fourth ventricle (▶ Fig. 11.3). A persistent Blake's-pouch cyst without fenestration is a consideration for a fourth ventricular outflow obstruction. It is known that patients with meningeal irritation/inflammation from meningitis can have impaired CSF resorption resulting in tetraventricular ventriculomegaly, and they may possibly also have prominence of the extra-axial space. This prominence is more common in the neonate because of the ability of the neonatal skull to enlarge (▶ Fig. 11.4).

Hydrocephalus with isolated enlargement of the subarachnoid space without signs of ventricular enlargement has been referred to as external hydrocephalus. This term is confusing and often mistakenly applied; most patients suspected of having this condition actually have normal pressures and instead have a condition known as benign enlargement of the subarachnoid spaces of infancy (BESSI) (further described below) (▶ Fig. 11.5).

Similarly, it is possible for a patient to have enlarged ventricles (ventriculomegaly) without having any abnormal CSF pressures or imbalance in CSF production/transit/resorption. The most common setting in which this is encountered is that of juxtaventricular parenchymal volume loss, which results in ex-vacuo enlargement of the ventricular system (▶ Fig. 11.6). This is a situation in which ventriculomegaly can exist without hydrocephalus, a condition that would not benefit from procedures for diverting CSF flow, such as the placement of a

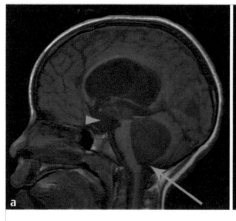
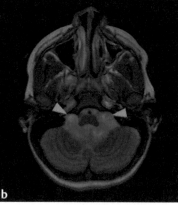

Fig. 11.3 Fourth ventricular outflow obstruction. (a) Sagittal T2W image shows dilation of the third ventricular recesses (*blue arrowhead*) and prominent cerebrospinal fluid flow artifact within the third and fourth ventricles. The foramen of Magendie appears patent, but flow voids did not traverse this (*blue arrow*), and (b) an axial T2W image shows membranes bowing through the foramina of Luschka (*blue arrowheads*). This represents membranes causing a fourth ventricular outflow obstruction and tetraventricular hydrocephalus. Although the sylvian aqueduct is patent with respect to the communication between the ventricular system and the subarachnoid space, this represents a noncommunicating tetraventricular hydrocephalus.

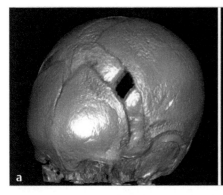
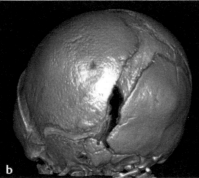

Fig. 11.4 Suture splaying. Three-dimensional reconstruction of the skull, from (a) anterior oblique and (b) posterior oblique projections, of a 3-month-old male with progressive macrocephaly, showing widening of the coronal, sagittal, squamosal, and lambdoid sutures.

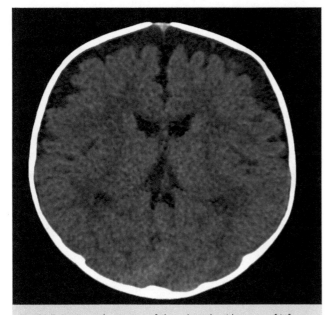

Fig. 11.5 Benign enlargement of the subarachnoid spaces of infancy (BESSI). Axial computed tomographic image in a 7-month-old with macrocephaly shows a normal appearance of the brain parenchyma and prominence of the subarachnoid space overlying both frontal lobes. Cortical veins are seen coursing through the subarachnoid space, and there is no visible extra-axial collection or mass effect on the brain parenchyma, which in the setting of macrocephaly is consistent with BESSI.

ventriculoperitoneal (VP) shunt. However, a common cause of parenchymal volume loss in children is prior germinal matrix hemorrhage and/or white-matter disease of prematurity, which themselves can result in hydrocephalus. Therefore, a patient can have hydrocephalus superimposed upon ex-vacuo ventriculomegaly. Differentiation between the conditions can be challenging; however, it is important to be aware that because pure ex-vacuo ventriculomegaly is associated with normal intraventricular pressures, there will be no evidence of abnormal splaying of the third ventricular recesses and the sylvian aqueduct should be patent.

An additional and more complicated type of hydrocephalus is complex posthemorrhagic hydrocephalus, which is commonly encountered in premature infants. In addition to obstruction of the sylvian aqueduct, this condition may include loculated membranes and adhesions within the lateral ventricles, possi-

bly requiring either cyst fenestration or the placement of separate shunt catheters within each lateral ventricle (▶ Fig. 11.7).

11.3 Treatment of Hydrocephalus

11.3.1 Shunts

Treatment of hydrocephalus is predominantly related to the diversion of CSF. The most common type of diversion is through a VP shunt, in which a catheter is placed into the ventricular system and drains into the peritoneal cavity. The shunts used for diverting CSF can have pressure valves that regulate the flow of CSF, with fluid passing through the catheter only when pressures exceed a certain value. Some shunt catheters even have the ability to readjust the pressure setting, which is done noninvasively through a magnetic device. The programmable shunt valves used for this produce an artifact on magnetic resonance imaging (MRI) (▶ Fig. 11.8), and the valve settings need to be confirmed and rechecked after an MRI to prevent over- or undershunting.

Overshunting occurs when intracranial pressures for which a shunt has been inserted become too low. It typically occurs with small lateral ventricles and a prominent subarachnoid space overlying both cerebral hemispheres, and it may predispose to the formation of subdural collections. Low CSF pressures also produce smooth, diffuse pachymeningeal enhancement on imaging, related to engorgement of the epidural venous plexus.

Although VP shunts are the most common type of shunt, the distal end of the shunt catheter can be placed in locations other than the peritoneum, such as within the pleural space (ventriculopleural shunt) or within the superior vena cava/right atrium (ventriculoatrial shunt).

Shunt catheters can become obstructed, resulting in hydrocephalus. The most common type of shunt malfunction is related to obstruction of the intraventricular portion of a shunt, typically from growth of the choroid plexus into the sideholes of a catheter. Obstruction in this location is referred to as a proximal shunt malfunction. Another type of proximal shunt malfunction is dislodgement of the catheter from the ventricular system. A kink in or disruption of the catheter can also impair the drainage of CSF; this can result from dislodgement of the catheter tubing from the shunt reservoir (▶ Fig. 11.9).

Obstruction of the distal end of a shunt catheter is another type of shunt malfunction (i.e., distal shunt malfunction). This can be related to adhesions around the distal end of the catheter resulting in a loculated fluid collection, known as a

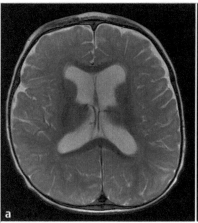
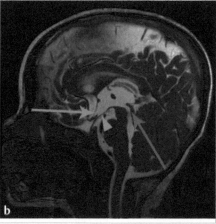

Fig. 11.6 Ex-vacuo enlargement of the ventricular system. (a) Axial T2 W image of the head of a 10-month-old shows mild ventriculomegaly of both lateral ventricles, but with preservation of the cerebrospinal fluid space within sulci overlying the cerebral hemispheres. (b) Sagittal image made with fast imaging employing steady-state acquisition shows a patent sylvian aqueduct (*red arrow*) and a normal position of the lamina terminalis (*blue arrow*) and floor of the third ventricle (*blue arrowhead*), without splaying of the chiasmatic or infundibular recesses of the third ventricle. This confirms an ex-vacuo basis for the patient's ventriculomegaly, as the result of a mild loss of cerebral white matter volume, without any relation to hydrocephalus.

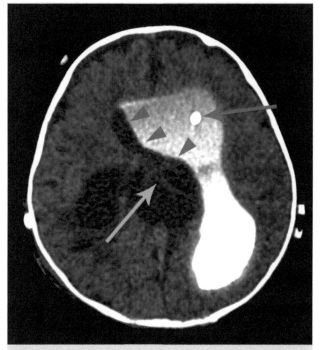

Fig. 11.7 Posthemorrhagic loculated hydrocephalus. Image made with axial computed tomographic ventriculography in a 4-month-old infant born at 26 weeks' gestation. The image was obtained after the injection of iodinated contrast material through the infant's shunt catheter (*red arrow*). There is contrast opacification of the left lateral ventricle, but the membrane (*red arrowheads*) is seen between the left lateral ventricle and the nonopacified right lateral ventricle. There is lack of opacification of a multiloculated midline conglomeration of cystic changes (*green arrow*) in this infant with loculated posthemorrhagic hydrocephalus.

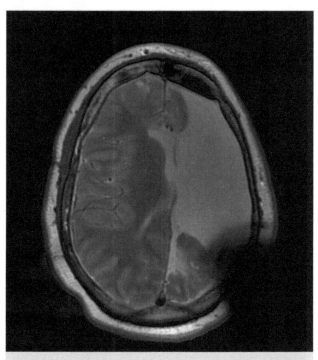

Fig. 11.8 Shunt artifact. Axial T2 W image in an adolescent 17-year-old female with a history of left-sided functional hemispherectomy shows a left posterior parietal area of signal dropout caused by artifact from a programmable shunt reservoir. When this problem is identified, it is important to ensure that the patient has appropriate follow-up, so that the shunt can be reprogrammed, as the settings may be reset in the magnetic field of the magnetic resonance imaging scanner.

pseudocyst or "CSFoma," around the catheter tip (▶ Fig. 11.10). A distal obstruction can also occur if the catheter tip becomes lodged against an anatomic or other structure, such as the liver, but this is less common.

Infection can be a further reason for shunt malfunction. An infected shunt may require removal of parts or all of the shunt tubing.

Some patients with hydrocephalus do not need a permanent shunt catheter. In the case of a patient in the immediate postoperative setting, or a patient with meningitis who needs a temporary catheter. To achieve temporary drainage, it is possible to insert a catheter that is intracranially identical to a VP shunt but whose extracranial portion does not terminate within a part of the patient's body, but in an external reservoir.

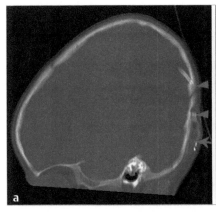
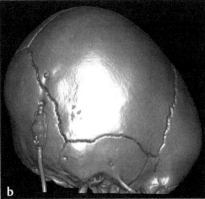

Fig. 11.9 Disconnection of shunt tubing. (a) Sagittal bone algorithm computed tomographic image shows a discontinuity in the extracranial portion of this patient's shunt catheter (between the *red arrowheads*). This is proximal to the shunt reservoir (*red arrow*). (b) A three-dimensional reformatting of the computed tomographic scan shows the relationship between the different portions of the catheter and the skull.

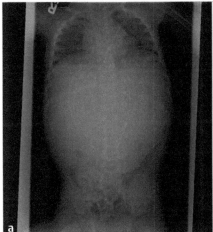
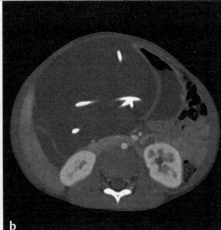
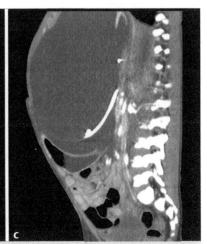

Fig. 11.10 CSFoma. (a) Frontal radiograph of the abdomen of a 3-year-old male with a shunt malfunction shows the distal shunt tubing coiled in a gasless portion of the abdomen. (b) Axial and (c) sagittal computed tomographic images show the tubing coiled within a collection of CSF (CSFoma, or CSF pseudocyst).

This is known as an external ventricular drain (EVD). Both an EVD and shunt catheter can be appropriately referred to as a ventriculostomy catheter. A surgeon may at times want to transform a VP shunt into an EVD, such as for preventing the intracranial spread of infection in a patient with peritonitis. It is possible to keep the intracranial portion of a shunt intact, but to connect the shunt tubing in such a manner as to have it function like an EVD. This procedure is known as externalization of a shunt catheter.

11.3.2 Other Treatments

Beyond shunts, there are other forms of treatment for hydrocephalus. In a patient with an obstruction at the level of the sylvian aqueduct, the primary abnormality is transit of CSF, with the production and resorption of CSF presumably being normal. An alternative to placing a permanent catheter, which carries the risk of subsequent failure, is an endoscopic surgical technique that creates a hole in the floor of the third ventricle, allowing the free passage of CSF between the third ventricle and the suprasellar cistern (▶ Fig. 11.11). This procedure, known as an endoscopic third ventriculostomy (ETV), can be curative if aqueductal obstruction is the only pathologic process

causing hydrocephalus. An ETV is often performed in conjunction with a biopsy in patients with pineal masses that cause hydrocephalus.

A newer technique than shunting or ETV, used more commonly in areas that lack full medical resources, is coagulative ablation of the choroid plexus in the lateral ventricles, to reduce the production of CSF. Although this surgical procedure is more challenging than shunt placement, it reduces the risk of shunt malfunction. A child in a rural area of a Third World nation may have only a single opportunity to have an ablative procedure on the choroid plexus and is unlikely to have direct access to brain imaging and shunt-revision surgery if or when shunt failure occurs. With maturation of the technique of coagulative ablation of the choroid plexus, it may be used more extensively in developed nations, either as a primary treatment for hydrocephalus or as an adjunct to shunting.

11.4 Interpreting a Post-shunt Study

When interpreting a computed tomographic or magnetic resonance scan of the brain in a patient with a shunt, it is important

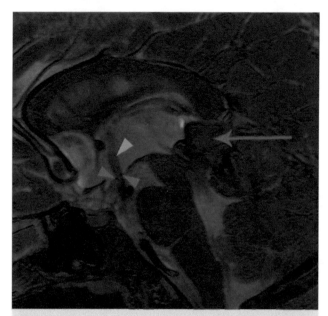

Fig. 11.11 Endoscopic third ventriculostomy (ETV). Sagittal image made with fast imaging employing steady-state acquisition of the head of a 7-year-old boy with a tumor in the pineal region (*red arrow*). The patient underwent biopsy of the tumor with simultaneous ETV. The defect in the floor of the third ventricle is visible (between the *red arrowheads*), and there is a void in CSF pulsation flow (*blue arrowhead*), confirming patency of the ETV. This lesion was a pineoblastoma.

the ventricle. The course of the catheter should be followed via a computed tomographic scan throughout its intracranial and visible extracranial course, ideally with the use of bone algorithm images reformatted in the sagittal and coronal planes.

It is important to compare in detail the size of all four ventricles. It is also very important to be careful about considering ventricular size as a "gestalt" entity, because subtle changes in size and other properties of the ventricles can be easily missed without close attention. Ventricular measurements can be made on an absolute basis or by using ratios. Absolute measurements are more accurate if an identical technique is used in all of the studies in which ventricular size and dimensions are being measured; this can be difficult if there is a difference in the position of the patient's head in different studies. Absolute measurements that can be used include the transverse dimension of the body of a lateral ventricle at the caudothalamic grooves or frontal horns (▶ Fig. 11.12); the dimensions of portions of the lateral ventricle, such as the frontal horn, temporal horn, or atrium; and the transverse dimension of the third ventricle. The transverse dimension of the third ventricle is very reproducible and is affected less than transverse measurements of the lateral ventricles when there is patient head tilt, especially if coronal images are available. Even minor changes in the transverse dimension of the third ventricle can be clinically relevant, to document both worsening hydrocephalus and the response to appropriate shunting.

At times, linear ventricular dimensions can be difficult to reliably compare, in particular in ultrasonographic images. Accordingly, it is sometimes easiest to compare ratios, such as the ratio of the transverse dimension of the frontal horns of the lateral ventricles to the transverse dimension of the calvarium at that same level, known as Evans' ratio. Although this is a commonly used technique, it can be insensitive to changes in ventricular size (both increases and decreases) in children with patent sutures, in whom the change in ventricular size can be associated with a corresponding change in head size. Therefore, close attention to other aspects of ventricular morphology and to the absolute measurements used to calculate Evans' ratio is

to perform a detailed analysis of the images produced by the scan and to compare them with the images made in prior studies of the patient. With regard to a shunt catheter, the location of the catheter tip has to be assessed. If the catheter tip is not within the ventricle, there may be impaired drainage. However, it is important to be aware that the tip of the catheter is not the sole access point for CSF, but that the sideholes along the distal-most portion of the catheter also permit drainage of CSF from

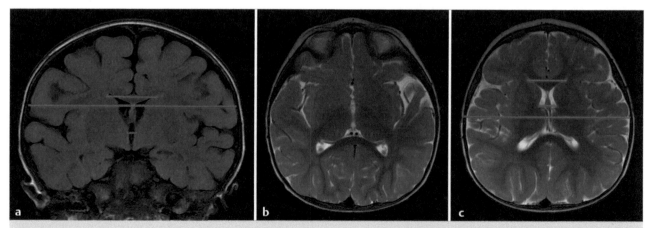

Fig. 11.12 Measurements in hydrocephalus, (a) Coronal fluid-attenuated inversion recovery image shows various measurements that can be made in hydrocephalus, such as the transverse dimensions of the bodies of the lateral ventricles, transverse measurement of the cranium, and transverse dimension of the third ventricle (superior to inferior). (b) Axial T2 W image shows a transverse measurement of the third ventricle. (c) Axial T2 W image shows (anterior to posterior) the transverse measurement of the frontal horns of the lateral ventricles, of the bodies of the lateral ventricles, and of the cranium.

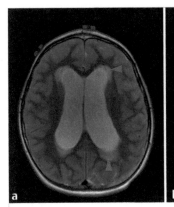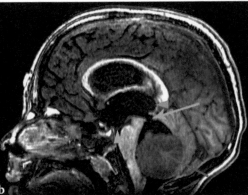

Fig. 11.13 Periventricular interstitial edema. (a) Axial T2 W image in a 6-year-old male with a new presentation of a fourth ventricular tumor shows enlargement of the lateral ventricles, with a hyperintense signal in the white matter adjacent to the frontal horns and atria of the lateral ventricles (*arrowheads*), consistent with periventricular interstitial edema. (b) Sagittal T1 W image shows the obstructing mass (*red arrow*) causing dilation of the sylvian aqueduct (*green arrow*) and the superior aspect of the fourth ventricle, as well as anterior bowing of the lamina terminalis (*red arrowhead*), inferior bowing of the floor of the third ventricle (*green arrowhead*), and splaying of the suprapineal recess of the third ventricle (*blue arrowhead*). This is a medulloblastoma with resulting acute hydrocephalus.

required. If the patient's medical chart is available, reviewing it to see whether there have been changes in the head circumference can help in gaining a better understanding of the patient's condition.

Because of the dynamic nature of the sutures in the young pediatric population, acute changes in ventricular size may result in suture splaying (see ▶ Fig. 11.4). Comparing ventricular size in subsequent studies in this population requires careful measurements. Simple comparison of the ratio of the size of the ventricles to the transverse dimension of the calvarium, on either a qualitative or quantitative basis, can miss changes in ventricular size. Accordingly, reliance on ratios like Evans' ratio will fail to detect worsening of (or improvement in) hydrocephalus if there are corresponding and proportionate changes in head size.

There are instances in which the surgeon attempts to remove a malfunctioning shunt but the shunt catheter does not appropriately retract, possibly because of adhesions, requiring the surgeon to cut the catheter at the calvarium and leave the intracranial portion intact. This is known as an "abandoned" shunt. When reporting a study of a patient with more than one shunt catheter, it is important to follow each catheter and its tubing. However, an abandoned catheter should not be mistaken for an unexpectedly disconnected shunt. When there is uncertainty about this, it can be helpful to study different examinations of the patient for shunt stability, review operative notes in the patient's chart, and possibly confer with the patient's neurosurgeon.

11.5 Acute Hydrocephalus

Acute hydrocephalus in children can cause symptoms ranging from headaches, nausea, and emesis to lethargy and bradycardia. One sign suggesting an acute hydrocephalus is periventricular interstitial edema (▶ Fig. 11.13), which first occurs adjacent to the frontal and occipital horns of the lateral ventricles. Relative to normal adjacent white matter, this will appear hypodense on computed tomographic images and hyperintense on T2 and fluid-attenuated inversion recovery (FLAIR) images. This has previously been referred to as "transependymal flow of CSF," but this term is an inaccurate description of the process responsible for periventricular interstitial edema and should be

avoided. It is now known that there is normally flow of CSF into the parenchyma. Because the central nervous system does not have a lymphatic system, resorption of CSF occurs directly from the interstitial space into the venous system. In acute hydrocephalus, there is compression of the venous system within the parenchyma and reduced resorption of CSF. Accordingly, recent evidence indicates that the edema in acute hydrocephalus is related to reduced resorption of CSF from the interstitial space, and not to the increased entry of CSF into the interstitial space. For this reason, "periventricular interstitial edema" is felt to be a more accurately descriptive term for this condition than "transependymal flow of CSF" or "transependymal edema."

11.6 Benign Enlargement of the Subarachnoid Spaces of Infancy

Benign enlargement of the subarachnoid spaces of infancy (BESSI) is a condition occurring in early childhood in which brain growth is normal but the growth of the skull is slightly accelerated. Children with this condition will therefore present with macrocephaly at approximately 5 to 6 months of age. The brain will appear approximately normal in volume, and there will be prominence of the subarachnoid space overlying both cerebral hemispheres. Benign enlargement of the subarachnoid spaces of infancy should be a bilaterally symmetric process without a midline shift or mass effect on the brain parenchyma, in which blood vessels will normally traverse the subarachnoid space (see ▶ Fig. 11.5). If blood vessels do not traverse this space, subdural collections of CSF (hygromas and/or chronic hematomas) must be suspected. There may be mild ventricular prominence in BESSI. Benign enlargement of the subarachnoid spaces of infancy will typically be a self-limiting condition, with the circumference of the head normalizing between 1 and 2 years of age.

Although BESSI is not hydrocephalus, it is included in this chapter for two reasons. First, it is often diagnosed in patients 5 or 6 months old on studies done for macrocephaly, and hydrocephalus is one of the primary concerns in the setting of macrocephaly. Second, BESSI has at times been referred to as external hydrocephalus, although this is probably an incorrect description. Some theories relate BESSI to the development of normal pressure hydrocephalus later in adulthood; this concept has not been widely accepted but is being actively studied, and more may become known as research continues.

It is also important to note that although BESSI is typically diagnosed at approximately 6 months of age in studies done for macrocephaly, a milder version that has not yet manifested as macrocephaly may be incidentally detected in a patient who has a study done for other reasons at 3 or 4 months of age (such as for seizure or trauma).

11.7 Imaging Techniques

In the neonatal period, ultrasonography through the anterior fontanelle is the primary means of diagnosing and following both hydrocephalus and associated abnormalities, such as germinal matrix hemorrhage. Magnetic resonance imaging can be performed as a troubleshooting technique, particularly for shunt planning in patients with loculated hydrocephalus (see ▶ Fig. 11.7) or associated congenital abnormalities. Computed tomography is not commonly needed in the neonatal population other than for emergent evaluation or characterization of a shunt catheter position.

Ultrasonography does not perform well as a technique for imaging the fontanelles beyond 3 or 4 months of age because the anterior fontanelle begins to close. At this time, computed tomography and magnetic resonance imaging become the mainstays of evaluation for hydrocephalus. Computed tomography has historically been used for emergent evaluation in children with hydrocephalus, as well as for evaluating the position and integrity of catheters. Magnetic resonance imaging avoids the use of ionizing radiation and provides improved soft tissue detail. It can be used for thin-section imaging to evaluate patency of the sylvian aqueduct and/or prior ETV, and cardiac-gated phase-contrast studies of CSF flow can also be performed. Current MRI scanners can identify most shunt catheters on T2W or gradient echo images, which was not possible with earlier MRI instruments. Magnetic resonance imaging instruments with rapid hydrocephalus protocols, using partial Fourier T2W images (e.g., half-Fourier-acquisition single-shot turbo spin-echo [HASTE] or single-shot T2 W), can provide imaging of the brain in approximately 10 to 20 seconds per imaging sequence. The images can be acquired in multiple planes, and the imaging can be done without patient sedation; if the patient moves, a given sequence can be repeated.

11.8 Cerebrospinal Fluid Dynamics and the Monro–Kellie Hypothesis

The Monro–Kellie hypothesis is an important concept with which to be familiar when discussing CSF physiology. It assumes that the cranium has a fixed volume, and within it are brain parenchyma, blood, and CSF. Because none of the components is compressible, a volume of CSF equal to the expansion of blood vessels must be displaced during systole, when blood vessels enlarge because of the increased pressure exerted on them by cardiac systole. The two main locations in which this displacement occurs are the spinal cord and sheaths of the optic nerves, each of which are surrounded by fat and/or a compressible venous plexus, allowing expansion that was not provided by the cranium. This is the source of the pulsations that cause the dynamic flow of CSF across the foramen magnum, which becomes obstructed in a Chiari type I malformation. Note that before closure of the cranial sutures, and particularly during the first 6 months of life, the Monro–Kellie hypothesis does not directly apply, because of the dynamic calvarial volume afforded by open sutures. Therefore, an evaluation of CSF flow during this period of life may not detect flow at the velocities typically expected in patients with a more mature cranium, and in this very young patient population, it is possible to erroneously identify aqueductal stenosis on CSF flow imaging.

11.9 Suggested Reading

[1] Flannery AM, Mazzola CA, Klimo P Jr et al. Foreword: Pediatric hydrocephalus: systematic literature review and evidence-based guidelines. J Neurosurg Pediatr 2014; 14 Suppl 1:1–2

[2] Mazzola CA, Choudhri AF, Auguste KI et al. Pediatric hydrocephalus: Systematic literature review and evidence-based guidelines. Part 2: Management of posthemorrhagic hydrocephalus in premature infants. J Neurosurg Pediatr 2014; 14 Suppl 1:8–23

[3] Nikas DC, Post AF, Choudhri AF, Mazzola CA, Mitchell L, Flannery AM. Pediatric hydrocephalus: Systematic literature review and evidence-based guidelines. Part 10: Change in ventricle size as a measurement of effective treatment of hydrocephalus. J Neurosurg Pediatr 2014; 14 Suppl 1:77–81

[4] Goeser CD, McLeary MS, Young LW. Diagnostic imaging of ventriculoperitoneal shunt malfunctions and complications. Radiographics 1998; 18(3):635–651

[5] Sivaganesan A, Krishnamurthy R, Sahni D, Viswanathan C. Neuroimaging of ventriculoperitoneal shunt complications in children. Pediatr Radiol 2012; 42 (9):1029–1046

12 Vascular Abnormalities

12.1 Introduction

The intracranial vasculature can have congenital and acquired abnormalities that result in injury to the brain parenchyma. Understanding the normal anatomy of the intracranial vasculature (▶ Fig. 12.1), developmental abnormalities that commonly affect it, and acquired conditions that affect it, can help identify possible causes of brain injury and may allow treatment before injury to the brain becomes irreversible.

12.2 Normal Anatomy

12.2.1 Arterial

The arterial blood supply to the brain passes predominantly through four vessels: two internal carotid arteries comprising the anterior circulation of the brain and two vertebral arteries comprising the posterior circulation. The internal carotid arteries traverse the petrous temporal bone, pass through the cavernous sinus, give rise to the ophthalmic arteries, have communication with the posterior cerebral artery (PCA) through the posterior communicating arteries (PCOM), give rise to the anterior choroidal arteries, and then split into the anterior and middle cerebral arteries at the carotid terminus (▶ Fig. 12.2). The segments of the anterior cerebral artery are referred are referred to sequentially as A1, A2, and A3. The A1 segment

extends from the origin to the anterior communicating artery (ACOM). The A2 segment extends from the ACOM to the origin of the frontopolar artery, and the A3 segment extends from the frontopolar artery to the origin of the callosomarginal artery. At this last point, the anterior cerebral artery (ACA) gives off the callosomarginal and pericallosal arteries, which course respectively along the superior and inferior margins of the cingulate gyrus.

The branches of the middle cerebral artery (MCA) are likewise numbered sequentially, based largely upon the direction of each branch. The M1 segment is directed horizontally and begins at the terminus of the internal carotid artery. The M2 branches of the MCA extend superiorly along the insular surface within the sylvian fissure. The M3 branches travel horizontally to exit the sylvian fissure, and the M4 branches extend superiorly over the over the lateral surface of the parietal and posterior frontal lobes (▶ Fig. 12.2). This naming convention originated largely through catheter angiography, and there is marked variability in the branching pattern of the MCA.

The V4 segments (the intradural segments) of the vertebral arteries give rise to the posterior inferior cerebellar arteries (PICA), which supply the inferior aspect of the cerebellar hemispheres. The two vertebral arteries combine to form the basilar artery. The midbasilar artery may give rise to anterior inferior cerebellar arteries (AICA) supplying the midportion of the cerebellum, but this is highly variable. The distal basilar artery

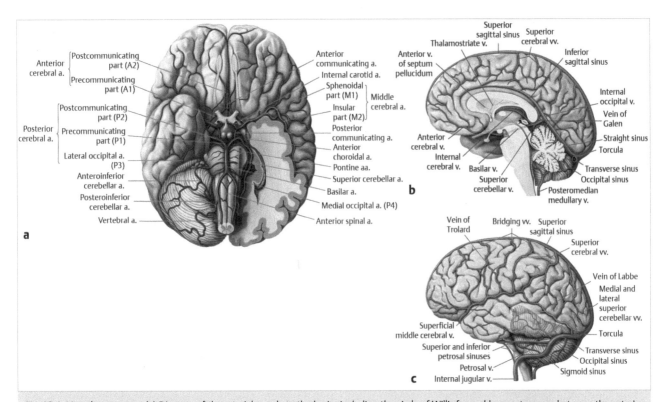

Fig. 12.1 Vascular anatomy. (a) Diagram of the arterial supply to the brain, including the circle of Willis formed by anastomoses between the anterior circulation (i.e., the anterior and middle cerebral arteries, arising from the internal carotid artery) and the posterior circulation (the basilar artery and posterior cerebral arteries, supplied by the vertebral arteries). (b) Midsagittal venous anatomy showing the major venous sinuses and the contributing veins. (c) Surface venous anatomy depicted from a lateral projection. From Atlas of Anatomy, © Thieme 2012, Illustration by Karl Wesker.

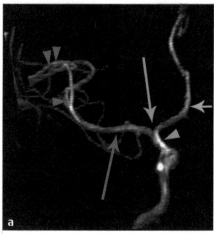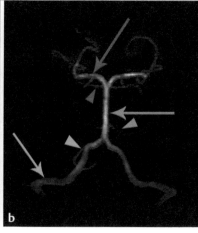

Fig. 12.2 Arterial anatomy. (a) Maximum-intensity projection (MIP) of the anterior circulation from magnetic resonance angiography (MRA) shows the supraclinoid internal carotid artery (*blue arrowhead*) bifurcating at the carotid terminus (*blue arrow*). Medially there is the anterior cerebral artery (*green arrow*), and laterally the middle cerebral artery, including its M1 (*red arrow*), M2 (*red arrowhead*), and M3 (*red arrowheads*) segments. (b) An MIP of the posterior circulation from MRA shows the distal vertebral artery (*green arrow*), which gives rise to the posterior inferior cerebellar artery (*green arrowhead*). The basilar artery (*blue arrow*) gives rise to the anterior inferior cerebellar artery (*blue arrowhead*). From the distal basilar artery arise the superior cerebellar arteries (*red arrowhead*) and the posterior cerebral arteries (*red arrow*).

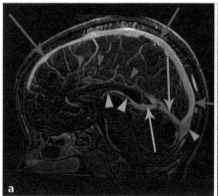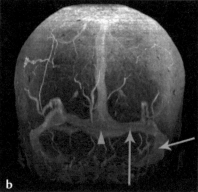

Fig. 12.3 Venous anatomy. (a) Sagittal T1 W subtraction image (precontrast image subtracted from postcontrast image) shows the internal cerebral veins (*green arrowheads*) from the vein of Galen (*green arrow*), which meets with the inferior sagittal sinus (*red arrowheads*) to form the straight sinus (*blue arrow*). The straight sinus meets the superior sagittal sinus (*red arrows*) at the torcula (*blue arrowhead*). (b) Posterior maximum intensity projection from magnetic resonance angiography shows the torcula (*blue arrowhead*), which drains thorough the transverse sinuses (*blue arrow*), which in turn become the sigmoid sinuses (*green arrow*).

gives rise to the superior cerebellar arteries, supplying the superior aspect of the cerebellum. The basilar artery terminates in the prepontine cistern, dividing into two posterior cerebral arteries (PCA) that extend posteriorly around the midbrain, along the crural and ambient cisterns (▶ Fig. 12.2). The segment of the PCA that extends from the origin of the PCA to the insertion of the PCOM is known as the P1 segment, with the next segment known as P2 as the PCA travels in the ambient cistern. The P3 and P4 segments of the PCA are more distal branches that extend through the quadrigeminal cistern and occipital region.

12.2.2 Veins

The major venous sinus in the head is the superior sagittal sinus, which is located along the calvarial margin of the falx cerebri, with blood flow extending posteriorly and eventually inferiorly toward the torcula (▶ Fig. 12.3). In this location, blood flow through the straight sinus joins the blood flow from the superior sagittal sinus, and two laterally directed, transverse sinuses carry the blood away. The transverse sinuses extend inferiorly behind the mastoid air cells as the sigmoid sinuses, and then extend into the jugular foramina and continue caudally within the neck as the internal jugular veins.

The right transverse/sigmoid sinus system is typically dominant, responsible for a larger percentage of venous drainage than the left.

The deep gray nuclei drain into the thalamostriate veins. These join an anterior septal vein (which courses along the anterior septum pellucidum in each cerebrum) to form the internal cerebral vein. The internal cerebral veins extend posteriorly, and are joined by the basal veins of Rosenthal, which follow the course of the hippocampi. These four veins, along with a superiorly directed vermian vein, form the vein of Galen. The vein of Galen joins with the inferior sagittal sinus, and this becomes the straight sinus. As described above, the straight sinus joins with the superior sagittal sinus in the torcula, from which blood flow is directed laterally within the transverse sinuses.

The head contains two paired cavernous sinuses, which receive inflow of blood from both the superficial middle cerebral vein (sylvian vein) and the superior ophthalmic vein. The outflow of blood from the cavernous sinus on each side of the head is into the superior petrosal vein, which connects to the proximal sigmoid sinus, and the inferior petrosal vein, which joins the jugular bulb. The jugular bulb is the venous structure extending through the jugular foramen at the junction between the sigmoid sinus and the internal jugular vein.

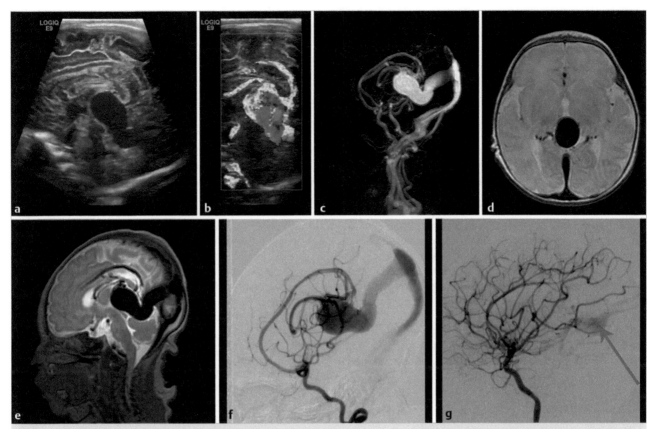

Fig. 12.4 Vein of Galen aneurysmal malformation (VGAM) as seen with ultrasonography. (a) Sagittal ultrasound (US) image through the anterior fontanelle of a newborn shows a cystic-appearing structure in the region of the quadrigeminal cistern. (b) Doppler US image shows that the lesion is vascular and has superior feeding vessels, confirming the diagnosis of a VGAM. (c) Sagittal maximum intensity projection of dynamic contrast-enhanced magnetic resonance angiographic image in the arterial phase shows prominent anterior cerebral/pericallosal arteries (persistent limbic arch) feeding the aneurysmally dilated venous structure, with contrast seen within the venous system in the arterial phase, without identification of parenchymal branches. (d) Axial and (e) sagittal T2 W images show enlarged flow voids from the dilated arterial and venous structures. (f) Lateral-projection cerebral angiogram from an injection of contrast medium into the internal carotid artery shows arterial-phase opacification of the dilated venous structure as a result of shunting, with few parenchymal vessels identified. (g) Lateral-projection angiogram acquired approximately 10 months later after sequential endovascular treatments shows only minimal opacification of the midline venous structure (*red arrow*), with markedly improved visualization of parenchymal branches.

Multiple superficial veins overlie the cerebral hemispheres, and are highly variable in their anatomy. There is typically one dominant, superiorly directed vein, known as the superior anastomotic vein (or vein of Trolard) overlying the lateral surface of both cerebral hemispheres and extending to the superior sagittal sinus, with multiple tributary veins. There is one posteriorly directed vein, known as the inferior anastomotic vein (or vein of Labbe), that connects with the distal transverse sinus bilaterally.

12.3 Imaging Techniques

12.3.1 Ultrasonography

Although ultrasonography has a limited role in evaluation of the intracranial vasculature, it does have some important applications. Doppler ultrasonography can have a role in imaging the neonatal central nervous system (CNS), such as suggesting the diagnosis of a vein of Galen aneurysmal malformation (VGAM) (▶ Fig. 12.4). Vascular waveform analysis of the

branches of the ACA in neonates may provide an indication of intracranial pressure (see Chapter 5). Transcranial Doppler ultrasonography plays an important role in the follow-up of patients with sickle-cell disease in helping to determine the timing of transfusions; increased flow velocities though the MCA have been shown to be associated with an increased risk of stroke, which decreases with transfusion.

12.3.2 Computed Tomographic Angiography

Computed tomographic angiography requires an iodinated contrast material and ionizing radiation. Images made with this technique are obtained shortly after administration of the contrast material, which remains predominantly within the arterial system. This allows the evaluation of luminal abnormalities, stenosis, and occlusions. There is typically some degree of venous opacification, and allowing a slightly longer lapse after injection of the contrast material allows a more directed computed tomographic venogram. Multiplanar reformattings and three-dimensional (3D) reconstructions can be done, but 3D reconstructions in some projections may be limited by the osseous base of the skull.

12.3.3 Magnetic Resonance Angiography

Magnetic resonance angiography (MRA) is most commonly performed without intravenous contrast material, using a technique known as 3D time of flight. This provides information about flowing blood, but because the acquisition of images with the technique can take several minutes, it is susceptible to artifacts caused by patient motion. Turbulent flow and high-grade stenosis can also create artifacts. Advantages of MRA include the lack of ionizing radiation and excellent depiction of vessels adjacent to, or surrounded by, bone. Contrast-enhanced MRA can be done with less artifact from turbulence or slow flow than imaging without contrast enhancement, but it provides prominent visualization of veins, which can be both a liability and a benefit. Dynamic MRA can be performed during the administration of contrast medium, and constitutes a non-invasive, radiation-free technique that provides some of the dynamic information of conventional catheter angiography, albeit with lower spatial and temporal resolution and without the ability to use vessel-selective injections.

12.3.4 Magnetic Resonance Venography

Techniques exist for evaluating the intracranial venous structures (magnetic resonance venography). These include flow-sensitive non-contrast-enhanced techniques, such as two-dimensional (2D) time-of-flight as well as phase-contrast imaging. Both techniques are susceptible to turbulent flow and

problems with stenosis, and given the slower flow in veins than in arteries, these techniques have more artifacts than MRA. When detailed venous characterization is required, postcontrast magnetic resonance venography provides additional information.

12.3.5 Digital Substraction Angiography

The traditional gold standard for evaluation of the vasculature is digital subtraction angiography (DSA), also known as catheter angiography or conventional angiography. This is an endovascular invasive technique, requires ionizing radiation, will almost always have to be done with sedation in children, and has risks of stroke and other vascular complications. However, the spatial and temporal resolution provided by DSA are unparalleled by any existing noninvasive technique, as is the ability to perform vessel-selective injections. The DSA technique is an excellent adjunct to endovascular therapy; it is typically used only for procedure planning or troubleshooting, and should not be a primary diagnostic tool.

12.3.6 Perfusion Imaging

Perfusion imaging techniques allow evaluation of blood flow to the brain. The most established procedure for investigating cerebral perfusion is a nuclear medicine study that evaluates the distribution of an injected radiotracer substance. This can be done in the evaluation of vascular disorders like moyamoya; in seizure patients, to identify ictal hyperperfusion or interictal hypoperfusion (see Chapter 9); and in the evaluation of cerebral blood flow in the setting of suspected brain death (▶ Fig. 12.5).

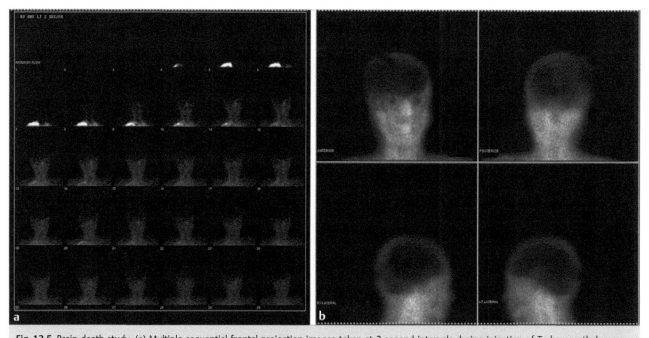

Fig. 12.5 Brain-death study. (a) Multiple sequential frontal-projection images taken at 2 second intervals during injection of Tc-hexamethylpropyleneamineoxime (HMPAO) show no signs of cerebral perfusion in this 11-year-old male status posttraumatic head injury. (b) Multiple planar acquisitions show no accumulation of HMPAO within the cerebral parenchyma, with identification of the soft tissues of the face and scalp. In the appropriate clinical setting, these findings are consistent with brain death.

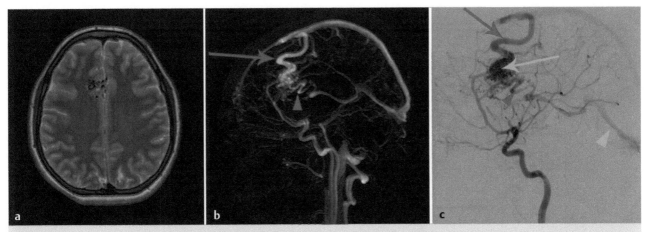

Fig. 12.6 Arteriovenous malformation. (a) Axial T2 W image shows prominent serpentine right-frontal parasagittal flow voids. (b) Sagittal maximum-intensity projection from dynamic contrast-enhanced magnetic resonance angiography shows an enlarged right anterior cerebral artery feeding the nidus. Venous drainage is predominantly through an enlarged vein directed toward the superior sagittal sinus (*red arrow*), with a smaller component extending to the internal cerebral veins (*red arrowhead*). (c) Lateral projection digital subtraction angiogram confirms that drainage from the nidus (*green arrow*) is predominantly superficial (*red arrow*), but with a deep component (*red arrowhead*) that extends to the internal cerebral vein (*blue arrowhead*), vein of Galen (*blue arrow*), and straight sinus (*green arrowhead*).

Recently, additional techniques for investigating cerebral perfusion have been developed. Computed tomographic perfusion imaging has been widely studied in the workup of acute stroke and vasospasm in adults, although the technique is not widely used in the pediatric setting because of differences in the disease processes seen in children and adults, and the high radiation dose required with the technique.

Three separate magnetic resonance imaging (MRI) techniques exist for examining perfusion. Dynamic susceptibility contrast (DSC) MRI uses the T2* effect of high-dose gadolinium during a first-pass injection to estimate blood-flow parameters. This has been used in the evaluation of stroke and other vascular disorders, as well as in characterizing tumors. Dynamic contrast enhancement (DCE) imaging is a dynamic T1-weighted (T1 W) technique most widely used for tumor imaging, in which sequential T1 images are acquired during the administration of a contrast agent. Arterial spin labeling (ASL) is an MRI technique that does not require intravenous contrast enhancement. It has been most widely used in the study of vascular disorders, including acute stroke, atherosclerotic disease, vasospasm, and moyamoya disease, with additional studies done to examine acute attacks of migraine.

12.4 Intracranial Vascular Abnormalities and Sequelae

12.4.1 Arteriovenous Malformations

An arteriovenous malformation (AVM) is a dysplastic "tangle" of vessels through which there is high blood flow and that results in arteriovenous shunting (▶ Fig. 12.6). An AVM can have one or more arterial feeding vessels and one or more draining veins; within its tangle of vessels are low-resistance connections that facilitate shunting. The central portion of the dysplastic vessels in an AVM, where shunting occurs, is called the nidus. There is typically no normal brain parenchyma within the nidus.

Treatment of an AVM can include endovascular obliteration through the injection of liquid embolic agents, surgical excision, and radiosurgery. Many AVMs are treated in a multimodal manner. A scoring system exists to determine the amenability of an AVM to surgical excision, based on the size of the AVM, whether there is deep or superficial drainage, and whether the lesion involves/is adjacent to eloquent areas of the brain (▶ Table 12.1). The lower the score, the more amenable an AVM is to surgical resection. It is important to note that the scoring system is a surgical grading scale and does not directly predict the risk of hemorrhage or stroke. Features of an AVM that increase the risk of hemorrhage include a larger nidus, growth of the nidus over time, stenosis in the venous outflow tract of the AVM, and a venous aneurysm and/or intranidal varix.

An AVM can be identified as an incidental finding, can present in relation to seizures, and at times presents with hemorrhage.

12.4.2 Arteriovenous Fistula

An arteriovenous fistula (AVF) is a lesion that causes arteriovenous shunting. It has a single arterial supply, a single venous drainage, and a single point of contact of the two, wherein there

Table 12.1 Spetzler–Martin scoring system for arteriovenous malformations

Feature of arteriovenous malformation	Scoring
Size of nidus	< 3 cm = 1 point
	3–6 cm = 2 points
	> 6 cm = 3 points
Eloquence of adjacent parenchyma	Eloquent = 1 point
	Noneloquent = 2 points
Venous drainage	Superficial only = 0 points
	Deep drainage = 1 point

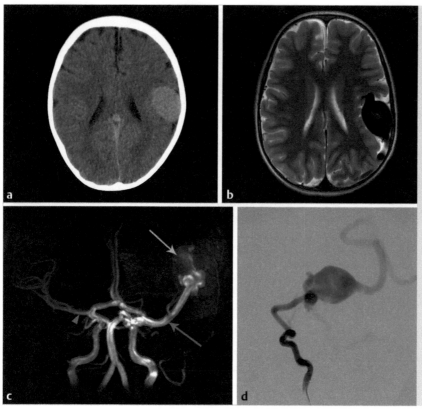

Fig. 12.7 Arteriovenous fistula (AVF). (a) Axial computed tomographic image of the head of a 7-year-old boy shows an ovoid, hyperdense, extra-axial mass without a dural tail, overlying the region of the left inferior parietal lobule. (b) Axial T2 W magnetic resonance image shows a diffuse hypointense appearance of the lesion, representing a large vascular flow void. (c) Frontal-projection maximum-intensity projection from magnetic resonance angiography shows asymmetric enlargement of the left middle cerebral artery (MCA) (*red arrow*) in comparison to the right MCA (*red arrowhead*), and arterialized flow within the fusiform aneurysm (*green arrow*). (d) Lateral-projection digital subtraction angiography shows arterial-phase filling of the venous pouch with subsequent venous drainage, without identification of parenchymal vessels, indicating a "steal" phenomenon. Because a single artery feeds a single draining vein with a "single hole" connection, without an intervening capillary bed or nidus of an arteriovenous malformation, this represents an AVF.

is a fistulous communication. This is sometimes called a "single hole" fistula (▶ Fig. 12.7). Blockage of the fistula, either by surgery, endovascular techniques, or both, is typically curative. Arteriovenous fistulae can also have multiple fistulous connections, which may be more difficult to identify. An AVF can be supplied by extracranial vessels with intracranial venous drainage, in which case it is known as a dural AVF (dAVF).

12.4.3 Aneurysms

Intracranial aneurysms in children are much less common than in adults, and most commonly are seen in the setting of connective tissue disorders and vascular dysplasias, such as neurofibromatosis type 1 and Loewys–Dietz syndrome.[1] Aneurysms are seen with increased frequency in the setting of an AVM or AVF, and include venous aneurysms from increased pressure within the venous system. Patients with sickle-cell disease are also at increased risk for intracranial aneurysms. Patients with systemic infections can have infectious aneurysms (mycotic aneurysms), and dissecting aneurysms (pseudoaneurysms) can follow trauma.

12.4.4 Vein of Galen Aneurysmal Malformation

The vein of Galen aneurysmal malformation (VGAM) is a developmental abnormality resulting in arteriovenous shunting and drainage into venous structures of the posterior midline (▶ Fig. 12.4).[2] Although it is called a VGAM, the veins themselves in this malformation are innocent bystanders; the

abnormality is the shunting lesion that results in an excessive blood flow that dilates the vein of Galen and straight sinus.

There are two subtypes of VGAM, one in which there is an AVM of the choroidal vasculature ("choroidal type"), and the second in which there is an AVF ("mural type"). Choroidal type VGAMs often present in the perinatal period as symptomatic abnormalities from high-output cardiac failure, whereas VGAMs of the mural type may present later in childhood. The mural type of VGAM can have a single fistula or multiple fistulae; the more and larger the fistulae, the earlier the child will become symptomatic.

The choroidal vascular supply to a VGAM can include not only the anterior choroidal arteries but also lesser known posterior choroidal arteries that branch from the PCA and distal ACA. There can also be a blood supply from the distal ACA/pericallosal arteries through persistent posterior superior choroidal arteries, creating what is known as a persistent limbic arch. Although the blood supply to a VGAM can come from the distal ACA, PCA, and anterior choroidal artery (which arises from the internal carotid artery [ICA]), the MCA will be uninvolved.

The shunting caused by a VGAM results in engorgement of the draining veins. In fact, the draining veins may not be the vein of Galen itself, but rather its precursor, the median prosencephalic vein of Markowski, which, because of the excess flow through it, fails to mature into the vein of Galen and straight sinus. Endovascular therapy, typically through the arterial side of a VGAM, has revolutionized the treatment of VGAM, with mortality rates of ~ 40% before the advent of endovascular therapy for this malformation falling to ~ 8% with endovascular therapy, and a normal neurodevelopmental trajectory for a third to half of children in whom this malformation now occurs.

The treatment of VGAM is a balance between decreasing the shunting caused by the malformation and waiting to provide treatment, because treatment of the malformation becomes easier as the affected child grows larger. Planned, staged therapy is the most common approach to treating a VGAM, with guidance on the appropriate timing of treatment based on the Bicêtre criteria,[2] which provide objective means for balancing the risks and benefits of early/emergent intervention and observation with those of delayed planned intervention.

In addressing a VGAM, it is important to be aware that children with this malformation may develop ventriculomegaly and hydrocephalus. The pathophysiology is complex, but in part it is related to increased production of CSF by hypervascular choroid and decreased resorption of CSF because of elevated venous pressures. Placement of a ventriculostomy catheter does not relieve either of these two abnormalities, but the resulting reduction in CSF pressures in the presence of the high venous pressures from a VGAM creates a very high risk of catastrophic hemorrhage. Therefore, a ventriculostomy catheter should never be used to treat hydrocephalus caused by a VGAM; rather, the VGAM itself should be treated, which will bring down venous pressures.

12.4.5 Developmental Venous Anomaly

A developmental venous anomaly (DVA) is, as its name suggests, a variant in venous development in which either the cerebral cortex drains focally to the deep venous system or the white matter drains to the cortical veins (▶ Fig. 12.8). The condition produces a characteristic caput medusa sign, but this is generally an incidental finding. Cavernomas (see below) are often present with a DVA, and may be symptomatic.

12.4.6 Cavernoma

A cavernoma is a dysplastic collection of veins that have a propensity for multiple microhemorrhages. Over time, this results in a peripheral rim of hemosiderin that causes hypointensity on T2W and susceptibility-weighted imaging (SWI) (▶ Fig. 12.8), although centrally there can be heterogeneous areas of hyperintense signal on T1W and T2W imaging. Cavernomas can be sporadic or familial, and patients with these malformations are predisposed to the formation of cavernomas after irradiation (such as for a prior brain tumor). The peripheral rim of hemosiderin in a cavernoma may result in cortical irritation, which can be the instigating factor for a seizure. Cavernomas are often seen in conjunction with a DVA (▶ Fig. 12.8).

12.4.7 Capillary Telangiectasia

A capillary telangiectasia is a tiny network of veins that is typically occult on conventional imaging, may have a hypointense appearance on SWI, and has a very faint blush of postcontrast enhancement (▶ Fig. 12.9). The pons is a common location for

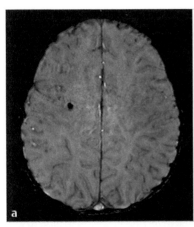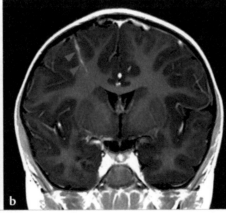

Fig. 12.8 Developmental venous anomaly/cavernoma. (a) Axial susceptibility-weighted image shows a focal area of hypointense signal in the right posterior frontal lobe in a 10-year-old male. (b) Coronal T1W image plus contrast shows a prominent vein extending to the periphery (red arrowheads), consistent with a developmental venous anomaly, with the hypointense area on susceptibility-weighted imaging representing a cavernoma.

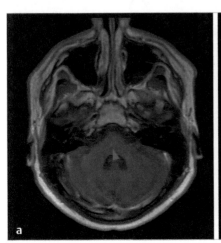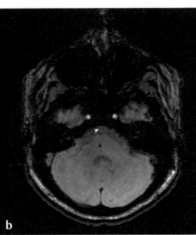

Fig. 12.9 Capillary telangiectasia. (a) Axial T1 plus contrast image of the brainstem in a 15-year-old boy shows a subtle focal blush of postcontrast enhancement (red arrowhead). (b) Axial susceptibility-weighted image shows a punctate area of hypointense signal in this location, which represents a pontine capillary telangiectasia.

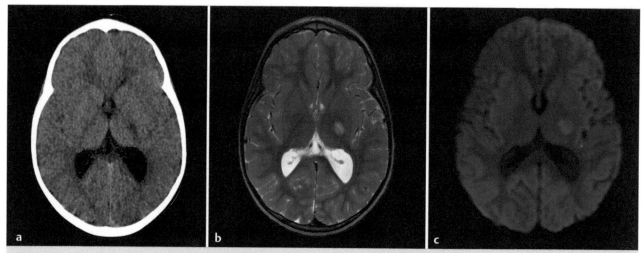

Fig. 12.10 Acute stroke. (a) Axial computed tomographic image of the head of a 3-year-old boy with right hemiparesis of acute onset shows a focal area of hypodensity in the left posterior limb of the internal capsule (PLIC) (*red arrowhead*). (b) Axial T2 W image shows a hyperintense signal in this location, which on (c) DWI was confirmed as restricting diffusion, and which represents an acute stroke. Although there is vascular variability, the PLIC is typically supplied by the anterior choroidal artery.

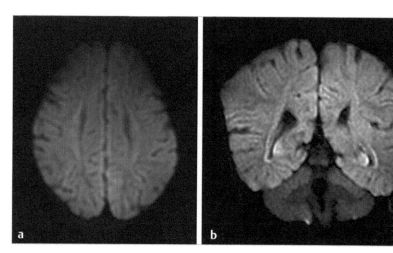

Fig. 12.11 (a) Diffusion-weighted images (DWI) in a 3-month-old girl who sustained posthypoxic injury from cardiac arrest shows a homogeneous appearance between the cerebral hemispheres. (b) Coronal DWI shows diffuse hyperintense signal throughout the supratentorial parenchyma relative to the infratentorial parenchyma, indicating cytotoxic edema throughout both cerebral hemispheres. The axial image represents a "superscan" and demonstrates a potential pitfall of interpreting studies in a purely qualitative manner.

this incidental finding. A capillary telangiectasia may have a pathophysiology similar to that of a small cavernoma.

12.4.8 Acute Stroke

Although atherosclerotic disease is less common in children than in adults, acute stroke can occur in children just as in adults, and diffusion-weighted imaging (DWI) is the gold standard for its rapid diagnosis (▶ Fig. 12.10). Strokes can occur in patients with congenital cardiovascular disease, status post drowning/episodes of near-drowning, trauma (and vascular dissections), vasospasm, moyamoya, and other conditions or experiences. In patients who have undergone resuscitation, in whom there may be global anoxic injury, coronal DWI can be helpful because the cerebellum may be spared, making it easier to detect extensive cerebral injury that may appear bilaterally symmetric on axial DWI ("DWI superscan") (▶ Fig. 12.11).

Hypoperfusion in low-pressure states can result in injury preferentially along the border zone between different vascular territories, a pattern referred to as watershed injury (▶ Fig. 12.12).

12.4.9 Moyamoya

Moyamoya is a constellation of disease processes related to vascular narrowing, with the resultant formation of collateral vessels, most commonly at the carotid terminus (▶ Fig. 12.13). Moyamoya disease is an idiopathic condition most frequent in patients of Japanese descent, whereas moyamoya syndrome is the occurrence of this phenotype either on an acquired basis or with a syndromic association. The name "moyamoya" itself arises from a Japanese word meaning "hazy" or "ethereal," as a description of the angiographic appearance of the collateral vessels in this disease or syndrome. Contrary to a commonly quoted mistranslation, moyamoya does not mean "puff of smoke."

Syndromic associations of moyamoya include neurofibromatosis type 1; trisomy 21, which can be accompanied either by unilateral or bilateral moyamoya or morning glory disc anomaly, in which there can be ipsilateral moyamoya. Patients with hemoglobinopathies, particularly sickle-cell disease, are predisposed to moyamoya. Patients who have

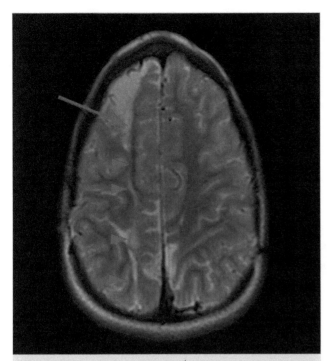

Fig. 12.12 Watershed injury. Axial T2 W image in a 7-year-old boy with sickle-cell disease and moyamoya syndrome shows a band of encephalomalacia (*red arrowheads*) along the border zone of the territories of the right anterior cerebral artery and middle cerebral artery, consistent with sequelae of prior watershed injury.

irradiation of the region of the central skull base, such as those with craniopharyngioma, can develop a radiation-induced moyamoya. Although not reported in children, atherosclerotic moyamoya is common in adults. Moyamoya can occasionally involve the posterior circulation and has rarely been described in the posterior fossa.

The evaluation of moyamoya through imaging involves parenchymal imaging to seek signs of prior stroke (focal vs. watershed) or hemorrhage. More recent work has used multidelay ASL perfusion to evaluate cerebrovascular reserve and possibly identify patients at risk for future stroke.[3] Vascular imaging characterizes the degree of narrowing and extent of collateral-vessel formation in moyamoya. Digital subtraction angiography with selective injections of contrast media can characterize collateral flow, including the presence of endogenous external-to-internal carotid collateral vessels, such as collaterals branching from the middle meningeal artery.

A surgical treatment option for moyamoya includes pial synangiosis, a procedure in which a branch of the superficial temporal artery (STA) is directed intracranially through a bur hole and there is a vascular pedicle that is sewn to the dura. Although the revascularization resulting from this takes several months to mature, it results in the development of multiple anastomoses to the territory of the MCA. This has benefits over a direct STA-to-MCA bypass, which is mature immediately but will not grow and the resultant blood flow is dependent entirely on a single anastomosis.

12.4.10 Vasculitis

Vasculitis is an inflammatory process involving the walls of blood vessels. This is a noninfectious inflammatory process that is more common in patients with connective tissue and/or autoimmune disorders. The diagnosis is often challenging. Digital subtraction angiography is more sensitive to the changes of vasculitis than are MRA or CTA, but may yield a normal result. Occasionally, a brain biopsy is performed to look for signs of vascular inflammation, but even when they are present, they do not necessarily confirm the diagnosis of vasculitis. The parenchymal changes in vasculitis can mimic those in ADEM and other noninfectious inflammatory processes.[4]

12.4.11 Vasospasm

Vasospasm refers to vascular narrowing related to secondary irritation. In adults, the most common reason for cerebral vasospasm is irritation caused by subarachnoid hemorrhage (SAH). Subarachnoid hemorrhage is less common in children than in adults, and the most common cause of vasospasm in children may be meningitis. Many children with meningitis have diffusion abnormalities/strokes in a vascular distribution, presumably from vasospasm in a given vessel. The luminal narrowing in an instance of vasospasm may be difficult to identify on imaging. Treatment typically focuses on treating the underlying infectious process.

Some subtypes of migraine headache may be related to vasospasm, which in turn may be mediated by the autonomic nervous system. Evidence of vasospasm in migraine attacks is based on the finding, through ASL, of perfusion deficits during the symptomatic phase of such attacks that reverse upon treatment.

12.4.12 Dissection

Arterial dissection in the head or spine is most commonly related to trauma. Dissection of the vertebral artery can occur in the V2 segment as the result of vertebral fracture or subluxation, and at the V3–V4 junction (the dural interface) in relation to an acceleration–deceleration injury (including chiropractic manipulation). Vertebral artery dissection can result in thromboembolic events in the posterior circulation.

The most common location for a dissection in the anterior circulation is at the entry of the internal carotid artery into the carotid canal. Intracranial dissections are less common without severe trauma, but can occur with shearing of the ACA along the free edge of the falx cerebri and/or of the PCA along the edge of the tentorium cerebelli. These shearing-related dissections can result in dissecting aneurysms (also known as pseudoaneurysms).

12.4.13 Venous Abnormalities

Venous sinus thrombosis can result from systemic hypercoagulable states, trauma to the involved vessels (including surgical manipulation), extrinsic vascular compression resulting in stasis, and thrombosis secondary to infection. Venous thrombosis

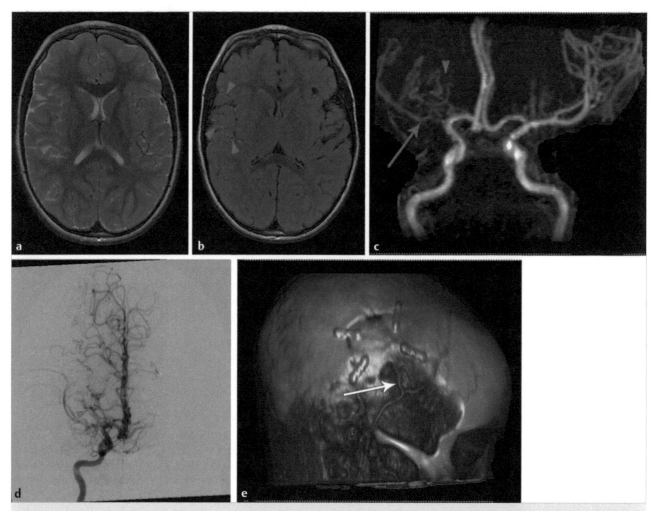

Fig. 12.13 Moyamoya. (a) Axial T2W image in a 6-year-old boy with headaches shows a paucity of middle cerebral arterial flow voids in the right sylvian fissure (*red arrowheads*). (b) Axial fluid-attenuated inversion recovery image shows hyperintense signal in the right branches of the middle cerebral artery (MCA, *red arrowheads*), representing slow flow within these vessels. (c) A frontal maximum intensity projection from magnetic resonance angiography shows a diminuitive M1 segment of right MCA (*red arrow*) with prominent lenticulostriate collaterals (*red arrowhead*). (d) A frontal projection digital subtraction angiogram in the arterial phase after injection of contrast medium into the right internal carotid artery shows an ill-defined network of right lenticulostriate vessels (*red arrowhead*) representing the hazy collaterals of moyamoya. (e) A lateral-projection three-dimensional rendering from a computed tomographic angiogram made after a revascularization procedure shows an enlarged posterior branch of the right superficial temporal artery (*white arrow*), extending toward a bur hole, and providing evidence of a mature pial synangiosis (indirect extracranial–intracranial bypass).

can result in venous infarction, which can often be hemorrhagic (▶ Fig. 12.14). A hemorrhagic venous infarction is one condition in which hemorrhage may be appropriately treated with anticoagulants, but this must be done with caution.

Patients with a high hematocrit related to dehydration or polycythemia rubra vera will have an increased vascular density and on CT will have a high density of the intracranial vasculature. When this is symmetric and involves all visible vessels equally, the increased density is unlikely to represent acute thrombosis.

12.4.14 Pseudotumor Cerebri

Pseudotumor cerebri, sometimes referred to as idiopathic intracranial hypertension, is a condition in which elevated intracranial pressures cause headaches and papilledema, with the papilledema causing blurry vision. It is now known that stenosis in the distal transverse sinuses can result in elevated intracranial venous pressures, which in turn result in elevated CSF pressures. The elevated venous pressures can result in unilateral or bilateral abducens nerve palsies (manifesting as esotropia and/or diplopia with lateral gaze) owing to the circumferential pressure on the abducens nerve as it travels within the cavernous sinus. The chronically elevated CSF pressures and pulsations of pseudotumor cerebri often result in flattening of the pituitary gland ("partial empty sella"), although this can also occur as a normal variant. Additionally, acute venous sinus thrombosis can result in a clinical presentation with features similar to pseudotumor cerebri.

Treatment of exacerbations of pseudotumor cerebri is focused on reducing CSF pressures. This can be achieved through therapeutic lumbar puncture, with the goal of reducing

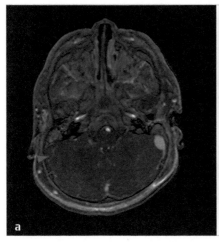 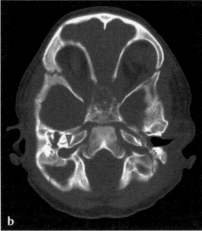

Fig. 12.14 Venous thrombosis (right sigmoid). (a) Axial postcontrast magnetic resonance angiography/venography image of the head of a 17-month-old male with leukemia shows non-filling of the right sigmoid sinus (*arrowhead*), consistent with thrombosis. It is important to differentiate a thrombosed from a congenitally hypoplastic vein. Apart from seeing the outline of the thrombosed vein on magnetic resonance imaging, (b) an axial bone algorithm computed tomographic image shows symmetric jugular foramina (*arrowheads*), indicating the right sigmoid sinus and jugular bulb developed, and the non-filling is not related to a congenitally hypoplastic right sigmoid/jugular system.

CSF pressures to approximately 16 to 20 cm H_2O. Because obesity is a primary risk factor for pseudotumor cerebri, lumbar puncture can be challenging to the inexperienced (or even the experienced) clinician working with an obese patient, and image-guided lumbar puncture may be required under such circumstances. Cerebrospinal fluid pressures can be reduced by fenestration of the optic nerve sheath by a neuro-ophthalmologist, or by neurosurgical shunting. Recent work has shown that stenting of a transverse sinus stenosis can alleviate symptoms of pseudotumor cerebri, but this is still being investigated and has not yet been established for use in children.

References

[1] Aeron G, Abruzzo TA, Jones BV. Clinical and imaging features of intracranial arterial aneurysms in the pediatric population. Radiographics 2012; 32(3): 667–681

[2] Lasjaunias PL, Chng SM, Sachet M, Alvarez H, Rodesch G, Garcia-Monaco R. The management of vein of Galen aneurysmal malformations. Neurosurgery 2006; 59(5) Suppl 3:S184–S194, discussion S3–S13

[3] Choudhri AF, Zaza A, Auschwitz TS, Klimo P, Mossa-Basha M. Noninvasive vascular imaging of moyamoya: Diagnosis, followup, and surgical planning. J Ped Neuroradiol 2014; 3(1):13–20

[4] Abdel Razek AAK, Alvarez H, Bagg S, Refaat S, Castillo M. Imaging spectrum of CNS vasculitis. Radiographics 2014; 34(4):873–894

13 Sella Turcica/Pineal Gland

13.1 Introduction

Both the pituitary gland and pineal gland are small structures that can have a variety of rare normal and abnormal conditions that can be difficult to interpret and diagnostically confusing. Understanding the normal anatomy and embryologic origins of these structures can aid in characterizing the pathologic conditions and physiologic variants they are likely to manifest.

13.2 Anatomy of the Pituitary Gland and Sella Turcica

The pituitary gland is an endocrine organ of dual origin; in fact, it may be easier to consider it as being two separate but adjacent organs. The anterior pituitary (adenohypophysis) is composed of glandular tissue, whereas the posterior pituitary is of neural origin (neurohypophysis). The pituitary sits within the sella turcica, within the central portion of the sphenoid bone (basisphenoid). The pituitary gland is bounded laterally by the cavernous sinuses (▶ Fig. 13.1), and is connected by a stalk (the pituitary stalk, also known as the pituitary infundibulum) to the hypothalamus.

The adenohypophysis arises from an evagination of nasopharyngeal mucosa, known as Rathke's pouch, through the basisphenoid bone within the craniopharyngeal canal. Rarely, there is a persistent craniopharyngeal canal; however, it is common to see the remnants of the obliterated craniopharyngeal canal (▶ Fig. 13.2). The adenohypophysis joins with the neurohypophysis, a caudal extension from the median eminence of the hypothalamus. The adenohypophsyis manufactures and secretes hormones under control by the hypothalamus. The

hypothalamus secretes releasing hormones (▶ Table 13.1) that traverse the hypothalamic–hypophyseal portal venous system within the pituitary stalk. Because of this vascularity, the adenohypophysis shows a rapid and homogeneous enhancement pattern.

13.3 Pituitary Lesions

Hypoenhancement within the pituitary gland raises the possibility of a neoplasm, typically a "microadenoma," although an intraglandular cyst will also appear as a hypoenhancing focus. The two types of intraglandular cyst are an inclusion cyst between the adenohypophysis and neurohypophysis, known as a pars intermedia cyst (▶ Fig. 13.3), and a Rathke's cleft cyst (▶ Fig. 13.4). Both types of cyst are incidental. A pars intermedia cyst is typically not a diagnostic challenge and requires no follow-up or intervention. A Rathke's cleft cyst can sometimes be difficult to differentiate from a cystic neoplasm, and occasionally can be enlarged and exert mass effect that may require surgical intervention.

In one variant appearance of the pituitary gland, it is flattened to the floor of the sella turcica (▶ Fig. 13.5). In the early days of computed tomography (CT) and magnetic resonance imaging (MRI), this was called an empty sella; however, with high-resolution imaging, it is known that the gland is present but flattened, making the term "partially empty sella" more appropriate for the appearance of this condition. This is typically a normal variant of pituitary shape, but is commonly seen in the clinical setting of pseudotumor cerebri, which should therefore be considered a possibility when a partially empty sella is found in an evaluation for headache or palsy associated with cranial nerve VI.

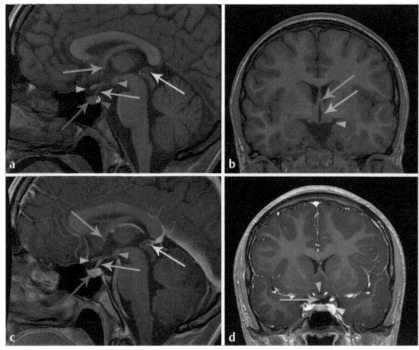

Fig. 13.1 Pituitary anatomy. (a) Sagittal and (b) coronal T1 W images of the pituitary gland show the adenohypophysis (*red arrow*) and neurohypophysis (*red arrowhead*) connected to the hypothalamus by the pituitary stalk (*green arrow*). Above the pituitary is the optic chiasm (*green arrowhead*). Also seen are the mammillary bodies (*blue arrowhead*), anterior commissure (*blue arrow*), and pineal gland (*yellow arrow*). (c) Sagittal and (d) coronal T1 plus contrast image shows normal enhancement of the adenohypophysis. Within the cavernous sinus, the carotid artery is seen (*yellow arrowhead*).

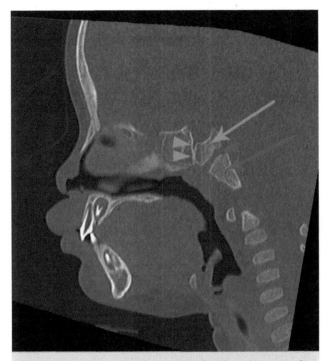

Fig. 13.2 Sagittal bone algorithm computed tomographic image of the sella turcica shows a persistent craniopharyngeal canal (*blue arrowheads*), which is a normal variant but provides insight into adenohypophyseal development. The clivus at this stage of development is in two parts, consisting of the basisphenoid (*blue arrow*), which contains the sella turcica, and the basiocciput (*red arrow*), joined by the spheno-occipital synchondrosis (*red arrowhead*).

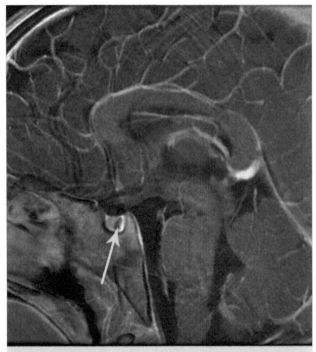

Fig. 13.3 Cyst in the pars intermedia. Sagittal T1 W plus contrast image in a 3-year-old boy shows a circumscribed hypoenhancing area between the adenohypophysis and neurohypophysis (*yellow arrow*), representing a cyst in the pars intermedia.

Primary pituitary tumors are much less common in children than in adults. As in adults, they nearly always arise from the adenohypophysis. Pituitary tumors are referred to as microadenomas (if smaller than 10 mm) and macroadenomas (if larger than 10 mm), but this distinction in size may be less important than determining why a given lesion is symptomatic. A microadenoma will not cause mass effect, and will therefore present only with endocrine abnormalities, such as elevated prolactin levels. Because microadenomas are typically secreting adenomas, their surgical resection optimally requires removal of the entire lesion.

Table 13.1 Hormones secreted by the anterior pituitary

Hormone	Stimulant	Target
Thyroid-stimulating hormone	Thyrotropin-releasing hormone	Thyroid gland
Growth hormone	Growth-hormone–releasing hormone	Viscera (growth)
Follicle-stimulating hormone	Gonadotropin-releasing hormone	Germ-cell maturation
Luteinizing hormone	Gonadotropin-releasing hormone	Triggers ovulation
Adrenocorticotropic hormone	Corticotropin-releasing hormone	Adrenal gland
Prolactin*		Milk production

*Prolactin is normally secreted without stimulation; its secretion is inhibited by dopamine.

Macroadenomas tend to present present with mass effect, most commonly on the optic chiasm, which can cause a bitemporal hemianopsia. An adenoma that reaches the size at which it exerts such an effect will typically be a nonsecreting adenoma, and the goals of its surgical management will primarily be to relieve its mass effect while preserving the function of adjacent structures. A subtotal resection of a nonsecreting macroadenoma may allow it to recur and require repeat surgery at a later date, but would appropriately address the patient's symptoms. In the case of some secreting macroadenomas, however, such as those that secrete growth hormone, a gross-total resection is preferred. Other tumors in the sellar region, particularly craniopharyngiomas, are addressed in Chapter 8.

An enlarged pituitary gland raises the possibility of a pituitary tumor, and in this situation, thin-section pre- and postcontrast imaging of the pituitary gland is warranted. However, this requires determination of what constitutes an enlarged gland. As a rough estimate, a glandular height of up to 6 to 8 mm can be considered normal, but focal irregularity or asymmetry should raise concern even with a smaller gland size. Because of the hormonal changes associated with menarche, a slight physiologic hypertrophy of the pituitary, of up to approximately 9 or 10 mm, can be seen in females during early adolescence (▶ Fig. 13.6). An additional situation in which there is physiologic pituitary glandular hypertrophy is in the newborn child, in whom the pituitary has a convex superior margin related to maternal hormonal stimulation (▶ Fig. 13.7); this typically reverses over the first two weeks of life, and the finding of a

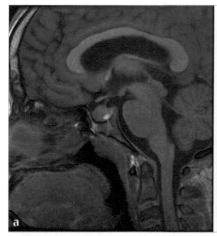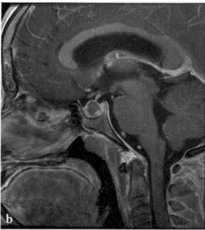

Fig. 13.4 Rathke's cleft cyst. (a) Sagittal T1 W image of the sella turcica in a 14-year-old boy shows enlargement of the pituitary gland, with a convex superior margin of the gland, and a focal area of T1 shortening within the pituitary (*red arrowhead*). (b) Sagittal T1 W plus contrast image shows that the area of T1 shortening is within a circumscribed hypoenhancing lesion, representing a Rathke's cleft cyst.

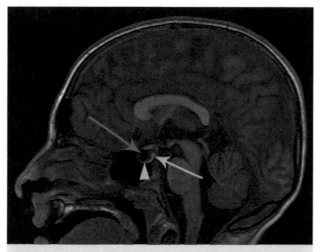

Fig. 13.5 Partially empty sella turcica. Sagittal T1 W image of the head of a 12-year-old boy shows the sella turcica predominantly filled with cerebrospinal fluid (*red arrow*), with a flattened adenohypophysis (*green arrowhead*) and neurohypophysis (*green arrow*) along the sellar floor. This represents a partially empty sella.

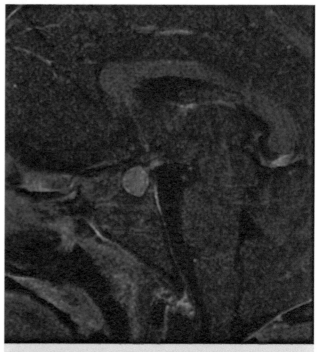

Fig. 13.6 Perimenarchal pituitary hypertrophy. Sagittal T1 W plus contrast image of the head of a 10-year-old girl shows a convex superior margin of the pituitary gland without a discrete intraglandular lesion. The gland measures 9 mm in craniocaudal dimension, and the enlarged size is related to perimenarchal glandular hypertrophy.

suspected pituitary mass in a newborn should therefore be regarded with extreme caution.

13.4 Neurohypophysis

The neurohypophysis, or posterior pituitary, is a completely distinct organ of different origin than the anterior pituitary. The neurohypophysis includes the distal axons of nerve cells that reside in the supraoptic and paraventricular nuclei of the hypothalamus. The bodies of these nerve cells create the peptide hormones vasopressin (antidiuretic hormone) and oxytocin (▶ Table 13.2). These peptide hormones travel along the axons of the cells as they traverse the pituitary infundibulum and are stored in secretory granules in the neurohypophysis while awaiting release. Because vasopressin and oxytocin are peptide hormones, they cause a characteristic T1 shortening seen in the neurohypophysis on precontrast imaging ("posterior pituitary bright spot").

In some instances, the neurohypophysis does not appropriately migrate caudally to the sella turcica during development, and instead is seen along the floor of the third ventricle. This is known as an ectopic neurohypophysis, and the pituitary stalk caudal to the ectopic neurohypophysis will either be absent or hypoplastic. The T1 shortening demonstrated by the ectopic neurohypophysis confirms the presence of posterior pituitary hormones and connection of the neurohypophysis with the hypothalamus, and patients in whom these findings are made typically have normal posterior pituitary function. However, because of their deficient pituitary stalk (and the

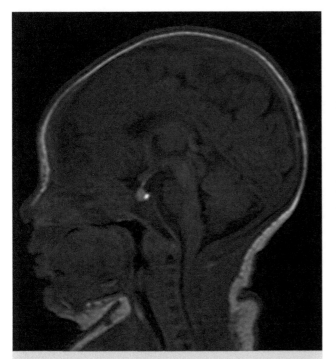

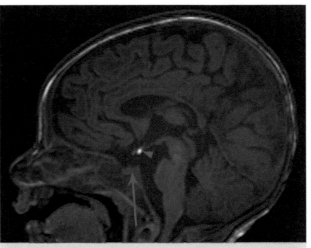

Fig. 13.8 Ectopic neurohypophysis. Sagittal T1 W image of the head of a 2-month-old child with impaired glucose metabolism shows a focus of T1 shortening at the expected location of the infundibular recess of the third ventricle (*red arrowhead*). There is a hypoplastic pituitary stalk, and there is no orthotopic neurohypophysis (*red arrow*), confirming that the focus of T1 shortening represents an ectopic neurohypophysis.

Fig. 13.7 Maternal hormonal stimulation of the pituitary. Sagittal T1 W image of the head of a 3-day-old infant shows a convex superior margin of the pituitary gland related to maternal hormonal stimulation; this typically regresses in the first 2 weeks of life.

maldevelopment of their hypothalamic–hypophyseal portal venous system), they often have adenohypophyseal dysfunction (most commonly growth hormone deficiency). An appropriate understanding of this relationship is important for accurately conveying information about this disorder to the endocrinologist, pediatrician, and the patient/family.

At times an ectopic neurohypophysis can be mistaken for a tumor, such as a germinoma, but the absence of an orthotopic area of neurohypophyseal T1 shortening, and the absence/hypoplasia of the pituitary stalk, provide further insight into the ectopic rather than neoplastic etiology of this finding (▶ Fig. 13.8).

One common indication for pituitary magnetic resonance imaging in children as opposed to adults is the evaluation of short stature. The reason for this evaluation is twofold; (1) to

identify any possible developmental abnormality within the pituitary gland or hypothalamus; and (2) to identify a pituitary tumor, which is a contraindication to growth hormone therapy. Care should be taken to avoid allowing incidental, nonpathologic pituitary lesions to become barriers to such treatment.

13.5 Pineal Gland

The pineal gland, also known as the epithalamus, is a circumventricular organ of diencephalic origin that is located along the posterior aspect of the third ventricle. The pineal gland has a stalk arising from the habenulae of both thalami (▶ Fig. 13.9). The exact function and importance of the pineal gland remain uncertain, but it is known to be related to circadian rhythms through the secretion of the hormone melatonin. The pineal gland in some animals has light-sensing capabilities and can detect the presence of daylight, and before the evolution of high-level visual capability, the gland functioned as a third eye, for which reason it has some embryologic similarities to the retina. These similarities appear to be the reason why children with a genetic predisposition to retinoblastoma may develop a pineal tumor related to retinoblastoma/primitive neuroectodermal tumor. When this occurs in the setting of bilateral retinoblastoma, the condition is referred to as "trilateral" retinoblastoma.

Pineal cysts are commonly encountered in the pediatric population, and can pose dilemmas in diagnosis and management (▶ Fig. 13.9). The chief concern with them is that particularly if large, they may be indicative of a pineal neoplasm. Autopsy studies have shown the presence of microscopic cysts within the pineal gland in the neonatal period, and even in utero.

Table 13.2 Hormones secreted by the posterior pituitary

Hormone	Secretion stimulated by	Target	Effect
Vasopressin (antidiuretic hormone)	Osmolar sensors	Collecting ducts of nephrons Arterioles Platelets	Water retention Vasoconstriction Platelet aggregation
Oxytocin	Hypothalamus	Uterus Mammary glands Other	Uterine contractions Letdown reflex of lactation Social behavior changes

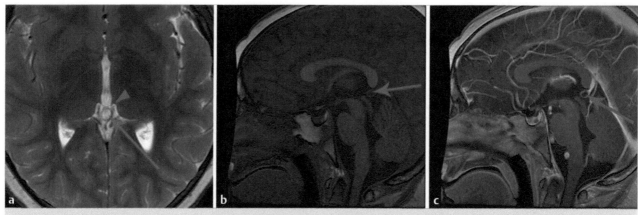

Fig. 13.9 Pineal anatomy. (a) Axial T2 W image of the head of a 7-year-old boy shows the pineal gland attached to the thalami by the habenulae (*arrowhead*). A cyst is seen within the pineal gland (*red arrow*), which is a physiologic finding. Sagittal T1 W image (b) without and (c) with contrast material shows no enhancement within the cyst (*red arrow*) and no mural nodularity, in accord with a physiologic cyst.

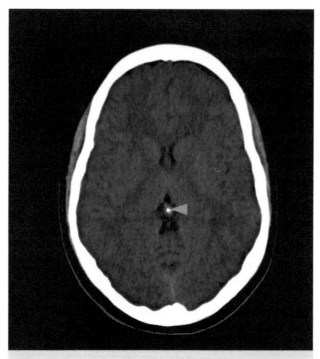

Fig. 13.10 Pineal calcifications. Axial computed tomographic image of the head of a 15-year-old girl shows calcifications within the pineal gland, which represent a physiologic finding after approximately 5 years of age.

Therefore, it is likely that pineal cysts are physiologic, and MRI studies have shown the presence of pineal cysts in more than 50% of children undergoing MRI at 3 teslas.[1] These cysts may have internal proteinaceous contents, evidenced by incomplete signal suppression on fluid-attenuated inversion recovery (FLAIR) images, and may show layering material. A general recommendation for pineal cysts is that those of 5 mm and smaller typically do not require description in a radiologic report. Cysts of 5 to 10 mm can be described in a radiologic report, but typically not in the impression of the report. It is commonly suggested that cysts larger than 10 mm should be described in the impression section of the study report, but follow-up recommendations for such cysts remain unclear. A contrast-enhanced MRI study done at 1 year of follow-up is often recommended for cysts larger than 10 mm, but with uncertain diagnostic yield. Asymptomatic cysts of any size that do not exert mass effect on the brainstem or other structures are likely to be incidental even if in the range of 10 to 15 mm, in the absence of suspicious features. Such features include a focal mural nodule or peripherally splayed calcifications ("exploding calcifications"), both of which raise concern about a neoplasm. When a pineal neoplasm is suspected, sampling of cerebrospinal fluid (CSF) for germ-cell markers is warranted.

During aging, a physiologic calcification occurs in the pineal gland, and by adolescence there is calcification detectable on CT in more than half of individuals (▶ Fig. 13.10). Early reports of findings on CT did not describe physiologic calcifications in persons younger than 6 years of age, suggesting that calcifications in patients younger than this should raise suspicion about a possible calcified pineal neoplasm. However, more recent reports, based on modern CT with thin collimation, have documented calcifications in children as young as 3 years of age.[2,3] Tumors of pineal origin have the potential to peripherally splay pineal calcifications, whereas pineal cysts and tumors of nonpineal origin will push on pineal calcifications without causing splaying (▶ Fig. 13.11).

When a pineal mass is encountered, diffusion-weighted imaging (DWI) can aid in differentiating tumors of pineal origin from germ-cell tumors, because the former tend to have lower apparent diffusion coefficient (ADC) values.[4,5] Exact prediction of the histologic characteristics of a pineal mass is difficult in the absence of other features, such as macroscopic fat suggesting a teratoma (▶ Fig. 13.12), or a new mass in a patient with known retinoblastoma. It is also important to be aware that germ-cell tumors of the pineal region show a strong (approximately 14:1) male predominance.

Tumors of pineal origin in children are more often high-grade lesions (pineoblastoma) than they are in adults (▶ Fig. 13.13). The treatment of tumors of pineal origin is typically maximal cytoreductive surgery. Because pineal germinomas respond

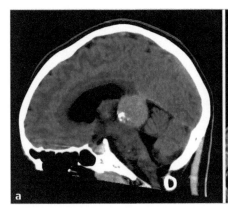
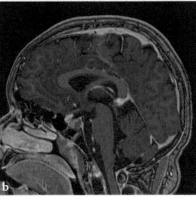

Fig. 13.11 Germinoma. (a) Sagittal computed tomographic image of the head of an 11-year-old boy shows a mass in the pineal region with a focal area of calcification within the anterior aspect of the lesion. Biopsy showed this to be a germinoma, and (b) a sagittal T1 W plus contrast image made 4 months after the image in (a) shows significant involution of the lesion due to radiation therapy.

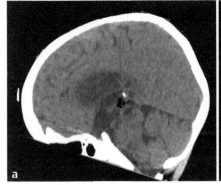
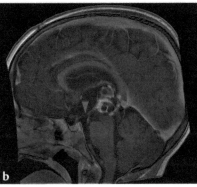

Fig. 13.12 Pineal teratoma. (a) Sagittal computed tomographic image of the head of a 4-year-old boy shows a heterogeneous mass in the pineal region with a focal area of calcification (*red arrow*) and other areas with fat density (*red arrowhead*). (b) Sagittal T1 W plus contrast image shows a heterogeneous multicystic lesion, and also a defect in the floor of the third ventricle due to prior endoscopic third ventriculostomy (*red arrowhead*). This represents a teratoma.

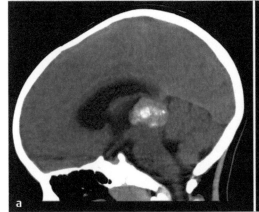
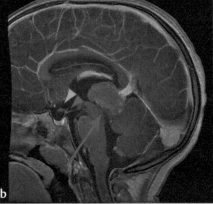
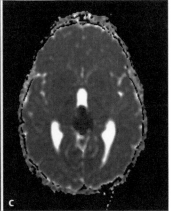

Fig. 13.13 Pineoblastoma. (a) Sagittal computed tomographic image of the head of a 3-year-old girl shows a large mass in the pineal region with heterogeneous internal calcifications. (b) Sagittal T1 W plus contrast image shows mild enhancement within the lesion, which effaces the sylvian aqueduct (*red arrow*), causing splaying of the chiasmatic and infundibular recesses of the third ventricle (*green and red arrowheads*, respectively). (c) Axial apparent diffusion coefficient (ADC) map indicates a hypointense appearance, with an ADC value of approximately 475×10^{-6} mm²/sec for this lesion, which was shown to represent a pineoblastoma.

well to nonsurgical adjunctive therapy, their diagnosis usually leads to radiation therapy rather than surgical resection. The diagnosis of germinoma may be based on the results of biopsy or suggested by an analysis of germ-cell markers in CSF. Pineal teratomas are treated with surgical resection, and when fully resected may not require adjunctive therapy.

When a pineal tumor of uncertain origin is encountered in a child, a biopsy may be performed to help determine an appropriate treatment algorithm. At the time of the biopsy, an endoscopic third ventriculostomy may be performed to either mitigate or prevent hydrocephalus caused by the tumor's effacing the sylvian aqueduct.

References

[1] Whitehead MT, Oh CC, Choudhri AF. Incidental pineal cysts in children who undergo 3-T MRI. Pediatr Radiol 2013; 43(12):1577–1583

[2] Zimmerman RA, Bilaniuk LT. Age-related incidence of pineal calcification detected by computed tomography. Radiology 1982; 142(3): 659–662

[3] Whitehead MT, Oh CC, Raju AD, Choudhri AF. Physiologic pineal region and choroid plexus calcifications in the first decade of life. Am J Neuroradiol 2015; 36(3):575–580

[4] Dumrongpisutikul N, Intrapiromkul J, Yousem DM. Distinguishing between germinomas and pineal cell tumors on MR imaging. AJNR Am J Neuroradiol 2012; 33(3):550–555

[5] Choudhri AF, Whitehead MT, Siddiqui A, Klimo P Jr, Boop FA. Diffusion characteristics of pediatric pineal tumors. Neuroradiol J 2015; 28(2):209–216

14 Metabolic Disorders

14.1 Introduction

Metabolic disorders are relatively rare conditions, but collectively and in most large pediatric centers are fairly frequent considerations in differential diagnosis. Findings on clinical examination and imaging are characteristic for some of these disorders, but are more nonspecific for most others. Familiarity with the key clinical and imaging features of different metabolic disorders, and with various imaging techniques, can aid in narrowing the differential diagnoses for these conditions (▶ Table 14.1). Because many of the conditions have a genetic basis, there may be regional predominances of otherwise rare metabolic disorders of which one should be aware in a given practice environment. Certain metabolic disorders with characteristic features are included in many multiple-choice examinations, even if the disorders themselves are rare. Ultimately, although this chapter provides appropriate familiarity with the basic aspects of metabolic disorders from the viewpoint of the role of imaging techniques and findings in their diagnosis and treatment, a more exhaustive reference source may be warranted when encountering cases of metabolic disorders on a clinical basis.

The number and variety of metabolic disorders and leukodystrophies are worthy of a book of their own, particularly because each of the entities can have highly varied clinical and imaging presentations. This chapter cannot therefore be exhaustive, and references are provided to additional sources of information about the etiologies and features of various metabolic disorders; however, it is hoped that this chapter provides the appropriate framework for seeking additional information when needed. Close communication with the clinical specialty groups that manage patients with metabolic disorders, including neurologists, geneticists, and other specialists, is often required to maximize the yield of diagnostic information about these disorders in the patients whom they affect. However, it is critical to recognize that even at tertiary care centers, barely half of all inborn errors of metabolism/leukodystrophies ever receive a specific diagnosis.

14.2 Terminology

Understanding the terminology for describing and characterizing metabolic disorders is important. A leukoencephalopathy is a pathophysiologic process affecting white matter (leuko) and can be of a wide variety of genetic or acquired etiologies. A poliodystrophy (not to be confused with poliomyelitis) is a condition that preferentially affects gray matter. A pandystrophy is one that affects both gray and white matter.[1]

A demyelinating disorder is a process in which there is injury or abnormality to neurons that are already myelinated. Demyelinating conditions related to noninfectious, immune-mediated inflammatory processes are discussed in Chapter 10.

A dysmyelinating condition is one in which there is abnormality in the process of myelination itself.

An inborn error of metabolism is one in which there is a defect in a metabolic pathway that results in the impaired creation of a particular substrate, or results in the impaired clearance and subsequent accumulation of a toxic substance, or both. Disorders resulting from such errors can take the form of organic acidemias, amino acidemias, or lysosomal or peroxisomal storage disorders.

A mitochondrial disorder is an abnormality that affects the function of the respiratory chain in mitochondria and results in the impared energy production within cells. Because of the greater metabolic demands of gray than of white matter, mitochondrial disorders tend to predominantly affect gray matter.

14.3 Imaging Tools

Magnetic resonance imaging (MRI) is the primary imaging technique used in evaluating metabolic disorders, although computed tomography (CT) may be the first modality used in an acute setting and is also helpful in confirming the presence of calcification. A technique that can be particularly helpful in evaluating suspected metabolic disorders is magnetic resonance (MR) spectroscopy. This technique resembles the nuclear magnetic resonance (NMR) spectroscopy used in organic chemistry (and perhaps is the only time in a medical career organic chemistry actually comes into play!). Magnetic resonance spectroscopy exists in the forms of single-voxel and multivoxel MR spectroscopy. Single-voxel spectroscopy provides high-resolution spectra from a single anatomic area, whereas multivoxel spectroscopy provides lower-resolution spectra from a larger area. Multivoxel spectroscopy is more helpful in tumor imaging and biopsy planning, and single-voxel spectroscopy is more important in the evaluation of metabolic disorders. Spectroscopy can also be performed with short (~ 35 msec), medium (~ 144 msec), and long (~ 288 msec) echo times (▶ Fig. 14.1), which refer to the durations of the pulses of resonant electromagnetic radiation used to refocus the spin magnetization of atomic nuclei within a chemical substance.

The three main metabolites identified on MR spectroscopy of the brain are choline (at 3.2 ppm), creatine (at 3.0 ppm), and *N*-acetyl aspartate (NAA) (at 2.0 ppm). Choline, an organic cation, is present in cell membranes in the form of phosphatidylcholine and sphingomyelin, and is present in elevated concentrations in proliferative tumors. Creatine is related to energy metabolism, and NAA is a marker of neuronal integrity. At birth, the concentration of NAA in the brain is low, after which it increases over the first 6 months to 1 year of age. Eventually, there is a progressive increase in height of the peaks of the MR spectra for choline, creatine, and NAA, leading to an increased angle of ascent of a straight line connecting these peaks, an angle known as Hunter's angle. Additional metabolic peaks of which to be aware include that of lactate, seen as a double peak at 1.33 ppm, and myoinositol (myoI), seen as a single peak at 3.55 ppm. Detailed evaluation of spectra of additional metabolites requires a highly calibrated MR system and is beyond the scope of this chapter. Magnetic resonance spectra can also be obtained with voxels centered in the deep gray nuclei and the deep white matter (either frontal or parieto-occipital) (▶ Fig. 14.1).

Table 14.1 Summary of major metabolic disorders

Disease	Major imaging features	Important points
Maple syrup urine disease	Myelinic edema in myelinated white matter. Especially around the PLIC and extending into the brainstem in newborns, more extensive distribution later in life. Magnetic resonance spectroscopy shows a peak at 1.9 ppm for the BCAAs (as well as lactate at 1.3 ppm)	Impaired metabolism of BCAAs. Toxic metabolites injure myelin. Brain changes may resolve with dietary restriction of BCAAs, acute episodes of neurologic dysfunction occur if diet not followed.
Canavan disease	Macrocephalic, nonenhancing, elevated peak for NAA	Macrocephlic dysmyelinating leukoencephalopathy, deficiency of aminoacylase-2
Alexander's disease	Macrocephalic, enhancing, no peak for NAA	Macrocephalic dysmyelinating leukoencephalopathy
X-linked adrenoleukodystrophy	Splenium involved, confluent posterior to anterior progression	Inability to metabolize long-chain fatty acids
MLD	Sparing of U fibers, tigroid T2 signal, enhancement of cranial nerves/cauda equina	Dysmyelinating lysosomal storage disorder affecting children < 2 years old; urine tests for arylsulftase can have false-negative results
Pelizaeus–Merzbacher disease	Tigroid pattern, connatal form with arrested/absent myelination	Leukodystrophy with arrested myelin development; X-linked; presents within 2 years
Nonketotic hyperglycinemia	Restricted diffusion, glycine peak on MRS at 3.56 ppm	Elevated glycine present in plasma and urine
Glutaric aciduria type 1	Macrocephaly, hypoplastic frontoparietal operculum, arachnoid cysts	Resembles NAT (subdural hematomas), elevated lysine, hydroxylysine, and tryptophan
L-2-Hydroxyglutaric aciduria	Centripital and anterior-posterior gradient abnormality, involvement of dentate nuclei	Propensity for intracranial neoplasms, dentate nucleus involvement differentiates from other disorders
Menkes syndrome	Tortuous vessels, subdural hematomas, frontotemporal white matter	Can resemble nonaccidental trauma; kinked hair on examination, copper deficiency, X-linked transmission
Krabbe disease	Spares subcortical U fibers until late in the disease, dense thalami on CT, cauda equina/optic nerve enhancement	Globoid-cell leukodystrophy, giant cells, three clinical stages of disease, with seizures and eventual vegetative state
Fahr disease	Symmetric calcifications in deep gray nuclei	Movement disorders and psychiatric symptoms in teenage patients
Mucopolysaccharidoses	Multiple enlarged perivascular spaces, retinal abnormalities	Many subtypes, including Hunter syndrome, Hurler syndrome, and Sanfilippo syndrome; increased urinary excretion of dermatan and heparan sulfate, except in Morquio syndrome
Leigh disease	Restricted diffusion in deep gray matter; presence of lactate on MRS	Slowly progressive, leading to respiratory failure, refractory seizures; rate of progression correlates with age of onset
Zellwegger syndrome	Germinolytic cysts, arrested myelination, polymicrogyria and pachygyria; also affects liver and kidneys	Elevated concentrations of long-chain fatty acids in plasma, intrahepatic biliary dysgenesis, polycystic renal disease, jaundice, death within first year of life.
MELAS	Cortical/peripheral restricted diffusion	Mitochondrial disease, onset age 2–11 years
Wilson disease	Panda sign (substantia nigra and red nuclei are surrounded by T2 hyperintense signaling within the rest of the mesencephalon) (lentiform T2 signal)	Abnormal copper metabolism, dystonia, liver dysfunction, psychosis
Neuronal ceroid lipofuscinosis	Nonspecific features on imaging	Four types based on age of onset: type 1 (6 months –2 years), type 2 (2–4 years), type 3 (5–8 years), type 4 (adolescence to young adulthood)
Carbon monoxide	T2 hyperintense signal of globi pallidi	Clinical history of carbon monoxide poisoning may not be apparent

BCAAs = branched-chain amino acids; CT = computed tomography; MELAS = mitochondrial encephalopathy, lactic acidosis, and strokelike episodes; MLD = metachromatic leukodystrophy; MRS = magnetic resonance spectroscopy; NAA = N-acetyl aspartate; NAT = nonaccidental trauma; PLIC = posterior limb of internal capsule.

14.4 Patterns of Involvement

Differential diagnoses including metabolic disorders can be narrowed by evaluating the patterns of involvement of the central nervous system (CNS) (▶ Table 14.2). Although a given case of such a disorder may appear challenging, breaking down the findings according to sites and types of involvement can clarify its diagnosis and management, and allow a more intelligent interpretation than is possible with a random and haphazard approach. ▶ Table 14.3 lists the features that should be evaluated for the diagnosis of leukodystrophic disorders.

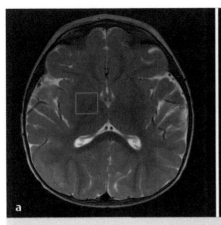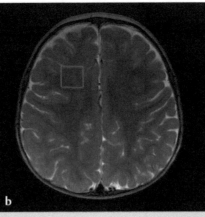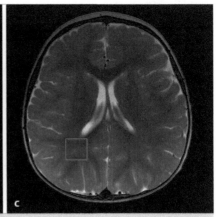

Fig. 14.1 Voxel placement. Three axial T2 W images showing potential locations for voxel placement for single-voxel magnetic resonance spectroscopy, including (a) a voxel in the right lentiform nucleus, (b) the right frontal white matter, and (c) the parietal white matter. Surrounding saturation bands must be located so as to null the signal from adjacent structures, in particular the calvarium, which has an abundance of lipid signal related to bone marrow within the diploic space.

Table 14.2 Imaging features and location of abnormalities in metabolic disorders

Central white matter predominant
Metachromatic leukodystrophy
X-linked adrenoleukodystrophy
Vanishing white matter disease
Neuronal ceroid lipofuscinosis
Phenylketonuria
Nonketotic hyperglycinemia
Gray and white matter abnormality (pandystrophy)
Canavan disease
Alexander's disease
Krabbe disease
Maple syrup urine disease
Leigh disease
Urea-cycle disorders
Glutaric aciduria
Anterior predominant
Alexander's disease
L-2-Hydroxyglutaric aciduria
Posterior predominant
X-linked adrenoleukodystrophy
Mucopolysaccharidoses
Enhancement
Krabbe disease (cranial nerves, cauda equina)
Metachromatic leukodystrophy (cranial nerves, cauda equina)
X-linked adrenoleukodystrophy
Alexander's disease
Restricted diffusion
Leigh disease
Mitochondrial disorders
Maple syrup urine disease
Canavan disease
Metachromatic leukodystrophy
X-linked adrenoleukodystrophy
Nonketotic hyperglycinemia

14.5 Metabolic Disorder—Specific Entities

14.5.1 Maple Syrup Urine Disease

Maple syrup urine disease (MSUD) is a disorder in which there is impaired metabolism of branched-chain amino acids (BCAAs; leucine, isoleucine, and valine) (▶ Fig. 14.2). The inability to metabolize BCAAs results in a buildup of neurotoxic metabolites, with injury to myelin and myelinic edema. Myelinic edema results from the trapping of water within the layers of myelin, markedly restricting diffusion across myelin and producing very low ADC values. Myelinic edema is one of the scenarios in which restricted diffusion does not necessarily mean stroke or cytotoxic edema.[2] Because myelinic edema must involve myelinated areas, an MRI of an infant with MSUD in the early postnatal period will show restricted diffusion corresponding with early areas of myelination, such as the posterior lentiform nucleus, ventrolateral thalamus, and posterior limb of the internal capsule (▶ Fig. 14.2). The myelinic edema in MSUD is treated and prevented with a specialized diet designed to avoid consumption of the BCAAs that cause this edema.[2,3]

14.5.2 Canavan Disease

Canavan disease is a macrocephalic dysmyelinating leukoencephalopathy of childhood related to a deficiency of the enzyme aminoacylase-2, the gene for which is located on chromosome 17, and whose deficiency causes the degeneration of myelin phospholipids. The disease presents with a diffuse T2 hyperintense signal in white matter of the anterior and posterior portions of the brain and posterior fossa, as well involvement of subcortical U fibers (▶ Fig. 14.3).[2,3] There is no abnormal postcontrast enhancement in Canavan disease. Markedly elevated levels of N-acetyl aspartate (NAA) are the characteristic feature of the disease on MR spectroscopy. Care is required in the evaluation of MR spectra in newborns with suspected Canavan disease because of the normally very low level of NAA in the newborn setting and because in a case of Canavan disease there will

Table 14.3 Analysis of features found on imaging for diagnosis of suspected leukodystrophies

Feature	Consideration
Symmetry	Does the abnormality involve both cerebral hemispheres relatively equally?
Anterior vs. posterior	Are the findings more pronounced anteriorly (frontal lobes), posteriorly (parietal lobes), globally, or in a somewhat random pattern?
Contiguous or discontiguous involvement	Are there multifocal areas of discontiguous involvement, or are the abnormalities confluent?
Gray matter, white matter, or both	Does the abnormality predominate in the gray matter, white matter, or both?
Subcortical U-fiber involvement	If the abnormality predominates in the white matter, is there involvement of the subcortical U fibers, or are these spared?
Diffusion	Is there reduced water diffusion or facilitated diffusion in the areas of signal abnormality?
Enhancement	Is there postcontrast enhancement, and if so, is there a specific pattern of enhancement?*
Cerebellar vs. cerebral	Is the cerebellum involved, are the cerebral hemispheres involved, or are both involved?
Macrocephaly vs. microcephaly	Does the patient have a large head, or small head, or is the child normocephalic?
Age of onset	At what age did the patient present (shortly after birth, or later in childhood)?
Progression	Has the abnormality progressed over sequential studies?
Delayed milestones vs. loss of milestones	If the patient does not have age-appropriate milestones, is this because of delayed milestones, or has the patient lost milestones that were previously present?

*See ▶ Fig. 14.4.

not have been a sufficiently long period for NAA to accumulate, yielding only mildly elevated peaks of NAA on MR spectroscopy. The elevated NAA levels in a newborn with Canavan disease result in peaks lower than a normal NAA peak in adulthood.

14.5.3 Alexander's Disease

Alexander's disease is a macrocephalic dysmyelinating leukoencephalopathy with a frontal predominance, and may show postcontrast enhancement.[2,3] The disease is related to a mutation in the glial fibrillary acidic protein (GFAP) gene on chromosome 17 and has an autosomal dominant pattern of inheritance. Brainstem involvement may precede supratentorial involvement in the juvenile/early adult-onset form of the disease. In contrast to Canavan disease (the other primary diagnostic consideration in the case of a macrocephalic dysmyelinating condition), there is no elevation of the NAA peak on spectroscopy in Alexander's disease.

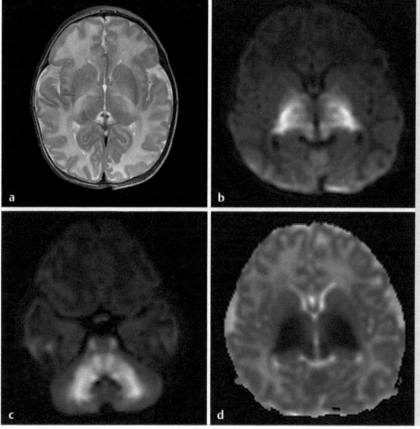

Fig. 14.2 Maple syrup urine disease (MSUD). (a) Axial T2 W image of the head of a 12-day-old boy with lethargy and abnormal muscle tone shows a hyperintense signal in the posterior limb of the internal capsule, posterior lentiform nucleus, and ventral posterolateral nucleus of the thalamus, corresponding to the expected areas of early myelination in the brain. (b) An axial diffusion-weighted image shows hyperintense signal in these areas, as well as (c) within the brainstem and cerebellum. (d) An axial apparent diffusion coefficient map shows a very hypo-intense appearance corresponding to the areas of hyperintense diffusion signal in (a), confirming profound diffusion restriction related to myelinic edema in this patient with MSUD.

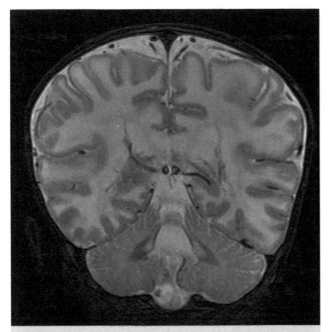

Fig. 14.3 Canavan disease. Coronal T2 W image of the head of an 18-month-old girl with developmental delay and macrocephaly shows a diffuse hyperintense appearance of the cerebral white matter in Canavan disease.

14.5.4 X-linked Adrenoleukodystrophy

X-linked adrenoleukodystrophy (X-ALD) is a congenital dysmyelinating condition whose inheritance pattern results in its being identified in young males (▶ Fig. 14.4).[2,3] The demyelination in the disease begins posteriorly, including characteristic involvement of the splenium of the corpus callosum, and has contiguous involvement as it extends anteriorly during disease progression. When the disease extends far enough anteriorly, it will commonly involve the anterior commissure.

There are three different zones of involvement in X-ALD, with the leading edges of areas of active myelin injury appearing as nonenhancing areas of T2 prolongation, seen anteriorly. Posterior to the leading edge of active myelin injury is a rim in which the degree of injury results in loss of integrity of the blood–brain barrier, with resulting postcontrast enhancement. Posterior to this are areas of nonenhancing gliosis. X-linked adrenoleukodystrophy results from the inability to metabolize very long–chain fatty acids, and treatment of the disease centers on a diet that avoids these fatty acids. The 1992 movie *Lorenzo's Oil* is based on the true story of a child with X-ALD.

14.5.5 Metachromatic Leukodystrophy

Metachromatic leukodystrophy (MLD) is a dysmyelinating lysosomal strorage disorder that typically presents between the first and second year of life (▶ Fig. 14.5).[2,3] The condition results in a deficiency of the enzyme arylsulfatase A. Urine tests for arylsulfatase A are noninvasive, relatively inexpensive, and a helpful diagnostic modality in patients with suspected MLD, but can occasionally yield false-negative results. The appearance of MLD on imaging is centered in the periventricular white matter and spares the subcortical U fibers. Horizontally oriented T2-weighted (T2W) striations may be seen and are described as a tigroid pattern. Postcontrast enhancement may be seen, including enhancement of cranial nerves and enhancement within the cauda equina.

14.5.6 Pelizaeus–Merzbacher Disease

Pelizaeus–Merzbacher disease is a leukodystrophy in which myelin development is arrested.[2,3] The disease can produce a diffuse T2 hyperintense signal abnormality in the cerebral white matter, which can have a tigroid pattern similar to that in MLD. There will be a loss of volume of cerebral white matter and resulting prominence of the sulci. The brainstem and cerebellum can be involved.

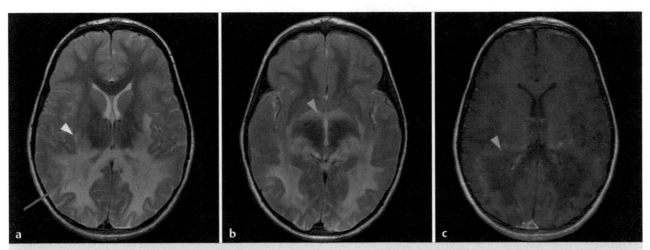

Fig. 14.4 X-linked adrenoleukodystrophy. (a) Axial T2 W image of the head of a 5-year-old boy shows a predominantly posterior area of T2-hyperintense signal (*red arrow*), which includes the splenium of the corpus callosum (*red arrowhead*) and extends anteriorly in the subinsular white matter (*white arrowhead*). (b) Axial T2 W image at a lower level shows a slightly expansile area of T2 hyperintense signal extending across the anterior commissure (*blue arrowhead*). (c) Axial T1 W plus contrast image shows a rim of enhancement along the periphery of the lesion, corresponding to areas of active inflammation with breakdown of the blood–brain barrier (*blue arrowhead*).

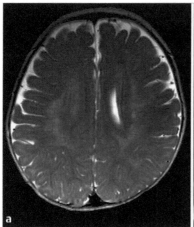
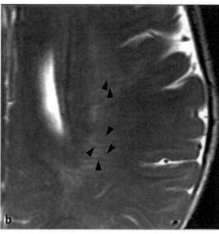

Fig. 14.5 Metachromatic leukodystrophy (MLD). (a) Axial T2W image of the head of an 8-month-old girl with developmental delay shows a hyperintense appearance of the cerebral white matter, with relative sparing of the juxtacortical white matter. (b) Magnified view shows horizontally oriented striations (*black arrowheads*) representing areas of spared involvement (tigroid pattern) in this patient with MLD.

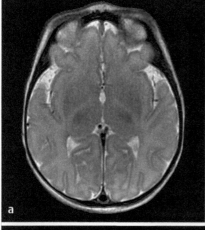
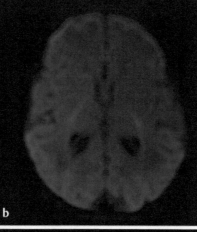
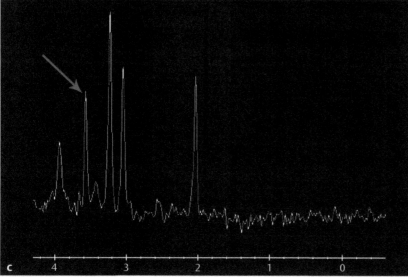

Fig. 14.6 Nonketotic hyperglycinemia. (a) Axial T2W image of the head of a 4-day-old infant with encephalopathy shows a nonexpansile hyperintense signal within the posterior limb of the internal capsule. (b) Axial DWI shows a hyperintense signal in the posterior limb of the internal capsule. (c) Single-voxel magnetic resonance spectroscopy of the right deep gray nuclei at an echo time of 144 msec shows an elevated peak at approximately 3.5 ppm (*red arrow*), corresponding to glycine accumulation in nonketotic hyperglycinemia.

14.5.7 Nonketotic Hyperglycinemia

Nonketotic hyperglycinemia is an autosomal recessive disorder in which the metabolism of glycine is impaired (▶ Fig. 14.6).[4,5,6] Excess glycine accumulates within the central nervous system (CNS) and is also detectable in the plasma and urine. The neurotoxic high levels of glycine result in restricted water diffusion in areas of myelination, particularly the posterior limb of the internal capsule. Magnetic resonance spectroscopy in nonketotic hyperglycinemia can show an increased peak for glycine at approximately 3.55 ppm, but this must be evaluated at long echo times to confidently make the diagnosis, because at short echo times the peak for glycine overlaps that for myoinositol.

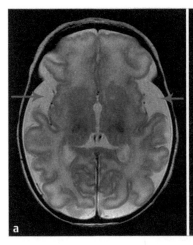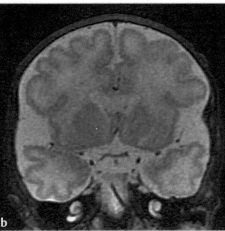

Fig. 14.7 Glutaric aciduria type 1 (GA-1). (a) Axial T2W image of the head of an 8-day-old girl with an abnormal result on neonatal metabolic screening shows widened sylvian fissures (*red arrows*) with uncovering of the insula. (b) A coronal short tau inversion recovery image shows that the widening of the sylvian fissures is related to underdevelopment of the frontal operculum in this patient with GA-1.

14.5.8 Glutaric Aciduria Type 1

Glutaric aciduria type 1 (GA-1) is a metabolic disorder that stems from impaired breakdown of the amino acids lysine, hydroxylysine, and tryptophan. The characteristic features of GA-1 on imaging are macrocephaly and underdevelopment of the frontoparietal opercula, with resulting prominence of the sylvian fissures and uncovering of the insula (▶ Fig. 14.7).[7] Individuals with GA-1 also are prone to developing multiple intracranial arachnoid cysts, including intraventricular cysts. In the setting of macrocephaly, patients with GA-1 can develop subdural hematomas, possibly at variable ages, and GA-1 is a consideration in the differential diagnosis of suspected abusive head trauma.

14.5.9 Menkes Syndrome

Menkes syndrome is an X-linked recessive disorder of copper transport that results in copper deficiency.[2,3] A characteristic manifestation of this disorder is a coarsened appearance to the hair, including colorless or steel-colored hair with a brittle, "kinked" texture, for which reason the syndrome is sometimes referred to as "Menkes kinky hair disease." Patients with Menkes syndrome are predisposed to develop subdural hematomas, and along with GA-1, Menkes syndrome is a consideration in the differential diagnosis for multiple subdural hematomas and suspected abusive head trauma, although it can typically be excluded by evaluation of hair on physical examination.

14.5.10 Krabbe Disease

Krabbe disease, also known as globoid cell leukodystrophy, is a leukodystrophy related to a dysfunction in sphingolipid metabolism.[2,3] The dysfunction is caused by a deficiency in the enzyme galactosylceramidase, which is encoded by the *GALC* gene on chromosome 14. On MRI, Krabbe disease is marked by a diffuse T2 hyperintense signal involving the periventricular white matter, and which spares the subcortical U fibers until late involvement with the disease. Computed tomography may show increased density within the deep gray nuclei, especially the thalami, and the cerebellum. There is no associated postcontrast enhancement. The onset of Krabbe disease is

typically within the first 2 years of life, but there is a late-onset form of the disease.

14.5.11 Fahr Disease

Fahr disease is a congenital disorder that can result in dystrophic calcification in the deep gray nuclei, as well as in the cerebral white matter and cortex, and within the cerebellum. The pattern of calcification is variable, but is typically symmetric within a given patient.[2,3,8] Although Fahr disease most commonly occurs in adulthood, it can present in adolescence.

14.5.12 Mucopolysaccharidoses

The mucopolysaccharidoses (MPS) are a group of metabolic disorders caused by the dysfunction or absence the lysosomal enzymes that are required to catalyze the breakdown of the carbohydrate substances known as glycosaminoglycans, which are important in the synthesis of bone, skin, connective tissue, and the cornea, among other structures. Mucopolysaccharidoses can have varied effects, but the presence of multiple prominent Virchow–Robin spaces should raise suspicion for a disorder belonging to this group of diseases.[9,10] The mucopolysaccharidoses have been grouped into different subtypes on the basis of their clinical features, and more recently according to their molecular and genetic features. Hurler syndrome is a subtype of mucopolysaccharidosis type I (MPS-I), which causes brain atrophy with resultant ventriculomegaly and produces signal abnormalities on MRI. The imaging findings in other subtypes of MPS are highly variable.

14.5.13 Leigh Disease

Leigh disease, also known as subacute necrotizing encephalomyelopathy, is a neurodegenerative disorder resulting from mitochondrial dysfunction and has variable genetic etiologies and imaging patterns, but is progressive and eventually fatal (▶ Fig. 14.8).[2,3] Different forms of Leigh disease have different inheritance patterns, including some mutations in mitochondrial DNA. Imaging abnormalities in Leigh disease will typically be bilateral, and include areas of restricted diffusion and

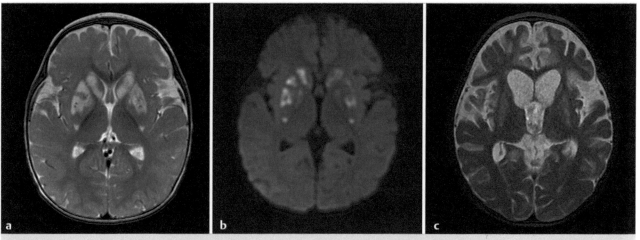

Fig. 14.8 Leigh disease. (a) Axial T2 W image of the head of an 8-month-old child female with developmental delay shows a symmetric, patchy, T2 hyperintense appearance of the putamen, caudate, and globi palladi. (b) Axial diffusion-weighted image (DWI) shows multifocal areas of reduced water diffusion. (c) Axial single-shot T2 W image made 1 year after the axial DWI in (b) shows marked volume loss, which is most pronounced in the areas that were previously abnormal. This represents Leigh disease.

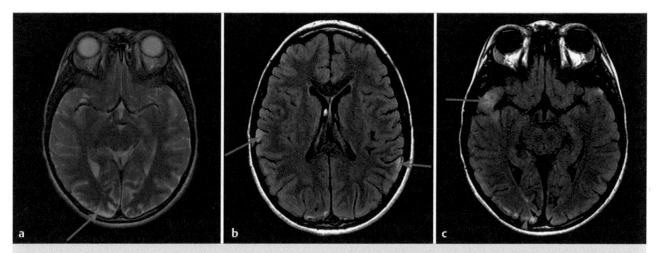

Fig. 14.9 Mitochondrial encephalopathy, lactic acidosis, and strokelike episodes (MELAS). (a) Axial T2 W image of the head of an 8-year-old boy with a history of seizures shows right occipital volume loss (*red arrow*). (b,c) Axial fluid-attenuated inversion recovery images show multifocal areas of hyperintense signal (*red arrows*), representing cortical edema from ongoing seizure activity/metabolic abnormality, and also show a hyperintense signal in the right occipital pole (*red arrowhead*), corresponding to gliosis from prior injury. This is related to MELAS.

associated hyperintense signaling on T2 W imaging and a hypo-dense appearance on CT. Areas of involvement eventually result in necrosis and volume loss.

14.5.14 Zellweger Syndrome

Zellweger syndrome is a peroxisomal disorder with dysfunction of the CNS, liver, and kidneys, also known as cerebrohepatore-nal syndrome. Patients with this condition may have hypomye-lination of the cerebral white matter (T2 prolongation) with associated ventriculomegaly with prominent periventricular germinolytic cysts.[11] The syndrome includes malformations of cortical development, including perisylvian-predominant poly-microgyria and perirolandic pachygyria.[12]

14.5.15 Mitochondrial Encephalopathy, Lactic Acidosis, and Stroke-like Episodes

Mitochondrial encephalopathy, lactic acidosis, and stroke-like episodes (MELAS) is a mitochondrial disorder (▶ Fig. 14.9) with a maternal (mitochondrial) inheritance pattern. It is marked by a multiphasic course of occasional flare-ups with intermittent times of quiescence. The areas involved during exacerbations may recover fully, partially, or not at all. The flare-ups are characterized by stroke-like episodes that occur in a nonvascular pattern. Patients will be encephalopathic, may have seizures, and will have lactate accumulation within the blood and CSF. Severe involvement can result in dementia. The condition has variable penetrance, based on the percentage of mitochondria with abnormal DNA. In acute flare-ups, the cerebral gyri are swollen and show T2 hyperintensity and and may show post-contrast enhancement. As in most mitochondrial disorders, MELAS preferentially involves gray matter (cortex), although subcortical white matter may also be involved. During acute flare-ups, there may be a hyperintense signal on diffusion-weighted imaging (DWI), but there is typically no reduction in the apparent diffusion coefficient (ADC). A reduced ADC in this setting would indicate cytotoxic edema, reflecting an actual stroke as opposed to a "stroke-like" condition.

14.5.16 Wilson Disease

Wilson disease is an autosomal recessive disorder of copper metabolism that involves the lentiform nuclei and liver, and is therefore also known as hepatolenticular degeneration. Patients with Wilson disease will have dystonia, symptoms resembling those of Parkinsonism, cerebellar dysfunction, and psychiatric abnormalities. Computed tomography will typically not show any appreciable abnormality, but MRI will show a T2 hyperintense signal within the lentiform nucleus. Within the midbrain in Wilson disease is an appearance known as a "panda sign," in which the substantia nigra and red nuclei are surrounded by T2 hyperintense signaling within the rest of the mesencephalon.

14.5.17 Neuronal Ceroid Lipofuscinosis

Neuronal ceroid lipofuscinosis (NCL) is a set of related lysosomal storage disorders with neurodegenerative effects and variable genetic etiologies and clinical presentations (▶ Fig. 14.10). The different forms of NCL each have typical ages of onset and may be more common in certain geographic regions than in others. It is worth noting that the four originally described subtypes of NCL, which are also the most commonly encountered, were classified according to their age of onset, with type I (infantile NCL) having an onset in the first 2 years of life, type II (late infantile NCL) having an onset between 2 and 4 years of age, type III (juvenile NCL, or Batten disease) having an onset between ages 4 and 8 years, and type IV (adult NCL) having its onset in adolescence or early adulthood. Neuronal ceroid lipofuscinosis is marked by an abnormal accumulation of lipofuscin, which can be neurotoxic. Historically, NCL has been associated with a hypointense appearance of the thalami on T2 W imaging, but this may not be a reliable sign of the disease. Instead, on imaging NCL will have nonspecific features of a neurodegenerative disorder (parenchymal volume loss) and the diagnosis will be made on clinical and/or genetic grounds.

14.5.18 L-2-Hydroxyglutaric Aciduria

L-2-Hydroxyglutaric aciduria is an organic acidopathy and leukoencephalopathy that predisposes to the development of cerebral neoplasms, often consisting of high-grade tumors, such as anaplastic astrocytoma, glioblastoma, and primitive neuroectodermal tumors.[13,14,15,16] If, therefore, L-2-hydroxyglutaric aciduria is known or suspected, the patient should be closely scrutinized to detect possible neoplasms, perhaps with the use of advanced imaging techniques.[17] The imaging features of L-2-hydroxyglutaric aciduria are a T2 hyperintense signal with a

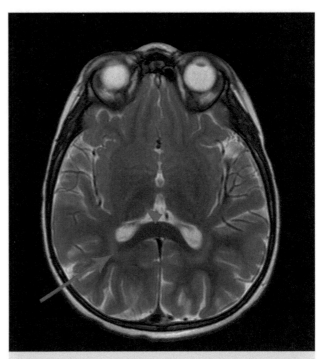

Fig. 14.10 Neuronal ceroid lipofuscinosis (NCL). Axial T2 W image of the head of a 3-year-old boy with seizures and profound developmental delay shows diminished volume of the thalami (*red arrowhead*) and hypomyelination in the periatrial white matter (*red arrow*). Although these findings on imaging were nonspecific, genetic analysis confirmed a diagnosis of NCL.

centripetal and anteroposterior gradient, with symmetric involvement of the globi palladi, caudate nucleus, and putamen. Additionally, there is involvement of the dentate nuclei bilaterally, which is a characteristic feature that alerts to the possibility of L-2-hydroxyglutaric aciduria and should prompt confirmatory laboratory tests. The dentate involvement, as well as involvement of the caudate nucleus and putamen, can help differentiate this disease from Canavan disease.

14.6 Acquired Metabolic Disorders

Although not commonly included in discussions of metabolic disorders in children, acquired metabolic findings are far more common than congenital lesions and inborn errors of metabolism. Familiarity with these entities will allow the prospective identification of processes that may have not been clinically suspected.

14.6.1 Carbon Monoxide Inhalation

Carbon monoxide inhalation will result in edema (hypointense appearance on CT, hyperintense signal on T2/fluid-attenuated inversion recovery [FLAIR]) and diffusion restriction in the globi palladi.[18] This finding is often isolated to the globi palladi, and it is therefore important to avoid describing it as a signal abnormality of the basal ganglia. Abnormalities elsewhere in the basal ganglia should lead to consideration of other conditions.[19]

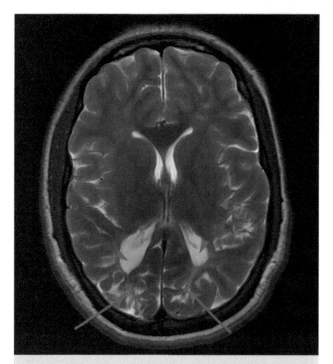

Fig. 14.11 Hypoglycemia. Axial T2 W image of the head of an adolescent shows bilateral occipital volume loss, with cortical thinning and loss of white-matter volume (*red arrows*) with resultant ex-vacuo prominence of the occipital horns of the lateral ventricles (*red arrowheads*), in a pattern consistent with sequelae of perinatal hypoglycemia.

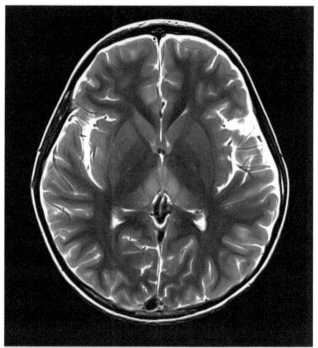

Fig. 14.12 Wernicke's disease. Axial T2 W image of the head of a 5-year-old child with a history of a brain tumor and with ataxia after prolonged parenteral nutritional support shows a symmetric hyper-intense signal abnormality in both thalami. This was confirmed to be Wernicke's encephalopathy related to a thiamine deficiency caused by the patient's parenteral nutrition regimen.

14.6.2 Hypoglycemia

Severe perinatal hypoglycemia shows a characteristically predominant involvement of the occipital lobes, which may result in edema and potentially diffusion abnormalities. (▶ Fig. 14.11).[20] Imaging of affected children later in life will show encephalomalacia in these regions.

14.6.3 Wernicke's Disease

Thiamine deficiency can result in a metabolic encephalopathy that on imaging manifests as a T2/FLAIR signal hyperintensity in the medial thalami, periaqueductal gray matter, and mammillary bodies (▶ Fig. 14.12). The deficiency is potentially treatable through the administration of thiamine (which should be given before glucose). Although thiamine deficiency disease is much more common in adults (in particular those who are malnourished and/or have alcoholism), it can occur in children. Given the nominal costs and risks of thiamine administration, it should be considered as a treatment possibility in any patient with unexplained bilateral thalamic abnormalities.

14.6.4 Medication-Related Metabolic Disorders

Myelinic edema in the globi palladi, hypothalami, and central tegmental tracts of the brainstem can be seen after administration of the antiepileptic medication vigabatrin. Recognizing this association is important so as to: (1) avoid mistaking this edema for an inborn error of metabolism or ischemic injury; and (2) alerting the neurologist to this finding so that the neurologist can assess whether vigabatrin is resulting in toxicity that requires reducing its dose or stopping its use (see Chapter 9).

14.6.5 Osmotic Myelinolysis

Rapid changes in serum osmolality, typically caused by the aggressive correction of hyponatremia or hypernatremia, can cause osmotic injury to myelin. The area most susceptible to this is the central pons ("pontine myelinolysis"); however, the supratentorial deep gray nuclei may also be involved ("extrapontine myelinolysis"). The signal abnormality in osmotic myelinolysis should be relatively symmetric areas that are minimally expansile to nonexpansile, nonenhancing, without diffusion restriction (likely facilitated diffusion). The clinical history is critical to making and/or confirming the diagnosis of osmotic myelinolysis.

14.6.6 Senescent Mineralization

Senescent mineralization in the globi palladi is commonly encountered in adult neuroradiology, with a subtle high density within the globi palladi. This finding is always abnormal in children and warrants evaluation for a metabolic disorder, such as Fahr disease, or for signs of prior stroke or infection. Calcifications of deep gray nuclei that are not located within the globi palladi are always pathologic at any age.

14.7 Suggested Reading

[1] Yang E, Prabhu SP. Imaging manifestations of the leukodystrophies, inherited disorders of white matter. Radiol Clin North Am 2014; 52(2):279–319

References

[1] Patay Z. Metabolic disorders. In: Tortori-Donati P, Rossi A eds. Pediatric Neuroradiology—Brain, Head, Neck, and Spine. New York, NY: Springer; 2005: 543–721

[2] Patay Z. Diffusion-weighted MR imaging in leukodystrophies. Eur Radiol 2005; 15(11):2284–2303

[3] Smith AB, Smirniotopoulos JG, Rushing EJ. From the archives of the AFIP: Central nervous system infections associated with human immunodeficiency virus infection: Radiologic–pathologic correlation. Radiographics 2008; 28 (7):2033–2058

[4] Khong P-L, Lam BCC, Chung BHY, Wong K-Y, Ooi G-C. Diffusion-weighted MR imaging in neonatal nonketotic hyperglycinemia. AJNR Am J Neuroradiol 2003; 24(6):1181–1183[Internet]

[5] Viola A, Chabrol B, Nicoli F, Confort-Gouny S, Viout P, Cozzone PJ. Magnetic resonance spectroscopy study of glycine pathways in nonketotic hyperglycinemia. Pediatr Res 2002; 52(2):292–300

[6] Mourmans J, Majoie CBLM, Barth PG, Duran M, Akkerman EM, Poll-The BT. Sequential MR imaging changes in nonketotic hyperglycinemia. AJNR Am J Neuroradiol 2006; 27(1):208–211

[7] Nunes J, Loureiro S, Carvalho S et al. Brain MRI findings as an important diagnostic clue in glutaric aciduria type 1. Neuroradiol J 2013; 26(2):155–161

[8] Lincoln CM, Bello JA, Lui YW. Decoding the deep gray: A review of the anatomy, function, and imaging patterns affecting the basal ganglia. Neurographics 2012;2(3):92–-102

[9] Kwee RM, Kwee TC. Virchow–Robin spaces at MR imaging. Radiographics 2007; 27(4):1071–1086

[10] Zafeiriou DI, Batzios SP. Brain and spinal MR imaging findings in mucopolysaccharidoses: A review. AJNR Am J Neuroradiol 2013; 34(1):5–13

[11] Unay B, Kendirli T, Ataç K, Gül D, Akin R, Gökçay E. Caudothalamic groove cysts in Zellweger syndrome. Clin Dysmorphol 2005; 14(3):165–167

[12] Stutterd CA, Leventer RJ. Polymicrogyria: A common and heterogeneous malformation of cortical development. In: Mirzaa GM, Paciorkowski AR (eds). Am J Med Genet C Semin Med Genet. 2014 May 28;166(2):227–239

[13] Patay Z, Mills JC, Löbel U, Lambert A, Sablauer A, Ellison DW. Cerebral neoplasms in L-2 hydroxyglutaric aciduria: 3 new cases and meta-analysis of literature data. AJNR Am J Neuroradiol 2012; 33(5):940–943

[14] Barbot C, Fineza I, Diogo L et al. L-2-Hydroxyglutaric aciduria: Clinical, biochemical and magnetic resonance imaging in six Portuguese pediatric patients. Brain Dev 1997; 19(4):268–273

[15] Steenweg ME, Salomons GS, Yapici Z et al. L-2-Hydroxyglutaric aciduria: Pattern of MR imaging abnormalities in 56 patients. Radiology 2009; 251(3): 856–865

[16] Steenweg ME, Jakobs C, Errami A et al. An overview of L-2-hydroxyglutarate dehydrogenase gene (L2HGDH) variants: A genotype–phenotype study. Hum Mutat 2010; 31(4):380–390

[17] Patay Z, Orr BA, Shulkin BL et al. Successive distinct high-grade gliomas in L-2-hydroxyglutaric aciduria. J Inherit Metab Dis 2015; 38(2):273–277

[18] Beppu T. The role of MR imaging in assessment of brain damage from carbon monoxide poisoning: A review of the literature. AJNR Am J Neuroradiol 2014; 35(4):625–631

[19] Ho VB, Fitz CR, Chuang SH, Geyer CA. Bilateral basal ganglia lesions: pediatric differential considerations. Radiographics 1993; 13(2):269–292

[20] Ma J-H, Kim Y-J, Yoo W-J et al. MR imaging of hypoglycemic encephalopathy: Lesion distribution and prognosis prediction by diffusion-weighted imaging. Neuroradiology 2009; 51(10):641–649

15 Skull and Scalp

15.1 Introduction

The brain is a critical organ for survival. Protection of the brain from physical injury is primarily provided by its osseous and soft tissue coverings, including the meninges, the skull, and the overlying soft tissues of the scalp. Developmental and acquired abnormalities of the skull and scalp can occur throughout childhood. Many of these abnormalities are not commonly encountered in adults, and many radiologists and clinicians may not be familiar with them.

15.2 Normal Skull

The skull and skull base arise from multiple bones, each of which has several parts. These bones are divided between the neurocranium, which consists of the:
- Ethmoid bone (cribriform plate)
- Frontal bone
- Occipital bone
- Parietal bone
- Sphenoid bone
- Temporal bone (petrous and squamous parts)

and the viscerocranium, which consists of the:
- Ethmoid bone
- Hyoid bone
- Inferior nasal concha
- Lacrimal bone
- Sphenoid bone (pterygoid process)
- Temporal bone
- Vomer
- Mandible
- Maxilla
- Nasal bone
- Palatine bone

Note that some of the bones named above are divided between the neurocranium and viscerocranium (e.g., the ethmoid bone is mainly in the viscerocranium, the sphenoid bone is mostly in the neurocranium, and the temporal bone is equally present in the neurocranium and viscerocranium). The embryology and development of the skull are important for the correct identification of pathologic conditions, and also for avoiding the diagnosis of a normal developmental pattern as pathologic.[1,2,3,4,5]

Understanding the anatomy of the developing skull may be easier when starting from knowledge of the mature skull (▶ Fig. 15.1). Early in life, the sutures between the bones of the skull are unfused (▶ Fig. 15.2), and typically mature in a symmetric pattern with a general order but some degree of variability. Three-dimensional (3D) computed tomographic reconstructions can greatly aid in understanding the anatomy of the skull, but familiarity with its anatomy in two-dimensional (2D) computed tomographic images (as well as on radiography) aids in detecting abnormalities.

Because the skull originates without a prominent diploic space, it appears on computed tomography (CT) as a single cortical layer at birth (▶ Fig. 6.9). As the skull matures, the diploic

space matures and a separate and distinct cortex develops for the inner cortex and another for the outer table, with trabeculae and marrow-containing spaces developing throughout the diploic space. The newborn skull is more susceptible to fracture than is the skull at later ages, partly because it is thin but also because it consists of a single layer of bone. The formation of two separate layers of cortical bone separated by an intervening trabeculated diploic space is more important than the increased thickness of the skull in providing improved stability as the skull grows. The support provided by the trabeculated diploic space is similar to the support provided by the central core in a sheet of corrugated cardboard, which is stronger than an equally thick layer of paper. Because of its susceptibility to fractures, close attention must be given to the newborn skull even in cases of seemingly minor trauma, and any fractures that do occur can be very difficult to detect without an understanding of the normal pediatric cranial anatomy.

Within the first 3 to 6 months of life, the metopic suture between the two frontal bones closes, and eventually, within the first 2 years, the anterior fontanelle disappears. The sagittal suture closes at a variable time, typically after 2 years of age. The remaining sutures have a somewhat variable pattern, but if the head is of normal circumference and shape, the maturation pattern of the sutures is likely to be normal.

15.3 Craniosynostosis

Early or abnormal closure of any cranial suture is referred to as craniosynostosis and can result in an abnormality of head shape (▶ Fig. 15.3).[6,7] The most common craniosynostosis is premature closure of the sagittal suture (sagittal craniosynostosis), which impairs widening of the skull and results in a compensatorily increased anteroposterior (AP) dimension of the skull. This calvarial configuration is known as scaphocephaly (also known as dolichocephaly) (▶ Fig. 15.4). If a case of scaphocephaly is symptomatic, surgery can be done to provide the cranial vault with the ability to expand. Expansion can both improve cosmesis and prevent elevated intracranial pressures. Isolated sagittal craniosynostosis is typically considered a sporadic finding; craniosynostosis of any other suture, alone or in conjunction with sagittal craniosynostosis, warrants a genetic evaluation.

Premature closure of the metopic suture gives the frontal bone a keel-like appearance known as trigonocephaly (▶ Fig. 15.5).[8] By itself, and in the absence of associated clinical signs of dysmorphism, the appearance of mild trigonocephaly on imaging can be a normal variant. Craniosynostosis of the coronal or lambdoid sutures can be unilateral or bilateral. Unilateral lambdoid craniosynostosis can result in asymmetric parieto-occipital flattening. Plagiocephaly, or flattening of one side of the head, can be related to pressure on that side, typically due to an affected child's always sleeping on that side, and the differentiation of positional plagiocephaly from an abnormality in skull shape caused by craniosynostosis is a common indication for skull radiography or CT in early childhood. In positional plagiocephaly, which is far more common than unilateral lambdoid craniosynostosis, there will be a normal suture-maturation pattern (▶ Fig. 15.6). Bilateral craniosynostosis of the coronal sutures

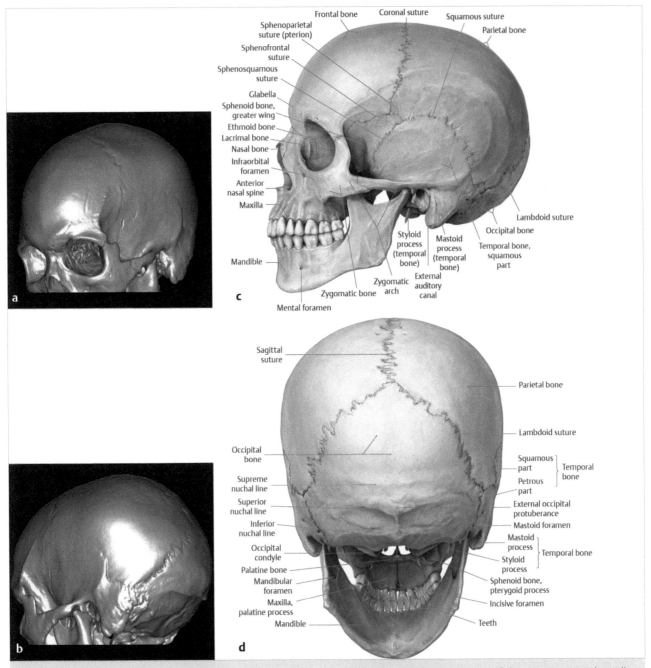

Fig. 15.1 (a,b) Mature normal skull. In this 17-year-old, the sutures have matured, and no visible remnant is seen of the metopic suture, the midline occipital fissure, or the mendosal fissures. (c) Artist's depiction of the skull in lateral projection, showing the bones and sutures of the skull and face. (d) Artist's depiction of the skull from a posterior projection, showing the relationship of the parietal bones and occipital bone. Parts "c" and "d" from Atlas of Anatomy, © Thieme 2012, Illustration by Karl Wesker.

is often associated with craniofacial syndromes like Apert syndrome and Crouzon syndrome, both of which are related to mutations in the *FGFR2* gene. The bilateral craniosynostosis in both syndromes prevents skull growth in the AP dimension, resulting in a skull of brachycephalic shape (▶ Fig. 15.7). Craniofacial syndromes and the *FGFR* gene are discussed in greater detail in Chapter 18.

The developing skull can normally have intrasutural ossicles (also known as wormian bones), most commonly in the lambdoid suture (▶ Fig. 15.8), and their presence has been detected with increased frequency through high-resolution CT scanning. An excess of intrasutural ossicles raises the possibility of a metabolic bone disorder, such as osteogenesis imperfecta (▶ Fig. 15.9).[9] Other abnormalities of the pediatric skull related to systemic and/or metabolic bone disorders include persistence of the metopic suture in patients with supernumerary teeth and absence of the clavicle in cleidocranial dysostosis.

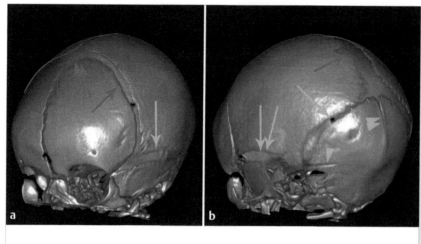

Fig. 15.2 Normal skull of a newborn. Three-dimensional (3D) reformattings of a computed tomographic scan of the skull (a) of a 1-day-old female shows a typical newborn suture pattern, with a patent metopic suture (*red arrowhead*), which meets the coronal sutures (*red arrow*) at the anterior fontanelle (*double red arrow*). Extending posteriorly between the parietal bone and squamosal temporal bone is the squamosal suture (*green arrow*). (b) Posterior 3D projection shows the squamosal suture (*double green arrows*). The sagittal suture extends posteriorly (*red arrow*) to meet the lambdoid sutures (*green arrow*). The midline occipital fissure is seen extending inferiorly from the junction of the sagittal and lambdoid sutures (*double green arrowhead*). The mendosal fissure (*green arrow-head*) extends from the lateral aspect of the occipital bone, separating the supraoccipital and interparietal portions of the occipital bone.

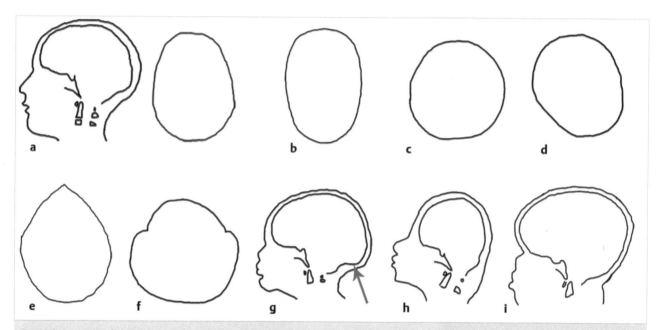

Fig. 15.3 Summary of abnormalities of head shape. (a) Normal shape of head (for comparison). (b) Scaphocephaly/dolichocephaly, with anteroposterior (AP) dimension of head exceeding transverse dimension (look for possible sagittal craniosynostosis on axial images). Sagittal craniosynostosis is typically sporadic. (c) Brachycephaly, with AP dimension of head approximately equal to transverse dimension; best seen on axial images (look for possible coronal craniosynostosis, can be a non-pathologic finding in some individuals). (d) Plagiocephaly, or flattening of the skull. This is typically best seen on axial images. When present in the parieto-occipital region in the absence of craniosynostosis, plagiocephaly is likely to be an effect of head positioning. The primary differential consideration for unilateral parieto-occipital positional plagiocephaly is unilateral lambdoid craniosynostosis. (e) Trigonocephaly, with a frontal keel due to craniosynostosis of the metopic suture, seen on axial images and typically diagnosed in the first few months of life because the metopic suture usually will close by approximately 6 months of age. (f) Kleeblattschädel, or "cloverleaf" skull, may have bilateral coronal and lambdoid craniosynostosis. Kleeblattschädel is best seen on axial images and in three-dimensional reconstructions, and is often associated with multiple additional osseous and CNS abnormalities. (g) Bathrocephaly, with focal prominence of the occipital region. This is best seen on sagittal images and may be sporadic. (h) Turricephaly, with a very tall skull ("towering" appearance). This is best seen on sagittal images. Bilateral coronal or bilateral lambdoid craniosynostosis should be sought in patients with turricephaly. (i) Frontal bossing. Protrusion of the frontal bone beyond the orbits and nasal bridge. This is best seen on sagittal images. It can be seen in skeletal dysplasias, and particularly in achondroplasia because of the midface hypoplasia in this condition.

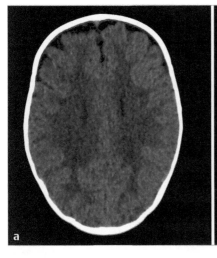
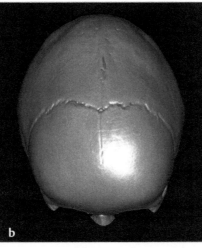

Fig. 15.4 Sagittal synostosis. (a) Axial computed tomographic image shows that the anteroposterior dimension of the skull is much larger than the transverse dimension, representing scaphocephaly. (b) Three-dimensional computed tomographic image of the head of an 8-month-old boy with scaphocephaly and early closure of the anterior fontanelle shows that the sagittal suture is fused, representing sagittal suture craniosynostosis.

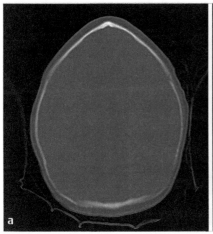
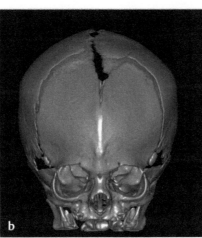

Fig. 15.5 Trigonocephaly. (a) Axial bone algorithm computed tomographic image of the head of a 1-day-old female with an irregularity of forehead contour shows midline fusion of the frontal bones with an angulated appearance, representing trigonocephaly in the setting of metopic craniosynostosis. (b) Three-dimensional computed tomographic rendering shows trigonocephaly with closure of the inferior half of the metopic suture.

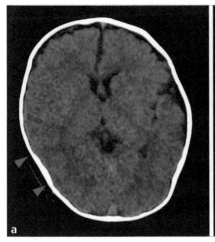
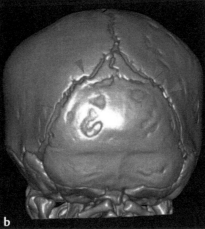

Fig. 15.6 Plagiocephaly. (a) Axial computed tomographic image of the head of a 2-month-old female made for evaluation of a head shape abnormality shows right parieto-occipital flattening (*red arrowheads*). (b) Posterior-projection three-dimensional computed tomographic image of the patient's skull shows patency of the lambdoid sutures (*red arrowheads*), indicating that the abnormality in head shape is related to positional plagiocephaly and not to unilateral lambdoid craniosynostosis.

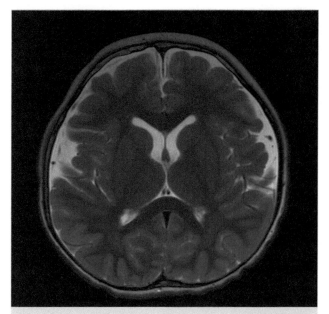

Fig. 15.7 Brachycephaly. Axial T2W image in a 4-year-old patient with seizures and microcephaly shows that the anteroposterior dimension of the skull is approximately equal to the transverse dimension, yielding the somewhat round appearance known as brachycephaly.

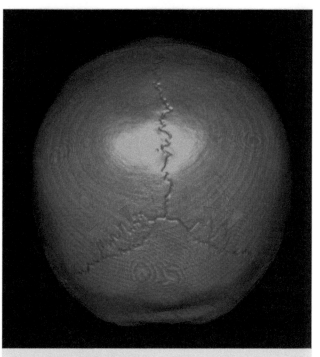

Fig. 15.8 Intrasuture ossicles. Three-dimensional rendering of the head of a 3-year-old boy shows several intrasuture ossicles (*red arrowheads*) in the superior portion of the lambdoid suture bilaterally, representing a normal variant.

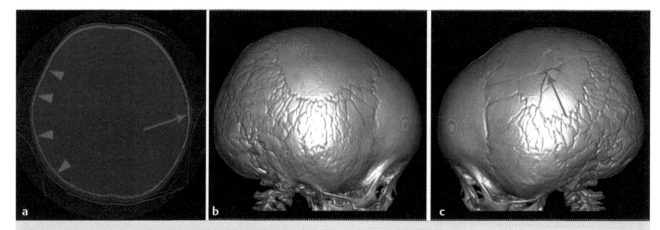

Fig. 15.9 Osteogenesis imperfecta. (a) Axial bone algorithm computed tomographic image in a 29-month-old girl shows a focal, minimally depressed fracture in the left parietal bone (*red arrow*), and multiple nondepressed lucencies in the right parietal bone (*red arrowheads*). (b) Right lateral projection of a three-dimensional computed tomographic rendering shows that the right-sided calvarial lucencies in (a) are related to innumerable intrasutural bones. (c) Left lateral projection shows a similar suture pattern with a superimposed, focally depressed fracture (*red arrow*) with additional fractures radiating outward.

Prominence of the frontal bone ("frontal bossing") and stenosis of the foramen magnum are features of skeletal dysplasias, and particularly of achondroplasia (▶ Fig. 15.10), which is also marked by midface hypoplasia and jugular foraminal stenosis. The jugular foraminal stenosis in achondroplasia can lead to intracranial venous hypertension and a communicating hydrocephalus.

15.4 Calvarial Defects

The protrusion of meninges and passage of cerebrospinal fluid (CSF) through a defect in the skull or vertebral column is known as a meningocele (▶ Fig. 15.11). A defect through which brain parenchyma protrudes is known as an encephalocele (▶ Fig. 15.12). The protrusion of brain parenchyma including

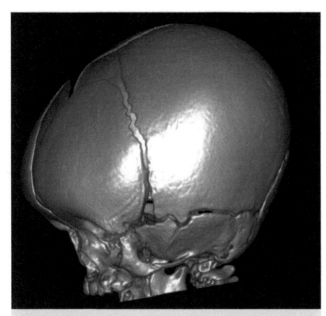

Fig. 15.10 Achondroplasia. Lateral projection three-dimensional computed tomographic image of the skull of a 3-month-old boy with achondroplasia shows midface hypoplasia and protrusion of the forehead (frontal bossing).

portions of the ventricular system through a defect is referred to as an encephalocystocele. Congenital encephaloceles are typically located in the midline, and in patients of Caucasian ancestry are most commonly posterior (occipital), whereas in patients of East Asian ancestry, anterior/frontal encephaloceles are more common (▶ Fig. 15.13). The most common reason for an encephalocele that is not located in the midline is a defect in the wing of the sphenoid bone (▶ Fig. 15.14).

An extracranial collection of CSF related to an acquired abnormality, possibly a postsurgical defect in which the collection is not lined by meninges, is referred to as a pseudomeningocele (▶ Fig. 15.15). A pseudomeningocele that results from trauma may prevent the healing of a fracture, in which case it is often referred to as a leptomeningeal cyst with a "growing fracture" (▶ Fig. 15.16).

Langerhans cell histiocytosis (historically also known as eosinophilic granuloma and Hand–Schüller–Christian disease) is a process in which the abnormal cells known as Langerhans cells, derived from bone marrow, migrate to other sites and proliferate. The condition can cause lytic lesions within the skull that ordinarily have smooth margins, sometimes with a bevel caused by variable involvement of the inner and outer tables of the skull, and without periosteal reaction (▶ Fig. 15.17).[10]

Cutis aplasia is a condition of varying severity in which there is focal agenesis of the skin covering overlying the skull, typically in the midline and over the posterior parieto-occipital region. The manifestation of the condition may be as mild as focal alopecia, but there can also be absence of the skin with exposure of the underlying soft tissues, and in some cases there can be a calvarial defect. Depending upon the severity of the condition, there may be no underlying neurologic deficits, and treatment is typically related to skin closure for cosmesis and the prevention of infection.

Focal failure of closure of the neural tube can result in a dermal sinus tract. This is most commonly a posterior occurrence (▶ Fig. 15.18), but anterior sinonasal defects can occur in varying locations (see ▶ Fig. 15.13). Frontal encephaloceles are more common in patients of East Asian ancestry. A dermal sinus tract may result in focal fenestration of the superior sagittal sinus, and can be associated with an extracranial collection of CSF (meningocele), dysplastic remnant tissue ("atretic cephalocele"), or an inclusion body (either dermoid or epidermoid) (▶ Fig. 15.18). Typically, these abnormalities can be evaluated through a combination of ultrasonography and magnetic resonance imaging (MRI), with the possible use of magnetic resonance (MR) venography to evaluate the superior sagittal sinus, and at times also with the use of CT to determine the extent of an osseous defect.

The head normally contains transcalvarial emissary veins, which drain into the venous system of the scalp. These are typically related to small cortical veins and do not result in significant enlargement of the veins of the scalp. However, a large intracranial vein or venous sinus sometimes extends through the calvarium and has predominantly extracranial drainage, a condition known as sinus pericranii.

As with other bones, the skull is a dynamic structure that can undergo remodeling as the result of chronic pressure, as can be

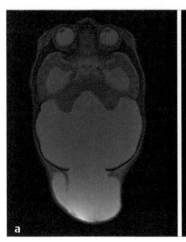
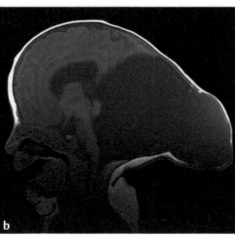

Fig. 15.11 Meningocele. (a) Axial T2 W and (b) sagittal T1 W images of the head of a 1-day-old girl show splaying of the cerebellar hemispheres with a hypoplastic uplifted vermis, consistent with a Dandy–Walker malformation. The cystically dilated posterior fossa has protruded through a calvarial defect, with cerebrospinal fluid and meninges but without neural elements also protruding through the defect, consistent with a meningocele.

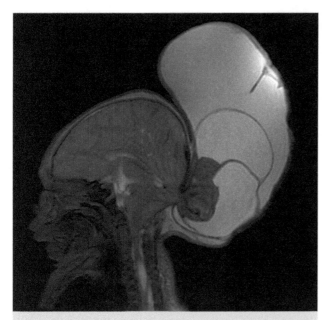

Fig. 15.12 Encephalocele. Sagittal T2W image of the head of a 1-day-old boy shows protrusion of brain parenchyma through a defect in the occipital bone, with a large surrounding collection of cerebrospinal fluid, representing an occipital encephalocele.

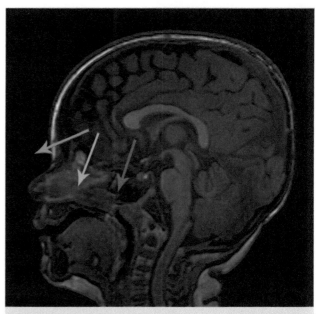

Fig. 15.13 Frontal encephalocele. Anterior midline encephaloceles can occur in the region of the anterior aspect of the crista galli anterior to the cribriform plate (*blue arrow*, frontonasal encephalocele), through the cribriform plate (*green arrow*, frontoethmoidal encephalocele), and through the planum sphenoidale (*red arrow*, frontosphenoidal encephalocele).

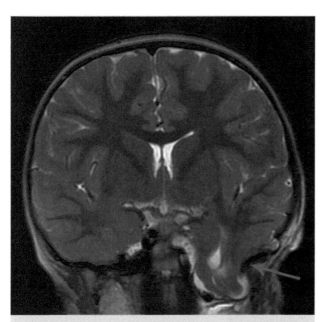

Fig. 15.14 Sphenoid encephalocele. Coronal short tau inversion recovery image of the head of a 4-year-old boy shows a deficiency in the left wing of the sphenoid bone, with caudal protrusion of the meninges and left temporal lobe through the defect, representing an encephalocele of the sphenoid wing.

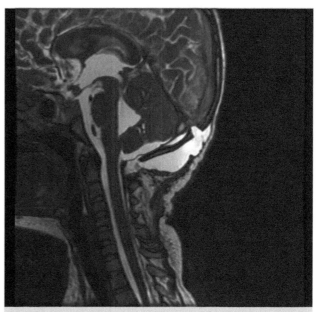

Fig. 15.15 Pseudomeningocele. Sagittal fast imaging employing steady-state acquisition image of the craniocervical junction in a 5-year-old girl with a prior suboccipital craniotomy for resection of a fourth ventricular medulloblastoma shows an extradural/extracranial fluid collection, representing a pseudomeningocele. There is also a nodular mass in the infundibular recess of the third ventricle, representing a metastatic deposit.

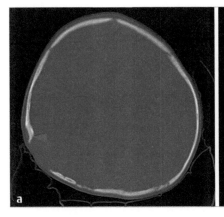

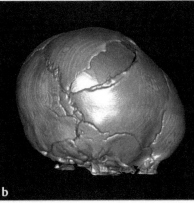

Fig. 15.16 Leptomeningeal cyst. (a) Axial bone algorithm computed tomographic image in a 6-month-old male with prior trauma shows a gap in the posterior right parietal bone with smooth margins, including the anterior margin of the bone gap, which flails outward (*red arrowhead*). (b) Lateral projection of a three-dimensional rendering shows a wide gap from this "growing fracture" related to a leptomeningeal cyst.

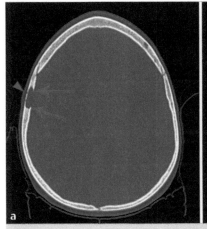

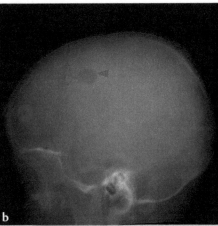

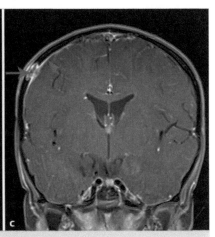

Fig. 15.17 Langerhans cell histiocytosis. (a) Axial bone algorithm computed tomographic image shows a lytic lesion within the right parietal bone that has extended through the inner table of the skull, with a sharp "beveled" margin (*red arrows*) and with early extension through the outer table (*red arrowhead*). (b) Sagittal thick-section reformatted image from a computed tomographic scan, simulating a lateral radiograph of the skull, shows a lytic lesion with circumscribed margins within the right parietal bone (*red arrowheads*). (c) Coronal T1 W plus contrast image shows an enhancing soft tissue component causing the lytic lesion (*red arrow*), and reactive dural thickening in the region (*red arrowhead*).

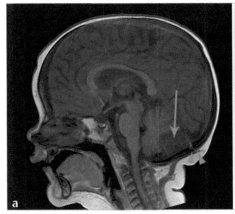

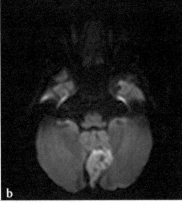

Fig. 15.18 Dermal sinus tract. (a) Sagittal T1 W image shows an extra-axial mass (*blue arrow*) adjacent to the occipital bone, with extension through a calvarial defect and connection with a dermal sinus tract (*blue arrowheads*). (b) Axial diffusion-weighted image shows that the lesion demonstrates restricted diffusion, representing an epidermoid inclusion body.

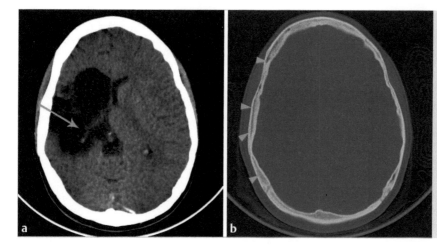

Fig. 15.19 Dyke–Davidoff–Masson phenomenon. (a) Axial computed tomographic image of the head of a 16-year-old girl shows encephalomalacia in the territory of the right middle cerebral artery (*blue arrow*). (b) Axial bone algorithm computed tomographic image shows ipsilateral prominence of the diploic space within the calvarium (*blue arrowheads*), consistent with a Dyke–Davidoff–Masson phenomenon.

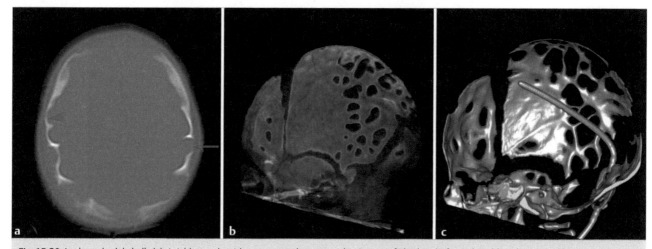

Fig. 15.20 Luckenschadel skull. (a) Axial bone algorithm computed tomographic image of the head of a 1-day-old male with a Chiari type II malformation shows multiple areas of scalloping of the inner table of the skull (*red arrowhead*), with areas of full-thickness nonossification (*red arrow*), consistent with a Luckenschadel skull with craniofenestra. (b) Surface reconstruction of the skull shows multiple craniolacunae. (c) Three-dimensional image of the skull from the inside shows the areas of craniofenestra and also a ventriculostomy catheter.

seen when there is an arachnoid cyst adjacent to it. Over time, the skull overlying areas of parenchymal volume loss will also focally thicken (▶ Fig. 15.19), a process known as the Dyke–Davidoff–Masson phenomenon, which gives a clue that the underlying volume loss is chronic.

In patients with a Chiari type II malformation, there is a high incidence (~ 80%) of membranous dysplasia of the inner table of the skull, resulting in what is known as a Luckenschadel skull (▶ Fig. 15.20). At times this also results in underdevelopment of the outer table of the skull, creating what are known as craniolacunae. Patients with longstanding hydrocephalus can have an acquired scalloping of the inner table of the skull that somewhat resembles that in a Luckenschadel skull, but is considered different because it is an acquired remodeling and not a developmental dysplasia. In this acquired situation, the convolutional markings in the skull give it the appearance known as a copper-beaten skull, because of its resemblance to the multifaceted appearance of hammered copper cookware.

Although benign enlargement of the subarachnoid spaces of infancy is felt to be related to a process of development of the skull, it is further discussed in Chapter 11 because it is most commonly encountered in the evaluation for macrocephaly and suspected hydrocephalus.

15.5 Suggested Reading

[1] Morón FE, Morriss MC, Jones JJ, Hunter JV. Lumps and bumps on the head in children: Use of CT and MR imaging in solving the clinical diagnostic dilemma. Radiographics 2004; 24(6):1655–1674

References

[1] Som PM, Naidich TP. Development of the skull base and calvarium: An overview of the progression from mesenchyme to chondrification to ossification. Neurographics 2013; 3(4):169–184

[2] Glass RBJ, Fernbach SK, Norton KI, Choi PS, Naidich TP. The infant skull: A vault of information. Radiographics 2004;24(2):507–522. Available from: http://radiographics.rsnajnls.org/cgi/doi/10.1148/rg.242035105

[3] Som PM, Naidich TP. Illustrated review of the embryology and development of the facial region, Part 1: Early face and lateral nasal cavities. AJNR Am J Neuroradiol 2013; 34(12):2233–2240

[4] Som PM, Naidich TP. Illustrated review of the embryology and development of the facial region, Part 2: Late development of the fetal face and changes in the face from the newborn to adulthood. AJNR Am J Neuroradiol 2014; 35(1):10–18

[5] Som PM, Streit A, Naidich TP. Illustrated review of the embryology and development of the facial region, Part 3: An overview of the molecular interactions responsible for facial development. AJNR Am J Neuroradiol 2014; 35(2):223–229

[6] Attaya H, Thomas J, Alleman A. Imaging of craniosynostosis from diagnosis through reconstruction. Neurographics 2011; 1(3):121–128

[7] Blaser SI. Abnormal skull shape. Pediatr Radiol 2008; 38 Suppl 3:S488–S496

[8] Meulen J. Metopic synostosis. Childs Nerv Syst 2012;28(9):1359–1367. Available from: http://link.springer.com/10.1007/s00381–012–1803-z

[9] Khandanpour N, Connolly DJA, Raghavan A, Griffiths PD, Hoggard N. Craniospinal abnormalities and neurologic complications of osteogenesis imperfecta: Imaging overview. Radiographics 2012; 32(7):2101–2112

[10] Zaveri J, La Q, Yarmish G, Neuman J. More than just Langerhans cell histiocytosis: A radiologic review of histiocytic disorders. Radiographics 2014; 34(7): 2008–2024

16 Skull Base and Cranial Nerves

16.1 Introduction

The cranial nerves have a critical role in neurologic function and have an intimate relationship with the skull base. Abnormalities in one can affect the other. The cranial nerves have characteristic functions, and dysfunction in them may present with specific or nonspecific clinical signs. Knowledge of the anatomy of the cranial nerves and the skull base can aid in determining a cause for many neurologic conditions. The function of each cranial nerve may involve a combination of afferent (sensation), special sensation (taste), efferent (motor), and parasympathetic function.

On a segmental basis (with minor variations), each cranial nerve has a nucleus (▶ Fig. 16.1), an intra-axial (fascicular) segment, a cisternal segment, an interdural segment, a foraminal segment, and an extraforaminal segment (▶ Fig. 16.2).[1,2,3] Some pathologic processes uniquely affect certain cranial nerves, whereas others are more nonspecific in the nerves they involve. This chapter discusses the function and anatomic features of each of the 12 cranial nerves together with characteristic pathologic conditions affecting them, and reviews conditions that affect the cranial nerves without specific predilections for one or another. The chapter begins with a brief review of the anatomy of the skull base.

16.2 Skull-Base Anatomy

The skull base is variably defined and comprises several bones, most prominently the sphenoid and temporal bones, with additional involvement of portions of the occipital and frontal bones (▶ Fig. 16.3).[4,5,6,7,8] The anterior skull base includes the cribriform plate (consisting of portions of the frontal and ethmoid bones), which is perforated by branches of the olfactory nerve (cranial nerve [CN] I) and roofs of the orbits (formed from portions of the frontal and sphenoid bones). The central portion of the sphenoid bone, the basisphenoid, contains the sella turcica. The basisphenoid and basiocciput are joined by a spheno-occipital synchondrosis, which eventually fuses and forms a structure known as the clivus. Between the basisphenoid and the lesser wing of the sphenoid bone is the optic canal (carrying CN II), and between the basisphenoid and the greater wing of the sphenoid is the superior orbital fissure (carrying CN III, IV, V_1, and VI). Within the greater wing of the sphenoid bone is an anteriorly directed canal known as the foramen rotundum (carrying V_2), and an inferiorly directed canal known as the foramen ovale. Posterolateral to the foramen ovale is the foramen spinosum, which carries the middle meningeal artery.

Within the petrous temporal bone is the internal auditory canal, which carries CN VIII to the structures of the inner ear and acts as a conduit for the facial nerve (CN VII). Between the portion of the temporal bone containing the inner ear and the clivus is the apex of the petrous temporal bone, a structure that can occasionally be pneumatized, with the possible development of an infectious/inflammatory process known as petrous apicitis (see Gradenigo's syndrome in the section of this chapter on CN VI). The pneumatized portion of the temporal bone can also, in the case of a cholesterol granuloma, contain a chronic accumulation of obstructed fluid and debris. On magnetic resonance imaging (MRI), asymmetric penumatization of the

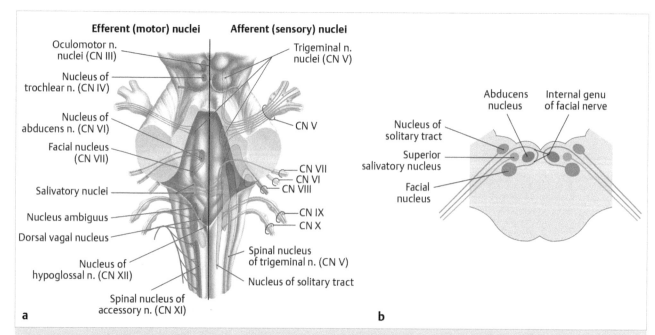

Fig. 16.1 Brainstem anatomy. (a) Schematic diagram showing the nuclei within the brainstem involved in various cranial nerves, with depiction of the efferent (motor) nuclei on one side and afferent (sensory) nuclei on the other. (b) Axial schematic image of the mid-pons shows the facial colliculi with underlying abducens nuclei. The motor nucleus of cranial nerve (CN) VII is seen ventral to this, with the motor fibers coursing around the nucleus of CN VI, and subsequently joining fibers from the solitary tract and superior salivatory nucleus. From Atlas of Anatomy, © Thieme 2012, Illustration by Karl Wesker.

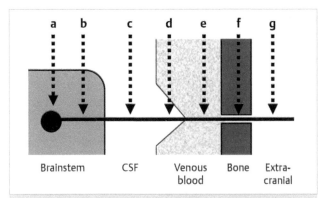

Fig. 16.2 Blitz segmentation. A segmental approach to the cranial nerves. Each cranial nerve has a nucleus (a), an intra-axial fascicular segment (b), a cisternal segment (c), a dural-cave segment (d), an extradural portion (e), a foraminal segment (f), and an extraforaminal segment (g). Although slight variations exist for different nerves, this segmental approach can help in understanding the components of various cranial nerves and how they may be affected by pathology. Used with permission from Blitz AM, Choudhri AF, Chonka ZD, et al. Anatomic Considerations, Nomenclature, and Advanced Cross-sectional Imaging Techniques for Visualization of the Cranial Nerve Segments by MR Imaging. Neuroimaging Clin. N. Am. 2014:241:1–15.

petrous apex can be mistaken for an enhancing lesion of the skull base because the marrow on the nonpneumatized side will appear bright on T1-weighted (T1 W) imaging as compared with precontrast imaging and fat-saturated imaging. When available, a CT scan can help confirm the diagnosis of a pseudo-lesion of the petrous apex and prevent unnecessary surgical intervention. The petrous temporal bone also contains the carotid canal.

The jugular foramen is located between the petrous and mastoid portions of the temporal bone and the occipital bone, and carries the jugular bulb, which is the transition between the sigmoid sinus and the internal jugular vein. The jugular foramen is parcellated into the posterior pars vascularis (carrying CN X and XI), and the smaller anteromedial pars nervosa (carrying CN IX). Within the exoccipital portion of the occipital bone are the hypoglossal canals, carrying the right and left hypoglossal nerve (CN XII).

16.2.1 Cavernous Sinus

The cavernous sinus is a network of venous structures along the lateral margins of the sella turcica bilaterally, and portions of the internal carotid artery course through this venous network.

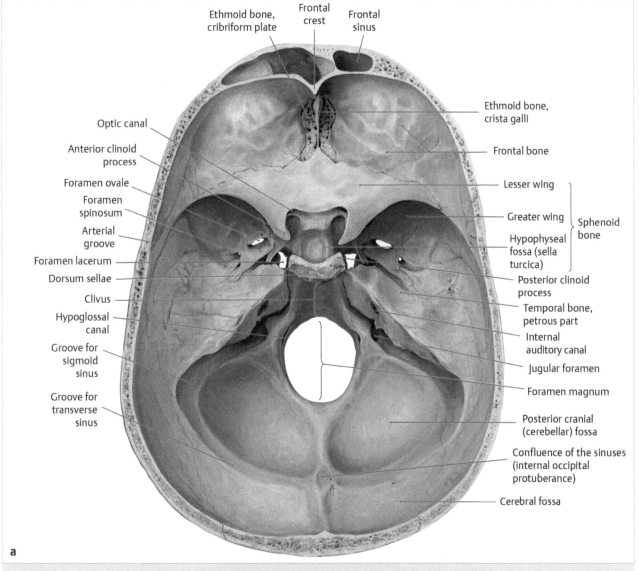

Fig. 16.3 (a-c) Skull base anatomy. From Atlas of Anatomy, © Thieme 2012, Illustration by Karl Wesker. (*continued*)

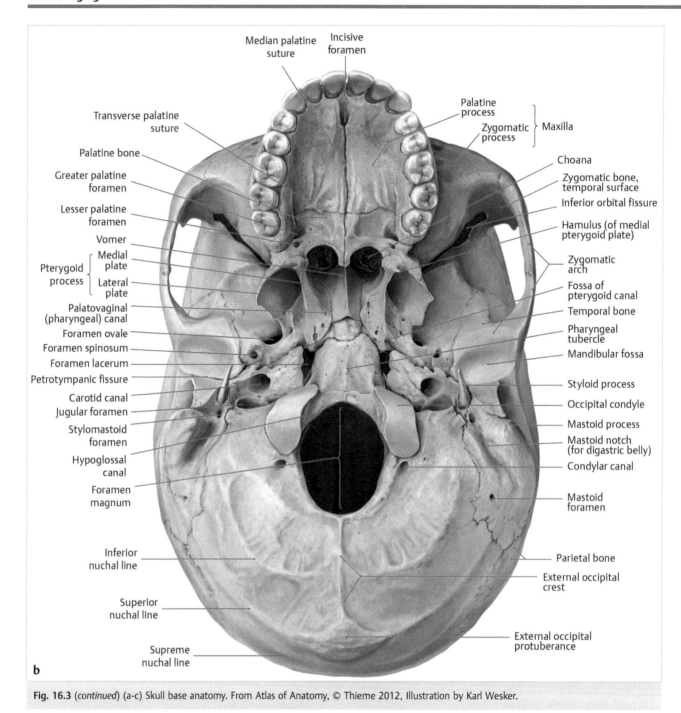

Fig. 16.3 (*continued*) (a-c) Skull base anatomy. From Atlas of Anatomy, © Thieme 2012, Illustration by Karl Wesker.

Along the lateral margins of the cavernous sinus course segments of CN III, IV, and the ophthalmic and maxillary branches of CN V. The abducens nerve (CN VI) courses within the cavernous sinus (▶ Fig. 16.4).

16.2.2 Pterygopalatine Fossa

An area of the skull base worthy of specific discussion is the pterygopalatine fossa, which is located between the greater wing of the sphenoid bone and the pterygoid process of the sphenoid bone (▶ Fig. 16.5). This is an area through which

multiple nerves and vessels pass, and it can be involved in the perineural spread of disease to distant parts of the face, skull base, and brain. The pterygopalatine fossa has two posterior access points, consisting of foramen rotundum, which carries CN V$_2$, and the vidian canal, which carries the vidian nerve. The vidian nerve is a combination of preganglionic parasympathetic fibers from the greater superficial petrosal nerve (GSPN) from CN VII, and postganglionic sympathetic fibers from the deep petrosal nerve. The parasympathetic fibers synapse in the pterygopalatine ganglion, with the postganglionic fibers ascending through the inferior orbital fissure into the posterior orbit. The

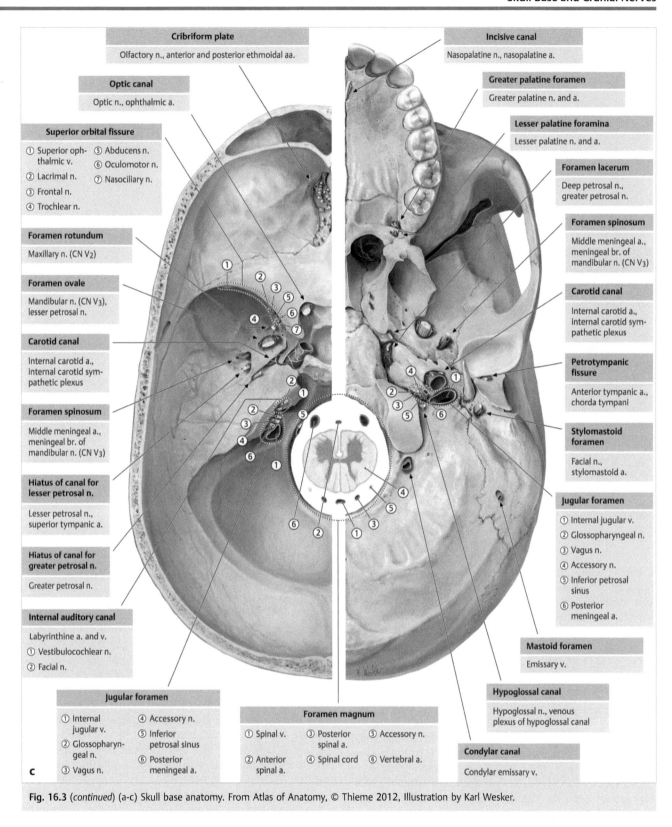

Cribriform plate

Olfactory n., anterior and posterior ethmoidal aa.

Optic canal

Optic n., ophthalmic a.

Superior orbital fissure

① Superior oph-   ⑤ Abducens n.
   thalmic v.   ⑥ Oculomotor n.
② Lacrimal n.   ⑦ Nasociliary n.
③ Frontal n.
④ Trochlear n.

Foramen rotundum

Maxillary n. (CN V$_2$)

Foramen ovale

Mandibular n. (CN V$_3$), lesser petrosal n.

Carotid canal

Internal carotid a., internal carotid sympathetic plexus

Foramen spinosum

Middle meningeal a., meningeal br. of mandibular n. (CN V$_3$)

Hiatus of canal for lesser petrosal n.

Lesser petrosal n., superior tympanic a.

Hiatus of canal for greater petrosal n.

Greater petrosal n.

Internal auditory canal

Labyrinthine a. and v.
① Vestibulocochlear n.
② Facial n.

Incisive canal

Nasopalatine n., nasopalatine a.

Greater palatine foramen

Greater palatine n. and a.

Lesser palatine foramina

Lesser palatine n. and a.

Foramen lacerum

Deep petrosal n., greater petrosal n.

Foramen spinosum

Middle meningeal a., meningeal br. of mandibular n. (CN V$_3$)

Carotid canal

Internal carotid a., internal carotid sympathetic plexus

Petrotympanic fissure

Anterior tympanic a., chorda tympani

Stylomastoid foramen

Facial n., stylomastoid a.

Jugular foramen

① Internal jugular v.
② Glossopharyngeal n.
③ Vagus n.
④ Accessory n.
⑤ Inferior petrosal sinus
⑥ Posterior meningeal a.

Mastoid foramen

Emissary v.

Hypoglossal canal

Hypoglossal n., venous plexus of hypoglossal canal

Condylar canal

Condylar emissary v.

Jugular foramen

① Internal   ④ Accessory n.
   jugular v.   ⑤ Inferior
② Glossopharyn-   petrosal sinus
   geal n.   ⑥ Posterior
③ Vagus n.   meningeal a.

c

Foramen magnum

① Spinal v.   ③ Posterior   ⑤ Accessory n.
                     spinal a.
② Anterior   ④ Spinal cord   ⑥ Vertebral a.
   spinal a.

Fig. 16.3 (*continued*) (a-c) Skull base anatomy. From Atlas of Anatomy, © Thieme 2012, Illustration by Karl Wesker.

anterior outlet of the pterygopalatine fossa is the infraorbital canal, which carries the infraorbital branch of CN V$_2$. Inferiorly are two canals for nerves innervating the palate, the greater and lesser palatine nerves, which traverse the greater and lesser palatine canals, respectively. Lateral access to the pterygopalatine fossa is from the pterygomaxillary fissure, through which the internal maxillary artery enters the pterygopalatine fossa. Medially is the sphenopalatine foramen, which is the communication between the pterygopalatine fossa and the sinonasal cavity, and where distal branches of the internal

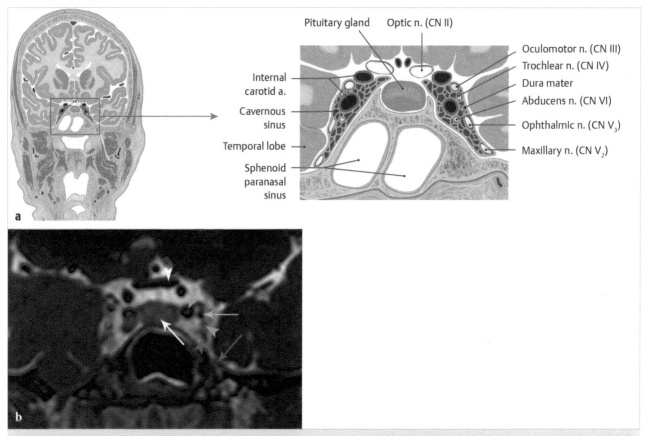

Fig. 16.4 Cavernous sinus. (a) Artist's rendering of the cavernous sinus, with (b) a companion coronal fast imaging employing steady-state acquisition after contrast administration image showing the cavernous sinus lateral to the pituitary gland (*white arrow*). Within the cavernous sinus is the internal carotid artery (*blue arrowhead*) and the abducens nerve (CN VI). Along the lateral margin are CN III (*green arrow*), CN IV (*green arrowhead*), CN V$_1$ (*red arrowhead*), and CN V$_2$ (*red arrow*). For reference, the optic chiasm is marked (*white arrowhead*); however, the optic nerve does not course within the cavernous sinus. "a" From Atlas of Anatomy, © Thieme 2012, Illustration by Karl Wesker.

maxillary artery extend to supply the nasal mucosa. The sphenopalatine foramen is also the location of the origin of a particular tumor known as a juvenile nasal angiofibroma, a highly vascular tumor that presents in adolescent males with recurrent unilateral epistaxis.

16.3 Anatomy and Nerve-Specific Pathology

16.3.1 Cranial Nerve I–Olfactory Nerve

The olfactory nerve is an afferent nerve involved in the sensation of smell. In formal terms, it is a tract and is part of the central nervous system (CNS), with its myelination produced by oligodendrocytes. The olfactory nerve courses within the olfactory groove along the superior aspect of the cribriform plate (▶ Fig. 16.6). The nerve is subject to traumatic injury in the case of fractures of the central skull base. Congenital absence of the olfactory nerve results in anosmia (inability to smell), and can be associated with hypogonadotropic hypogonadism in Kallman's syndrome. Hypoplasia of the olfactory nerve can be seen in patients with septo-optic dysplasia. Abnormalities in the olfactory pathway can present with dysgeusia (abnormality or loss of the sensation of taste).

16.3.2 Cranial Nerve II–Optic Nerve

The optic nerve carries afferent fibers involved in sight (▶ Fig. 16.7). The nerve begins in the optic disc in the posterior aspect of the globe of the eye, courses posteriorly in the orbit of the eye, passes through the optic canal, and reaches the optic chiasm. Within the chiasm, fibers of the optic nerve from the nasal retinal field (temporal visual field) of one eye decussate and join with fibers from the temporal retinal field (nasal visual field) of the contralateral eye, which do not decussate. At the optic chiasm, the tracts consisting of temporal retinal fibers of one eye and nasal retinal fibers of the contralateral eye extend posterolaterally as the right and left optic tracts, respectively, which then continue to the right and left lateral geniculate nuclei.

The optic nerve is formally a part of the CNS, with its myelination produced by oligodendrocytes rather than Schwann cells. Therefore, tumors of the optic nerve are gliomas rather than optic nerve schwannomas. Additionally, the optic nerve is susceptible to inflammatory and demyelinating processes (optic neuritis) that affect the CNS (e.g., multiple sclerosis, acute disseminated encephalomyelitis [ADEM], neuromyelitis optica [NMO]). A sellar/suprasellar mass like a pituitary macroadenoma or craniopharyngioma that impinges the optic chiasm

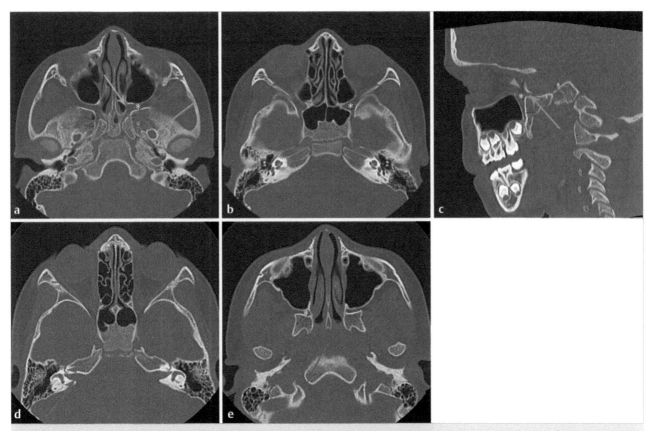

Fig. 16.5 Skull-base foramina and pterygopalatine fossa. (a) Axial computed tomographic image shows the pterygopalatine fossa (*white asterisk*), with communications posteriorly through the vidian canal (*red arrowheads*), laterally through the pterygomaxillary fissure (*red arrow*), and medially through the sphenopalatine foramen (*green arrow*). The foramen ovale (*blue arrow*) and foramen spinosum (*blue arrowhead*) are also seen. (b) Axial computed tomographic image shows the pterygopalatine fossa (*white asterisk*), with communications posteriorly through foramen rotundum (*blue arrowhead*). (c) Sagittal computed tomographic image shows the pterygopalatine fossa (*white asterisk*), with communications posteriorly through foramen rotundum (*blue arrow*), superiorly to the orbital apex through the inferior orbital fissure (*blue arrowhead*), and inferiorly through the palatine canal (*red arrowhead*). (d) Axial computed tomographic image shows the internal auditory canal (*red arrow*) and the fallopian canal, the latter of which carries the labyrinthine segment of the facial nerve (*red arrowhead*). (e) Axial computed tomographic image shows the hypoglossal canal (*red arrow*), as well as the pterygopalatine fossa (*white asterisk*) which is anterior to the pterygoid process of the sphenoid bone.

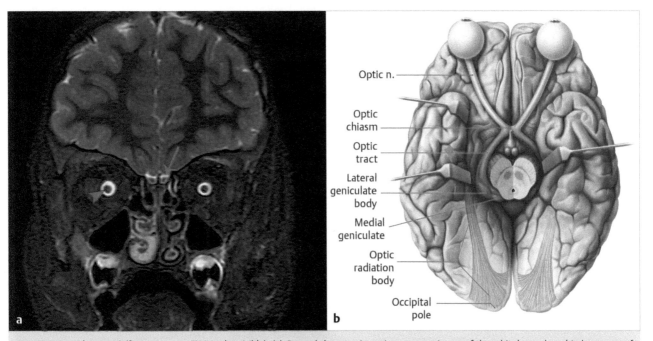

Fig. 16.6 Cranial nerve I (olfactory nerve; CN II is also visible). (a) Coronal short tau inversion recovery image of the orbit shows the orbital segment of the optic nerve (CN II, *red arrowhead*) surrounded by CSF within the optic nerve sheath. Along the superior margin of the cribriform plate the left olfactory nerve (CN I, *red arrow*) is seen. (b) Artist's rendering of the undersurface of the brain showing the optic tracts extending anteriorly from the lateral geniculate nuclei, and the optic nerves extending anteriorly from the optic chiasm. The olfactory nerves course adjacent to the gyrus rectus. "b" From Atlas of Anatomy, © Thieme 2012, Illustration by Karl Wesker.

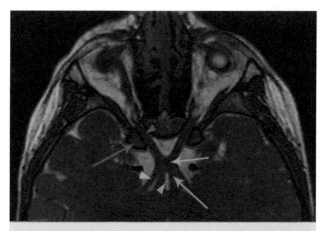

Fig. 16.7 Cranial nerve II (optic nerve). Axial fast imaging employing steady-state acquisition image shows the canalicular segment of the optic nerve (CN II, *red arrowhead*), which courses adjacent to the anterior clinoid process (*red arrow*). Posterior to this is the optic chiasm (*green arrow*). Extending posterolaterally from the optic chiasm are the optic tracts (*green arrowhead*). The hypothalamus contacts the chiasm (*blue arrow*) along the lateral aspect of the chiasmatic recess of the third ventricle (*blue arrowhead*).

will affect visual fibers decussating in the chiasm, resulting in a bitemporal hemianopsia.

16.3.3 Cranial Nerve III–Oculomotor Nerve

The oculomotor nerve has somatic motor and parasympathetic functions, with nuclei in the midportion of the mesencephalon (▶ Fig. 16.8). The nerve exits the mesencephalon along the medial margin of the cerebral peduncle, and the cisternal segment courses between the posterior cerebral and superior cerebellar arteries, parallels the course of the posterior communicating artery, and enters the superolateral wall of the cavernous sinus through its dural cave, the oculomotor cistern. From the cavernous sinus, the oculomotor nerve enters the orbit through the superior orbital fissure and innervates four of the six extraocular muscles (superior rectus, medial rectus, inferior rectus, and inferior oblique), and the levator palpabrae superioris, which raises the eyelid. The parasympathetic fibers of the oculomotor nerve innervate the ciliary ganglion, which controls pupillary and ciliary function. The cisternal segment of the

oculuomotor nerve is adjacent to the uncus of the temporal lobe, and a third nerve palsy is therefore often the first focal neurologic symptom of uncal herniation. A complete third nerve palsy results in inferolateral deviation of the affected eye, with pupillary dilation ("down, out, and dilated"). In adults, the primary concern in a case of third nerve palsy is an aneurysm of the posterior communicating artery, but this is rare in children. Parasympathetic fibers of CN III are peripheral within the nerve bundle, and tend to be preferentially impaired upon its extrinsic compression. Motor fibers of CN III are more central and are preferentially impaired by a diminished blood supply (e.g., is seen in diabetic ischemic neuropathy).

16.3.4 Cranial Nerve IV–Trochlear Nerve

The trochlear nerve is nearly impossible to see on MRI without the use of an exquisitely high-resolution technique or without very good luck (▶ Fig. 16.9). However, it is important to be aware of the course of the trochlear nerve. The trochlear nerve is the only cranial nerve to arise from the dorsal aspect of the brainstem, is the only cranial nerve to decussate, and has the longest cisternal course of any cranial nerve. Apart from the amenability of these three features to multiple-choice questions, there are practical reasons to be aware of the course of the trochlear nerve. The trochlear nerve arises from the dorsal midbrain, decussates, courses around the midbrain, and extends to the lateral wall of the cavernous sinus, just below the oculomotor nerve. Given its long cisternal course, the trochlear nerve is susceptible to injury in head trauma, either in the form of direct injury or from acceleration/deceleration injury. The trochlear nerve provides innervation to the superior oblique muscle (which has a reflection at the trochlea, leading to the name of the nerve), and a trochlear nerve palsy results in the inability to medially supraduct the eye (inability to look upward and inward), resulting in torsional misalignment of the eyes. An abnormality of the superior oblique muscle known as Brown's syndrome, which can be either congenital or acquired, limits the elevation of the affected eye. The acquired form of the syndrome may be due to scarring or fibrosis in the superior oblique muscle and/or its tendon.

16.3.5 Cranial Nerve V–Trigeminal Nerve

The trigeminal nerve (CN V) is the largest of the cranial nerves and has numerous nuclei within the brainstem (including some

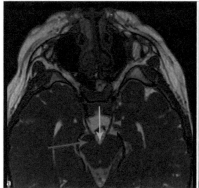
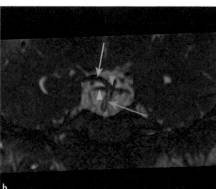

Fig. 16.8 Cranial nerve III (oculomotor nerve). (a) Axial fast imaging employing steady-state acquisition (FIESTA) image of the midbrain shows the cisternal segment of the oculomotor nerves (*red arrowheads*) arising from the margin of the cerebral peduncles (*red arrow*) and the interpeduncular fossa (*green arrow*). (b) Coronal FIESTA image shows the cisternal segment of the oculomotor nerves (*red arrowheads*) coursing between the posterior cerebral artery (*green arrow*) and the superior cerebellar artery (*green arrowhead*), which arise from the basilar apex (*blue arrowhead*) at the end of the basilar artery (*blue arrow*).

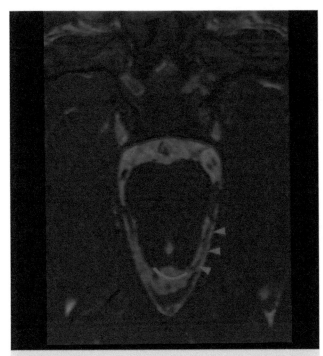

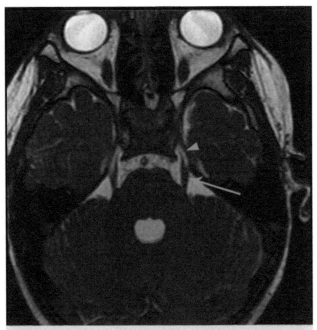

Fig. 16.9 Cranial nerve IV (trochlear nerve). Axial-oblique fast imaging employing steady-state acquisition image of the midbrain shows the cisternal segment of the left trochlear nerve within the left ambient cistern (*red arrowheads*). The proximal portion of the nerve cannot be seen in this image, but follows the expected course of the *thin red line*.

Fig. 16.10 Cranial nerve V (trigeminal nerve). Axial fast imaging employing steady-state acquisition image shows the cisternal segment of the trigeminal nerve (*blue arrow*) extending from the pons to Meckel's cave (*blue arrowhead*).

that extend caudally to the upper cervical spinal cord) (▶ Fig. 16.10). The trigeminal nerve has motor and sensory functions and has no intrinsic parasympathetic functions, although parasympathetic fibers from other cranial nerves follow portions of CN V. The trigeminal nerve exits the brainstem along the lateral aspect of the pons as a bundle of multiple small nerves. Within the cisternal course, these nerves start to separate into three separate bundles. The bundles enter Meckel's cave, the largest dural cave of any of the cranial nerves, through the porus trigeminus. From here, the three main nerve bundles originating from the trigeminal nerve separate. The ophthalmic nerve, or first division (V_1), of the three nerve bundles, courses along the lateral aspect of the cavernous sinus (below the trochlear nerve) and enters the orbit through the superior orbital fissure. The ophthalmic nerve provides sensation to the upper face and forehead. The maxillary nerve, or second division (V_2) of the three nerve bundles originating from the trigeminal nerve, courses along the lateral aspect of the cavernous sinus (below V_1) and traverses foramen rotundum to enter the pterygopalatine fossa. From the pterygopalatine fossa, multiple divisions branch from the maxillary nerve, but the largest is the infraorbital nerve, which extends through the infraorbital canal to reach the infraorbital foramen. The branches of the intraorbital nerve provide sensation to the mid-face. From the pterygopalatine fossa, additional branches extend caudally as the greater and lesser palatine nerves to provide sensation to the hard and soft palates. The third division of the trigeminal nerve, the mandibular nerve (V_3), extends from Meckel's cave to the foramen ovale without becoming associated with the cavernous sinus. From the foramen ovale, the

mandibular nerve enters the infratemporal fossa and divides into several branches, the largest being the inferior alveolar nerve, which extends through the infratemporal fossa to the medial aspect of the posterior mandibular body, and enters the mandibular canal. Within the infratemporal fossa, the lingual nerve is joined by the chorda tympani (arising from CN VII), which carries afferent taste fibers from the anterior two-thirds of the tongue. Other branches of V_3 innervate the muscles of mastication (temporalis, masseter, medial and lateral pterygoid muscles), and the accessory muscles of mastication (mylohyoid and the anterior belly of the digastric muscle).

As mentioned in Chapters 9 and 10, the gasserian ganglion of the trigeminal nerve, which rests within Meckel's cave, can be the site of reactivation of infections by herpes simplex virus type 1 (HSV-1), and the adjacent portions of the medial temporal lobe become preferentially involved in the early stages of HSV encephalitis. Branches of the trigeminal nerve provide sensory innervation to the meninges of the anterior and middle cranial fossae, and may be involved in some types of headaches.

16.3.6 Cranial Nerve VI–Abducens Nerve

The abducens nerve arises from a nucleus in the dorsal pons, subjacent to a irregularity in the contour of the posterior pons (or a "bump" along the floor of the fourth ventricle) known as the facial colliculus (▶ Fig. 16.11). The fibers of the abducens nerve travel anterolaterally and exit the brainstem at the pontomedullary sulcus (▶ Fig. 16.12). From there, the cisternal

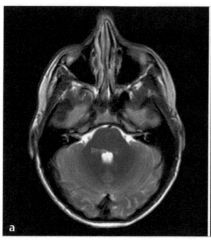
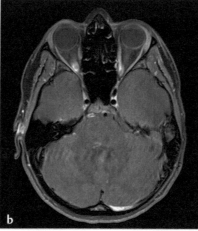

Fig. 16.11 Multiple sclerosis (MS) plaque at the facial colliculus. (a) Axial T2 W image of the head of a 15-year-old girl with MS with a right sixth-nerve palsy of new onset shows a focal area of hyperintense signal associated with the right facial colliculus (*red arrowheads*), which enhances on (b) a T1 W plus contrast image, consistent with an area of active demyelination.

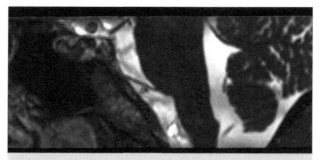

Fig. 16.12 Cranial nerve VI (abducens nerve). Sagittal oblique image made with constructive interference in steady-state imaging shows the cisternal segment of the abducens nerve (*red arrowhead*) extending from the pontomedullary sulcus to the dorsal aspect of the clivus.

segment of the abducens nerve follows an anterior and superolateral course, piercing the dura along the dorsal aspect of the clivus, following the course of the inferior petrosal sinus, and, after passing beneath the petrosphenoidal ligament ("Gruber's ligament") in a space known as Dorello's canal, traveling anteriorly within the cavernous sinus. From there, the nerve travels through the superior orbital fissure to innervate the lateral rectus muscles. Impairment of the abducens nerve results in the inability to laterally deviate the affected eye and presents clinically as esotropia (inward-turned eye), with the patient reporting diplopia (double vision) when looking toward the affected side. A congenital sixth nerve impairment is known as Duane syndrome. It is marked by difficulty in rotating one or both eyes inward or outward, and has very specific ophthalmologic criteria.

The course of the abducens nerve within the cavernous sinus subjects it to circumferential pressure in conditions in which there are elevated intracranial venous pressures, such as pseudotumor cerebri or venous sinus thrombosis. For this reason, pseudotumor cerebri may present with a clinical history of "sixth nerve palsy," "esotropia," or "diplopia." Congenital esotropia may be treated through surgical repositioning and/or shortening of the insertion of the lateral rectus muscle on the eye, by ophthalmologists who specialize in strabismus (typically pediatric ophthalmologists and/ or neuro-ophthalmologists).

The retroclival course of the abducens nerve is adjacent to the petrous apex, and a lesion of the petrous apex can result in an ipsilateral abducens palsy, whereas a lesion within the clivus has the potential to result in a bilateral abducens nerve palsy. An infection within a pneumatized petrous apex can cause an abducens nerve palsy (typically with associated pain and fever) in a triad of symptoms known as Gradenigo's syndrome, consisting of unilateral periorbital pain, diplopia, and otorrhea.

16.3.7 Cranial Nerve VII–Facial Nerve

The facial nerve has three separate nuclei within the brainstem (▶ Fig. 16.13), and as a result has motor, parasympathetic, and sensory functions. The motor nucleus of the facial nerve provides efferent function controlling the muscles of facial expression and is within the central pons, with fibers that course around the abducens nucleus at the level of the facial colliculus (hence the name "facial colliculus"). The superior salivatory nucleus of the facial nerve gives rise to parasympathetic efferent fibers, and the solitary-tract nucleus of the nerve is the origin of afferent taste fibers. These latter two groups of fibers join the visceral motor fibers of the facial nerve after they have hooked around the abducens nucleus. Thus, a lesion at the level of the facial colliculus will result in an ipsilateral abducens nerve palsy and facial motor weakness, but may not affect the taste or parasympathetic functions of CN VII.

The facial nerve leaves the brainstem and traverses the cerebellopontine angle cistern (cisternal segment) and travels through the internal auditory canal (IAC) (canalicular segment), where it is the anterosuperior resident. Along the anterior superior aspect of the fundus of the IAC, the facial nerve exits through the fallopian canal between the cochlea and vestibule (labyrinthine segment) to reach the geniculate ganglion. The parasympathetic fibers of the facial nerve from the superior salivatory nucleus pass through the geniculate ganglion without synapsing and course anteromedially adjacent to the carotid canal as the greater superficial petrosal nerve. The fibers join with postganglionic sympathetic fibers of the deep petrosal nerve to form the vidian nerve and enter the pterygopalatine fossa through the vidian canal. The parasympathetic fibers of the facial nerve then synapse in the pterygopalatine ganglion, and the postganglionic fibers ascend through the inferior

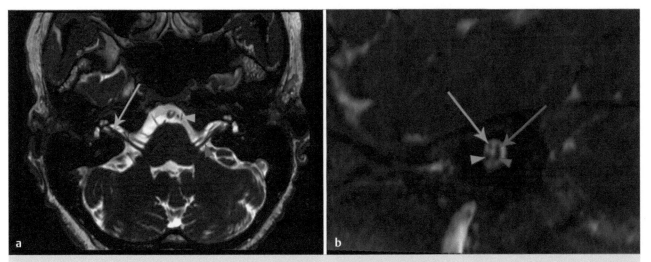

Fig. 16.13 Cranial nerves VII (facial nerve) and VIII (vestibulocochlear nerve). (a) Axial image of the internal auditory canal (IAC) made with CISS imaging shows the cisternal segments of the abducens nerve (*green arrowheads*), and the CN VII/VIII complex (*red arrowhead*). The canalicular segments of the nerves can also be seen (*green arrow*). (b) Sagittal oblique fast imaging employing steady-state acquisition image of the IAC shows the facial nerve in the anterior–superior portion of the canal (*blue arrow*) and the cochlear nerve in the anterior–inferior aspect of the canal (*blue arrowhead*). Posteriorly are the superior (*red arrow*) and inferior (*red arrowhead*) vestibular nerves.

orbital fissure, where they join fibers of V_2 traveling to the orbit to conduct functions like lacrimation.

The somatic motor fibers of the facial nerve synapse in the geniculate ganglion and course posteriorly along the superior aspect of the tympanic cavity (tympanic segment), after which they course caudally within the mastoid portion of the temporal bone (mastoid segment) and exit the skull through the stylomastoid foramen (between the tips of the mastoid and styloid processes). The extracranial portion of the facial nerve enters the parotid gland and branches to innervate the muscles of facial expression. Within the parotid gland, the facial nerve serves as the distinction between the nonanatomic parotid parcellations known as the deep and superficial lobes; because the nerve is difficult (yet not impossible) to see, the adjacent retromandibular vein is used as a surrogate marker for the location of the facial nerve.

From the descending mastoid segment, the nerves that provide taste sensation to the anterior two-thirds of the tongue break free, travel through the tympanic cavity as the chorda tympani, and eventually join fibers from the lingual nerve (a branch of the mandibular division of the trigeminal nerve [CN V_3]). Preganglionic parasympathetic fibers of the chorda tympani synapse in the submandibular ganglion before they enter the tongue via the lingual nerve (a branch of CN V_3). An additional small branch of the facial nerve arises from the descending mastoid segment of CN VII and innervates the stapedius muscle.

On contrast-enhanced MRI, there can be normal (yet inconsistent) enhancement of the geniculate ganglion as well as of the tympanic (and possibly the descending mastoid segments) of the facial nerve. The enhancement of the geniculate ganglion is due to the lack of a blood–brain barrier, and the apparent enhancement of the tympanic and mastoid segments is due to a surrounding venous plexus (and not to true nerve enhancement). Enhancement within any other segment of the facial nerve, or any of the other cranial nerves, is consid-

ered abnormal. (N.B.: Every type of scanner and imaging/contrast administration protocol provides images of differing appearances, making it important for users to confirm this on their own scanners.) A patient with a facial weakness can have an inflammatory activation of a virus within the facial nerve, known as Bell's palsy, which will commonly produce smooth enhancement (without thickening) of the labyrinthine segment and distal canalicular segments of the facial nerve. Although symptoms of Bell's palsy may be unilateral, the enhancement may be bilateral, suggesting contralateral subclinical disease (▶ Fig. 16.14).

A rare but interesting congenital condition of which to be aware is Möbius syndrome, in which patients have bilateral congenital absence (or hypoplasia) of CN VI and CN VII.

16.3.8 Cranial Nerve VIII–Vestibular and Cochlear Nerves

The eighth cranial nerve has two distinct components: (1) the cochlear nerve, which is involved in transmitting afferent auditory information from the cochlea to the brainstem; and (2) the vestibular nerve (typically with separate superior and inferior divisions), which is involved in balance (▶ Fig. 16.13). The cochlear nerve arises from the brainstem in the cerebellopontine angle cistern (cisternal segment), courses along the anterior–inferior aspect of the internal auditory canal (canalicular segment), and enters the cochlear aperture; the spiral ganglion of the cochlear nerve resides within the modiolus. A narrowed cochlear aperture (cochlear aperture stenosis, see Chapter 22), typically involving an aperture of less than 1 mm in diameter, is suggestive of either cochlear nerve hypoplasia or aplasia. This is important to recognize because a patient with cochlear nerve aplasia is not likely to benefit from an ipsilateral cochlear implant device.

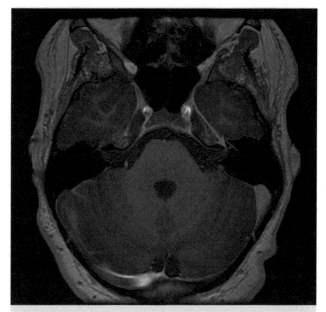

Fig. 16.14 Bell's palsy. Axial T1 W plus contrast image of the internal auditory canal in a 17-year-old boy with left-sided facial weakness shows abnormal enhancement within the labyrinthine segment of the left facial nerve (*red arrow*), representing the imaging findings in Bell's palsy.

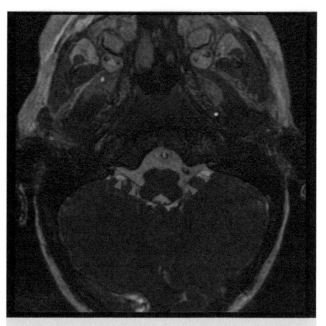

Fig. 16.15 Cranial nerves IX (glossopharyngeal nerve) and X (vagus nerve). Axial fast imaging employing steady-state acquisition image of the medulla oblongata shows the cisternal segments of cranial nerves IX and X (*red arrowheads*) extending toward the jugular foramen.

Like the cochlear nerve, the vestibular nerve arises from the brainstem at the cerebellopontine angle, but courses along the posterior aspect of the internal auditory canal. Ordinarily the cochlear nerve has two divisions, a superior and an inferior division, but these may appear as a single large vestibular nerve. Recognizing that the vestibule is posterior to the IAC helps in remembering that the vestibular nerve is posteriorly positioned within the IAC. Similarly, the cochlea is anterior to the IAC, and therefore the cochlear nerve is anteriorly positioned within the IAC. The labyrinthine segment of the facial nerve arises from the anterosuperior aspect of the fundus of the IAC, which should help the recognition that the facial nerve is superior to the cochlear nerve (also, because the cranial nerves are numbered in a superior to inferior order of location, it makes sense that CN VII is superior to CN VIII).

The vestibular nerves are predisposed to the development of schwannomas in patients with neurofibromatosis type 2 (NF2). These benign neoplasms are commonly referred to as "acoustic neuromas," but only rarely involve the "acoustic" (cochlear) nerve, and are related to the nerve sheath and not the nerve itself, and are therefore not truly neuromas. The occurrence of bilateral vestibular schwannomas meets the diagnostic criteria for NF2, as does a unilateral vestibular schwannoma in a patient who has a first-degree relative with confirmed NF2 (see Chapter 7).

16.3.9 Cranial Nerve IX–Glossopharyngeal Nerve

The glossopharyngeal nerve arises from the lateral aspect of the medulla oblongata, with the cisternal segment of the nerve traversing the lateral medullary cistern, and the nerve exits through the pars nervosa of the jugular foramen, which is the location where the inferior petrosal sinus joins the jugular bulb (▶ Fig. 16.15). The glossopharyngeal nerve has parasympathetic efferent fibers that control the parotid gland, and it provides efferent somatic motor fibers to the stylopharyngeus muscle, which is involved in swallowing. The glossopharyngeal nerve also has additional functions, including afferent taste sensation from the posterior third of the tongue, and somatic sensation (afferent) for the posterior third of the tongue, tympanic membrane, and oropharynx. Given the range of functions of the glossopharyngeal nerve, it has multiple nuclei within the brainstem. The glossopharyngeal nerve, together with the vagal nerve, contributes to the pharyngeal plexus innervating the oropharyngeal mucosa. Cranial nerves IX and X are involved in the gag reflex, and CN IX is involved with the carotid body reflex. Glossopharyngeal neuralgia presenting as ear pain, neck pain, and dysphagia can be caused by an elongated styloid process in the condition known as Eagle syndrome.

16.3.10 Cranial Nerve X–Vagus Nerve

The vagus nerve (CN X) arises from the lateral aspect of the medulla oblongata, immediately caudal to the origin of CN IX, and exits through the pars vascularis of the jugular foramen (▶ Fig. 16.15). The vagus nerve provides parasympathetic innervation to nearly the entirety of the neck, chest, abdomen, and pelvis. Additionally, it provides motor innervation for the palate, pharynx, and larynx, and carries somatic afferent sensation from the external auditory canal and tympanic membrane and meninges of the posterior cranial fossa, and taste sensation from the epiglottis. The recurrent laryngeal nerve, an important branch of the vagus nerve, extends caudally to the upper thorax and then ascends deep to the thyroid gland and provides laryngeal innervation. The right recurrent laryngeal nerve extends

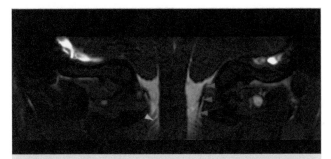

Fig. 16.16 Cranial nerve XI (spinal accessory nerve). Coronal image of the foramen magnum made with CISS imaging shows the ascending segment of CN XI (*red arrowheads*) prior to it and extending to the jugular foramen. Several nerve rootlets of the first cervical nerve are visible (*green arrowhead*).

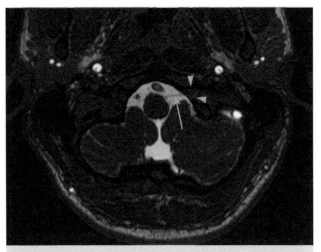

Fig. 16.17 Cranial nerve XII (hypoglossal nerve). Axial image of the medulla made with CISS imaging shows the cisternal segment of the left hypoglossal nerve (CN XII, *green arrow*) extending toward the hypoglossal canal (*green arrowheads*). The ascending portion of the spinal accessory nerve (CN XI, *red arrowhead*) is seen as it passes through the foramen magnum.

beneath the right subclavian artery, and the left recurrent laryngeal nerve extends beneath the aortic arch (in a patient with situs solitus and a left-sided aortic arch). Injury to the recurrent laryngeal nerve from mediastinal tumors (more common in adults) or surgery in the thyroid/parathyroid region (also more common in adults) can result in ipsilateral vocal-cord paralysis.

16.3.11 Cranial Nerve XI–Spinal Accessory Nerve

The spinal accessory nerve (CN XI) arises from the upper portion of the cervical spinal cord with fibers that ascend through the foramen magnum and then exit through the pars vascularis of the jugular foramen (▶ Fig. 16.16). The spinal accessory nerve is involved in innervation of the trapezius and sternocleidomastoid muscles. Dysfunction of the sternocleidomastoid muscle results in impaired contralateral turning of the head.

16.3.12 Cranial Nerve XII–Hypoglossal Nerve

The hypoglossal nerve (CN XII) arises from the ventrolateral aspect of the medulla oblongata, has a short cisternal course, and then traverses the hypoglossal foramen (▶ Fig. 16.17). The hypoglossal nerve innervates the intrinsic muscles of the ipsilateral half of the tongue, and hypoglossal dysfunction results in ipsilateral deviation of the tongue on protrusion. Acute hypoglossal denervation results in hemitongue edema, and chronic denervation results in fatty degeneration of the ipsilateral hemitongue.

16.4 Pathology (General)

Pathologic conditions other than those discussed in the preceding sections can occur in various cranial nerves. Infection with Lyme disease (caused by the spirochete *Borrelia burgdorferi*) can result in smooth enhancement of the cisternal segments of multiple cranial nerves. A similar appearance can occur in Miller–Fisher syndrome, an immune-mediated, noninfectious, postviral inflammatory process that represents the cranial

nerve variant of Guillain–Barré syndrome. The clinical context in which these conditions occur will tend to differentiate them. Any focal thickening or nodularity among the findings in these conditions raises concern about the existence of other processes, including granulomatous conditions (e.g., sarcoidosis) or neoplasia.

Although schwannomas of the vestibular nerve in the setting of NF2 are known entities, any of the cranial nerves myelinated by Schwann cells can have schwannomas. Patients with NF2 are predisposed to schwannomas in multiple cranial nerves, rather than of the vestibular nerve alone. It is important to be aware that the transition from myelination by oligodendrocytes in the CNS and by Schwann cells in the peripheral nervous system does not occur at the apparent origins of cranial nerves, but several millimeters distal to this. The transitional zone between these two locations is known as the Obersteiner–Redlich zone, and a schwannoma will not occur proximal to this. The Obersteiner–Redlich zone for CN VIII is the farthest from the brainstem (typically > 10 mm) of any of these zones, which is why a vestibular schwannoma will always involve the IAC and not involve the CP angle cistern in an isolated manner.

After hemorrhage, whether from trauma, germinal matrix hemorrhage, an aneurysm, a vascular malformation, or prior surgery, it is possible for hemosiderin to deposit on the cisternal (and possibly on the canalicular) segments of cranial nerves, resulting in nonspecific cranial neuropathies. This is known as superficial siderosis, and is best seen on susceptibility-weighted imaging (▶ Fig. 5.12e).

16.5 Suggested Reading

[1] Chandra T, Maheshwari M, Kelly TG et al. Imaging of pediatric skull base lesions. Neurographics 2015; 5(2):72–84http://dx.doi.org/10.3174/ng.2150106

[2] Razek AA, Huang BY. Lesions of the petrous apex: Classification and findings at CT and MR imaging. Radiographics 2012; 32(1):151–173

References

[1] Blitz AM, Choudhri AF, Chonka ZD et al. Anatomic considerations, nomenclature, and advanced cross-sectional imaging techniques for visualization of the cranial nerve segments by MR imaging. Neuroimaging Clin N Am 2014; 24(1):1–15

[2] Blitz AM, Macedo LL, Chonka ZD et al. High-resolution CISS MR imaging with and without contrast for evaluation of the upper cranial nerves: Segmental anatomy and selected pathologic conditions of the cisternal through extraforaminal segments. Neuroimaging Clin N Am 2014; 24(1):17–34

[3] Soldatos T, Batra K, Blitz AM, Chhabra A. Lower cranial nerves. Neuroimaging Clin N Am 2014; 24(1):35–47

[4] Choudhri AF, Parmar HA, Morales RE, Gandhi D. Lesions of the skull base: Imaging for diagnosis and treatment. Otolaryngol Clin North Am 2012; 45(6): 1385–1404

[5] Som PM, Naidich TP. Development of the skull base and calvarium: An overview of the progression from mesenchyme to chondrification to ossification. Neurographics 2013; 34:169–184

[6] Som PM, Naidich TP. Illustrated review of the embryology and development of the facial region, Part 1: Early face and lateral nasal cavities. AJNR Am J Neuroradiol 2013; 34(12):2233–2240

[7] Som PM, Naidich TP. Illustrated review of the embryology and development of the facial region, Part 2: Late development of the fetal face and changes in the face from the newborn to adulthood. AJNR Am J Neuroradiol 2014; 35(1): 10–18

[8] Som PM, Streit A, Naidich TP. Illustrated review of the embryology and development of the facial region, Part 3: An overview of the molecular interactions responsible for facial development. AJNR Am J Neuroradiol 2014; 35(2):223–229

Part 3

Head and Neck Imaging

3

17 Neck Soft Tissue

17.1 Introduction

The soft tissues of the neck can be an intimidating area to evaluate radiologically. However, children have numerous congenital and acquired abnormalities within the neck that are best characterized on cross-sectional imaging. Familiarity with the anatomy, disease processes, and clinical management of these conditions will facilitate a systematic approach to the imaging evaluation of the pediatric neck and soft tissues.

17.2 Anatomy

Much of the concern about interpretating studies of the soft tissues of the neck comes from uncertainty about the anatomy of the neck. A review of the normal anatomy of the neck as shown in different imaging modalities is a good start to alleviating this uncertainty. Many methods exist for parcellating the anatomy of the neck, including techniques summarized by description of the fascial planes of the neck, by surgical approaches, and by the relationship of anatomic structures of the neck to other structures. Head and neck anatomy can be (and is) the subject of entire textbooks; however, this chapter provides a brief summary of structures of the head and neck that are relevant to pediatric imaging (▶ Fig. 17.1).

Some textbooks separate the spaces of the neck into triangles based on anatomic boundaries, in many cases the musculature of the neck. In this system, the anterior triangle is defined by the midline of the neck anteriorly, the sternocleidomastoid muscle (SCM) posteriorly, the clavicle inferiorly, and the lower

border of the mandible superiorly. The posterior triangle is defined by the SCM, trapezius muscle, and clavicle. Both the anterior and posterior triangles are further divided into smaller triangles by the deeper neck musculature, notably the omohyoid and digastric muscles, which help to further define anterior subtriangles (submental, submandibular, carotid) and posterior subtriangles (subclavian, occipital). This system is descriptive, but as the triangles on which it is based have variable depths, they are not all that useful for cross-sectional imaging. A different anatomic classification localizes tissues and organs within the fascial planes, which for the most part run circumferentially in the neck, from superficial to deep.

17.3 Fascial Planes

The superficial fascia of the neck encloses the connective tissue, nerves, and blood vessels just beneath the skin. In the head and neck, unlike the rest of the body, the superficial fascia also envelops the muscles of facial expression and the platysma. Deep to the superficial fascia lies the most external layer of the deep cervical fascia, termed the investing fascia. The investing fascia completely surrounds the submandibular glands and sternocleidomastoid and trapezius muscles, and is contiguous with the masseteric–parotid fascia of the face. Deep to the investing fascia lies the carotid sheath, which encompasses the carotid artery, jugular vein, and vagus nerve. Deep and medial to the carotid fascia lies the visceral or pretracheal fascia, which encompasses the trachea, esophagus, and thyroid gland. Posteriorly, the vertebral fascia surrounds the spinal column

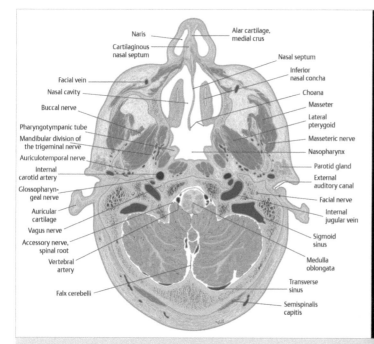
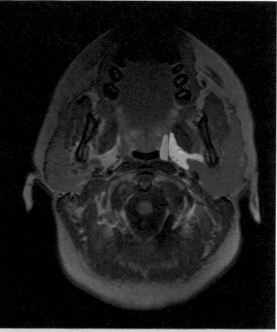

Fig. 17.1 (a) Axial artist's rendering of the neck at the level of the nasopharynx, and (b) axial T1 W plus contrast image at the same level (slightly different angulation) showing the parapharyngeal space (*green overlay*), pharyngeal mucosal space (*yellow*), parotid space (*red*), masticator space (*purple*), and retropharyngeal space (*gray*). "a" From THIEME Atlas of Anatomy, Head and Neuroanatomy, © Thieme 2010, Illustration by Marcus Voll.

Table 17.1 Structures originating from the branchial apparati

Branchial component	Muscle	Nerve	Vessel	Bone/soft tissue
First (mandibular arch)	Muscles of mastication, anterior belly of the digastric, mylohyoid, tensor tympani, and tensor veli palatini muscles	Trigeminal nerve (CN V)	Maxillary artery	Maxilla, mandible, zygomatic bone, incus, malleus
Second (hyoid arch)	Muscles of facial expression	Facial nerve (CN VII)	Stapedial artery, hyoid artery	Stapes, styloid process, hyoid bone (part)
Third	Stylopharyngeus muscle	Glossopharyngeal nerve (IX)	Common carotid, internal carotid artery	Hyoid bone (part), thymus, inferior parathyroids
Fourth	Cricothyroid muscle, muscles of soft palate (except tensor veli palatini)	Vagus nerve (CN X)	Subclavian artery (right), aortic arch (left)	Superior parathyroid glands, thyroid cartilage
Sixth	Intrinsic muscles of larynx (except cricothyroid muscle)	Vagus nerve (CN X), recurrent laryngeal nerve	Pulmonary artery, ductus arteriosus (left)	Cricoid cartilage, arytenoid cartilage

and associated muscles. A space between the prevertebral and visceral fascia is important in the spread of infection from the oral cavity to the mediastinum (discussed in Chapter 23).

Depending on the nature of a disease that affects the neck, it may make sense to refer to fascial planes, anatomic triangles, or specific structures, e.g., the carotid bifurcation, in imaging and describing the disease The radiologist can use the anatomic descriptors named above as a tool set when documenting the locations of radiologic findings in the soft tissues of the neck.

17.4 Congenital Lesions

The largest class of congenital lesions of which to be aware in the pediatric neck are congenital cysts of the branchial apparatus. These are more commonly encountered on standardized tests than in clinical practice. There are six branchial apparati (▶ Table 17.1). It is worth noting that some anatomic purists use the term "pharyngeal" instead of "branchial." The terms are essentially interchangeable, and "branchial" is encountered more often both in clinical practice and in the medical literature, for which reason it is used for the purposes of this chapter.

Of the six branchial arches, the first four can give rise to congenital cysts, which embryologically are related to entrapped cells that form a cyst. Associated with the cyst, there will usually be a sinus tract, which for cysts of the first and second branchial apparatus connects to the skin surface, and for the third and fourth branchial apparatus connects to the upper aerodigestive mucosa. In the presence of a congenital cyst, the sinus tract may be relatively obliterated and be evident only as a small cutaneous pit, or it may be in free communication with the cyst. Branchial cysts can present because of mass effect or palpable/visible swelling, or they may present with an infection. In the acute setting, it can be difficult to determine whether an abscess represents a suppurative lymph node, a soft tissue abscess, or an infected branchial cyst. An infected cyst can look like an abscess; however, it will typically have a more spherical shape and circumscribed margins than an abscess arising from a necrotic lymph node. Follow-up may be required to determine whether the lesion resolves after treatment of the infection.

Cysts of the first branchial apparatus are embryologically associated with the external auditory canal (EAC). The sinus tract may extend to the EAC itself (a type A cyst of the first

branchial apparatus) or to a preauricular pit (a type B cyst of the first branchial apparatus). The cysts can be intraparotid.

A cyst of the second branchial apparatus will have a cutaneous pit in the upper neck below the angle of the mandible, but its location is highly variable. The subclassification of second branchial cysts is based on their relationship to other structures, with the most common classification system having four subtypes. Although the subtypes of second branchial cyst are commonly described as types I through IV, I refer to them as types A through D. This avoids the confusion of describing a type I second branchial cyst as opposed to a type II first branchial cyst, by instead describing these two lesions as a type 2A and a type 1B cyst, respectively. Because cysts of the second branchial apparatus constitute nearly 95% of all branchial cysts, familiarity with the classification (and clarity in the description) of these entities is warranted.

The four subtypes of cyst of the second branchial apparatus (also referred to as the second branchial cleft) are based on the depth of the cyst from the skin, from the most lateral to the most medial, with a type A cyst being the most superficial and a type D cyst being the deepest (▶ Fig. 17.2). A type A cyst is deep to the platysma muscle and anterior to the sternocleidomastoid muscle. A type B cyst, the most common, abuts both the internal carotid artery and internal jugular vein. A type C is is located between the internal and external carotid arteries, and a type D cyst is medial to the internal and external carotid arteries and abuts the pharyngeal wall.

It is critical to be aware of conditions that mimic branchial cysts, in particular a cystic metastatic lymph node. Although metastatic lymph nodes are not common in children, they are more common in young adults and older individuals, particularly as a result of papillary thyroid cancer or carcinoma of the head and neck associated with human papillomavirus (HPV) infection. Therefore, diagnosing a cyst as a branchial apparatus cyst should be avoided in persons beyond adolescence, unless the cyst was known to be present in childhood. Additionally, other etiologies should be considered even for patients in their mid to late teenage years.

A cyst of the fourth branchial cleft develops together with the upper lobe of the thyroid gland, and the sinus tract of this cyst extends to the apex of the left piriform sinus. The most common presentation of a cyst of the fourth branchial cleft (albeit a rare entity) is an abscess within the upper pole of the left lobe

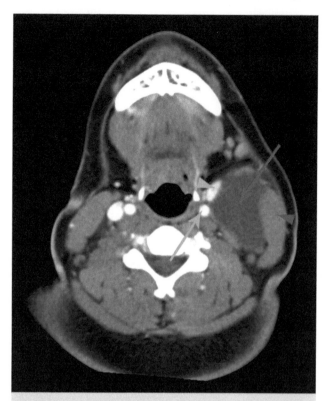

Fig. 17.2 Cyst of the second branchial cleft. Axial contrast-enhanced computed tomographic image of the head of a 17-year-old girl shows a circumscribed, low-density, nonenhancing cystic lesion (*red arrow*) deep to the sternocleidomastoid muscle (*red arrowhead*), and superficial to the internal jugular vein (*green arrowhead*) and common carotid artery (*green arrow*), consistent with a type B cyst of the second branchial cleft.

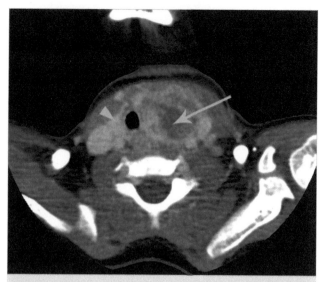

Fig. 17.3 Thyroid abscess. Axial contrast-enhanced computed tomographic image of the head of a 3-year-old boy shows a fluid collection in the left lobe of the thyroid gland (*green arrow*) with surrounding heterogeneous enhancement, consistent with a thyroid abscess. The right lobe of the thyroid gland is normal (*green arrowhead*). A left-lobe thyroid abscess should prompt an investigation for a third/fourth branchial cleft cyst with a sinus tract extending to the apex of the left piriform sinus.

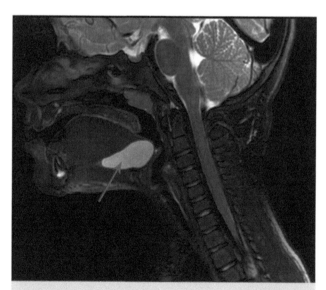

Fig. 17.4 Cyst of the thyroglossal duct. Sagittal T2 W fat-saturated image of the head of a 5-year-old girl shows a circumscribed cystic lesion at the posterior base of the tongue, representing a large cyst of the thyroglossal duct.

of the thyroid (▶ Fig. 17.3). When this diagnosis is suspected, evaluation of the apex of the piriform sinus can provide confirmatory information. This can be evaluated otolaryngologically by direct laryngoscopic visualization, or with a carefully performed barium study. Some authors have recently postulated that the intrathyroid cyst actually arises from the third branchial apparatus, as opposed to the fourth.

Awareness of three congenital cystic lesions of nonbranchial origin is important. The first is a duplication cyst. Duplication cysts can be of enteric or respiratory origin, with differentiation of the two being difficult without histologic analysis of the epithelial lining of the cyst. Collectively, duplication cysts can be referred to as upper aerodigestive duplication cysts when their exact origin is unclear. These cysts will be adjacent to the esophagus, pharynx, or tracheobronchial tree. They may be identified as incidental findings or may present when infected, in which case they appear to be abscesses. The cysts may have communication with the lumen of the aerodigestive tract, which can predispose to the accumulation of debris that can serve as a source of infection.

The thyroglossal duct is the embryologic canal extending from the foramen cecum at the posterior base of the tongue caudally, along the anterior aspect of the midportion of the hyoid bone, and inferiorly to the expected location of the thyroid gland. Cystic remnants of the thyroglossal duct may be identified at any point along its course (▶ Fig. 17.4). Above the hyoid bone the cyst will always be at the midline, but below the hyoid bone it may be slightly off midline. When a cyst is suspected, it is important to look for possible ectopic thyroid tissue, as well as to confirm the presence of orthotopic thyroid tissue having a normal appearance. If there is ectopic thyroid tissue within a cyst and no orthotopic thyroid tissue,

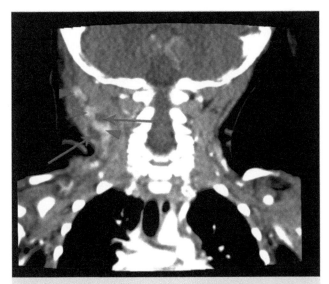

Fig. 17.5 Suppurative adenitis. Coronal contrast-enhanced computed tomographic image of the head and neck of a 4-month-old girl with neck swelling shows multiple right-sided enhancing lymph nodes (*red arrowheads*), and two low-density nodes (*red arrows*) representing suppurative lymph nodes. This does not yet represent an abscess.

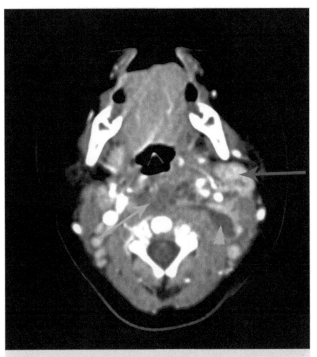

Fig. 17.6 Neck phlegmon. Axial contrast-enhanced computed tomographic image of the neck of a 5-month-old boy with neck swelling and fever shows thickening of the retropharyngeal space (*green arrow*), with fluid extending into the deep soft tissues of the neck (*green arrowhead*) with surrounding heterogeneous enhancement. Because there is no discrete fluid collection with an organized, enhancing rim, this represents a phlegmon instead of an abscess. Note the reactive sialadenitis of the left submandibular gland (*red arrow*).

removal of the cyst (and associated ectopic tissue) will result in permanent hypothyroidism. The presence and distribution of normal thyroid tissue can be determined with a ^{99m}Tc-sestamibi scan. When a cyst of the thyroglossal duct is to be surgically removed, the entire tract must be resected, along with the middle third of the hyoid bone, to prevent recurrence; this is known as the Sistrunk procedure.

A congenital thymic cyst can also be identified in the lower neck. This is typically an incidental finding, but it has the potential for superinfection. The congenital thymic cysts that develop in this location are most often unilocular and have thymic tissue along the cyst wall. If a multilocular cystic lesion is identified, without signs of an infectious etiology, a lesion of vascular origin, such as a lymphatic malformation (a.k.a., lymphangioma or cystic hygroma) or venous malformation (previously known as a cavernous hemangioma), should be suspected; refer to Chapter 19 for further description of these entities.

17.5 Acquired Conditions

Although congenital lesions of the neck are important in differential diagnoses, surgical planning, and for purposes of testing, by far the most common set of abnormalities encountered within the neck in most practice settings are acquired abnormalities, with infections in children an important group of such abnormalities. Although any structure within the neck can sustain trauma, this section focuses predominantly on infectious conditions.

With most infections of the neck, there will be reactive lymphadenopathy. The detailed measurement of reactive lymph nodes is a practice largely based on the staging of adult head and neck cancer and usually serves no purpose in the evaluation of pediatric head and neck infections. Additionally, numerical levels for the head and neck are more relevant for the staging and surgical planning of head and neck cancer and not directly relevant to the situation with infection.

Infected lymph nodes may undergo suppurative changes (▶ Fig. 17.5), in which they have a relatively spherical shape with a low central density; these do not represent abscesses, but rather suppurative adenitis. The infection in such nodes may break through the capsules of the nodes and result in a conglomeration of infected lymph nodes, known as a phlegmon (▶ Fig. 17.6). The phlegmon will be ill defined on imaging but will show areas of enhancement and poorly marginated areas of nonenhancing fluid, yet it is not considered to represent an abscess because there is no discretely drainable collection of fluid or organized rim. Eventually the phlegmon organizes, with a more discrete fluid collection, at which point it is considered an abscess. The distinction between a phlegmon and an abscess is important because the aspiration of, or drain placement within, a phlegmon will not result in appreciable drainage or a marked reduction in its size. Regardless of the stage of evolution at which an infectious process is encountered, it can affect adjacent structures. Thus, for example, infectious collections can cause partial (or complete) effacement of the internal jugular vein. In some cases infection can lead to septic thrombophlebitis of the internal jugular vein, often in association with the oropharyngeal anaerobic bacterium *Fusobacterium necrophorum*, putting the patient at risk for septic thromboemboli to the lung in the condition known as Lemierre's syndrome

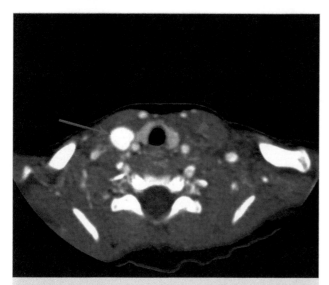

Fig. 17.7 Lemierre's syndrome. Axial contrast-enhanced computed tomographic image of the upper torso and neck of an 11-month-old girl shows a low-density area in the expected location of the left internal jugular vein (*red arrowhead*), and a widely patent right internal jugular vein (*red arrow*). This represents septic thrombophlebitis of the left internal jugular vein, or Lemierre's syndrome.

(▶ Fig. 17.7). Infectious collections adjacent to the carotid artery and its branches may result in vasospasm.

Retropharyngeal swelling can result in airway narrowing. When this is seen, sometimes initially identified on a lateral radiograph of the neck, identification of the etiology is important. At times this radiographic appearance can be an artifact caused by the phase of inspiration, patient swallowing, or underlying asymmetry of the soft tissues of the neck, but the primary concern when airway narrowing is seen is a retropharyngeal abscess. If a retropharyngeal abscess is identified, close attention should be given to bone algorithm images of the cervical spine for signs of osteomyelitis, disk space narrowing, or irregularities suggestive of diskitis. It may also be possible to see an epidural abscess (see Chapter 25). A retropharyngeal abscess will, like most abscesses, have an enhancing peripheral rim with central hypodensity. Retropharyngeal thickening can be seen with nonenhancing collections of low density, probably in relation to edema and/or cellulitis, which may be the precursor to an abscess.

Infection in the soft tissues overlying salivary glands may result in secondary sialadenitis (inflammation of a salivary gland) (▶ Fig. 17.6). An intramuscular abscess within the sternocleidomastoid muscle in relation to the caudal extension of coalescent mastoiditis with osseous dehiscence is known as a Bezold abscess; its treatment requires addressing both the intramuscular abscess and the mastoiditis.

An abscess centered in the poststyloid parapharyngeal space is a deep neck abscess and can be a management challenge. Direct surgical access to such an abscess is complicated by the overlying parotid gland (which carries the facial nerve), and a transoral approach does not provide direct access. An inferior approach can be used, but the major arterial and venous structures in the region make this complicated. Computed tomography guided drainage can be considered in this condition. An infection in the parapharyngeal space is sometimes referred to as a "peritonsillar" abscess, but the term "peritonsillar" does not appropriately recognize the location of such a condition in the deep neck space, and this inconsistently defined term should generally be avoided. Further description of infectious processes involving the palatine tonsils is given in Chapter 23.

17.6 Fibromatosis Colli

An idiopathic process seen in infants with torticollis is fibromatosis colli, which is thought to be related to a noninfectious inflammatory fibromatosis in the sterncleidomastoid muscle. If imaging of this condition is required, it is most appropriately done with ultrasonography. The latter will show thickening of the affected sternocleidomastoid muscle without a discrete mass (▶ Fig. 17.8). The torticollis will involve the patient's looking away from the side of involvement. When findings characteristic of fibromatosis colli are made with ultrasonography, no further imaging is required.

17.7 Thyroid Gland

The normal thyroid gland is located in the anterior aspect of the lower neck, with two lobes connected across the midline by an isthmus. The iodine sequestered in the gland will give it a high density on an unenhanced computed tomographic scan. Some patients have a congenital absence of the thyroid gland, usually in the setting of a lingual thyroid and/or thyroid tissue along

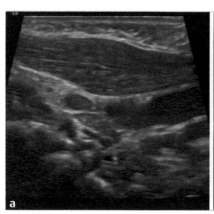
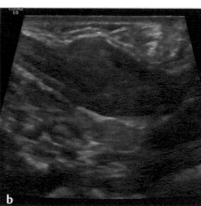

Fig. 17.8 Fibromatosis colli. Sagittal ultrasonographic images of the (a) right and (b) left sternocleidomastoid muscles demonstrates enlargement and heterogeneous internal characteristics on the left side, consistent with fibromatosis colli. Normal longitudinal muscle striations are seen on the right side.

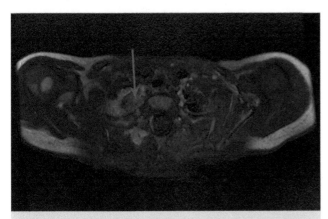

Fig. 17.9 Horner syndrome. Axial T1 W fat-saturated plus contrast image of the neck and upper torso of a 16-month-old male with right-sided Horner syndrome shows a mass at the apex of the right lung (*red arrow*), which was identified to be a nerve-sheath tumor. Evaluation of Horner syndrome requires imaging of the brain, cervical spine, neck, and upper chest to below the level of the aortic arch, because abnormalities along any portion of the sympathetic chain can cause the syndrome.

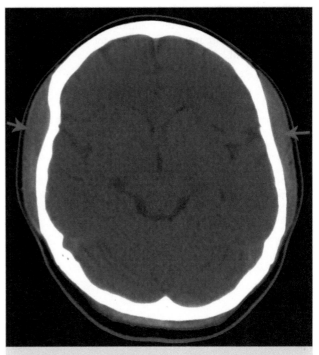

Fig. 17.10 Bruxism. Axial computed tomographic image of the head of a 16-year-old girl with headaches shows hypertrophy of the temporalis muscles bilaterally (*red arrows*), which is a finding associated with bruxism.

the course of the thyroglossal duct. Scanning with ^{99m}Tc-sesta-mibi can help determine whether functioning orthotopic thyroid tissue is present in a patient with ectopic thyroid tissue, although the finding of a morphologically normal thyroid gland on ultrasonography, computed tomography, or magnetic resonance imaging (MRI) may obviate the need for this test. Although small intrathyroid cysts and nodules are common in adults, they are rare in children, and focal lesions warrant thyroid function tests and probably also warrant follow-up imaging, with ultrasonography the modality of choice for evaluation of the thyroid parenchyma. Occasionally, Graves disease and Hashimoto's thyroiditis can be seen in children, with an imaging appearance and clinical presentation similar to that in adults.

17.8 Neoplasm

Other than a capillary (infantile) hemangioma in the first year of life, soft tissue neoplasms of the neck are rare in children (see Chapter 19). The possibilities for those that do occur include metastatic neuroblastoma, which will present as a soft tissue mass, often have calcifications visible on computed tomography (CT), and have restricted diffusion on MRI; rhabdoid tumors, which will be heterogeneous lesions with myriad appearances; and sarcomas which also will have a variety of appearances on imaging.

17.9 Horner Syndrome

Horner syndrome is the triad of clinical findings of ptosis, miosis, and anhidrosis related to impaired sympathetic innervation of an eye. Ptosis is drooping of the eyelid, in this case due to impaired function of the superior tarsal muscle, also known as Müller's muscle. Miosis is pupillary constriction from impaired function of the radial dilator muscles of the iris, and because the pupils are asymmetric, this represents a form of anisocoria. Anhidrosis in the setting of Horner syndrome is decreased sweating of the ipsilateral face, as this function is also mediated

by sympathetic fibers. The sympathetic fibers descend from the brainstem to the upper thoracic cord, where the preganglionic fibers join the sympathetic plexus. The fibers synapse, in this case in the stellate ganglion, and the postganglionic fibers ascend with the carotid artery. Some fibers of the deep petrosal nerve join the greater superficial petrosal nerve (preganglionic parasympathetic fibers originating with CN VII) to form the vidian nerve, and eventually reach the orbit by ascending from the pterygopalatine fossa through the inferior orbital fissure. Other fibers travel with the carotid artery to the cavernous sinus and extend to the orbit through the superior orbital fissure. An abnormality along any portion of the sympathetic chain can result in Horner syndrome, and the study of choice for evaluating this is therefore an MRI of the brain, neck/cervical spine, and upper chest (see appendix on MRI protocols) (▸ Fig. 17.9).

It should be noted that a third nerve palsy can also result in ptosis, owing to the innervation by this nerve of the levator palpebrae superioris muscle, as well as mydriasis, or pupillary enlargement, owing to impaired function of the circular fibers of the sphincter muscle of the iris. Additionally, third nerve palsies will typically result in an abnormal position of the eye (inferolateral deviation). These funcitons are mediated by parasympathetic fibers of CN III; sympathetic fibers do not play a direct role in eye movement.

17.10 Miscellaneous

Individuals who grind their teeth excessively (bruxism) can have hypertrophy of the temporalis and masseter muscles owing to excessive activity of these muscles (▸ Fig. 17.10). This can be the cause of headaches. Patients with bruxism are at risk for degenerative changes of the mandibular condyle and articular disk, which can result in severe pain of the temporomandibular joint.

17.11 Suggested Reading

[1] LaPlante JK, Pierson NS, Hedlund GL. Common pediatric head and neck congenital/developmental anomalies. Radiol Clin North Am 2015; 53(1):181–196

[2] Hegde SV, Armstrong LK, Ramakrishnaiah RH, Shah CC. A space-based approach to pediatric face and neck infections. Neurographics 2014; 4(1):43–52

[3] Warshafsky D, Goldenberg D, Kanekar SG. Imaging anatomy of deep neck spaces. Otolaryngol Clin North Am 2012; 45(6):1203–1221

[4] Kanekar SG, Mannion K, Zacharia T, Showalter M. Parotid space: Anatomic imaging. Otolaryngol Clin North Am 2012; 45(6):1253–1272

[5] Gamss C, Gupta A, Chazen JL, Phillips CD. Imaging evaluation of the suprahyoid neck. Radiol Clin North Am 2015; 53(1):133–144

[6] Johnson JM, Moonis G, Green GE, Carmody R, Burbank HN. Syndromes of the first and second branchial arches, Part 1: Embryology and characteristic defects. AJNR Am J Neuroradiol 2011; 32(1):14–19

[7] Johnson JM, Moonis G, Green GE, Carmody R, Burbank HN. Syndromes of the first and second branchial arches, Part 2: Syndromes. AJNR Am J Neuroradiol 2011; 32(2):230–237

[8] Ludwig BJ, Foster BR, Saito N, Nadgir RN, Castro-Aragon I, Sakai O. Diagnostic imaging in nontraumatic pediatric head and neck emergencies. Radiographics 2010; 30(3):781–799

[9] Meuwly J-Y, Lepori D, Theumann N et al. Multimodality imaging evaluation of the pediatric neck: Techniques and spectrum of findings. Radiographics 2005; 25(4):931–948

[10] Tumu AY, Chandra T, Maheshwari M, Kelly TG, Segall HD. Imaging of pediatric aerodigestive tract disorders. Neurographics 2014; 4(1):33–42

18 Craniofacial Abnormalities

18.1 Introduction

Acquired and congenital craniofacial abnormalities can be intimidating because of the complex anatomy and apparent overlap of the clinical and imaging features of many of these entities. Regardless of the diagnosis, the ability to recognize the specific features demonstrated in a particular case of craniofacial abnormality can complement clinical and genetic information in making its diagnosis.

18.2 Anatomy

Although understanding craniofacial embryology is not necessary to the understanding of anatomy, knowledge of craniofacial development can help in the interpretation of anatomic abnormalities and deformities. For example, the first branchial arch normally fuses with the frontonasal process at 4 to 6 weeks of gestation, and failure of this fusion results in cleft lip. Another good example of the relationship between embryology and craniofacial anomalies is seen in branchial cleft cysts, which are further discussed in Chapter 17. Although craniofacial embryology is not reviewed here, the relationship between embryology and anatomy should be appreciated, and the embryology relevant to a particular anomaly is referenced if pertinent.

Ultimately, both pre- and postnatal development lead to the familiar structures of the human head and face. This chapter primarily focuses on the osseous anatomy of these structures.

The main bones of the face are the mandible and maxilla (▶ Fig. 18.1a). The orbits are formed by multiple bones,

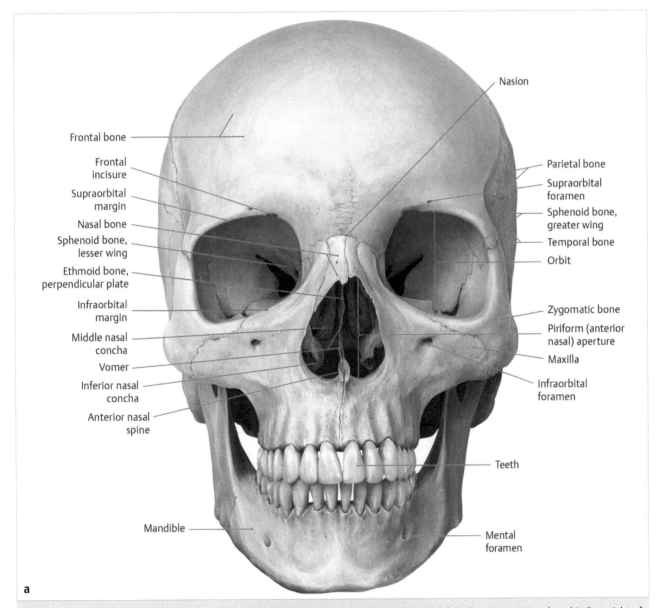

Fig. 18.1 (a,b) Facial bones. Artist's depiction of the bones forming the face, and a magnified view of the bones comprising the orbit. From Atlas of Anatomy, © Thieme 2012, Illustration by Karl Wesker. (*continued*)

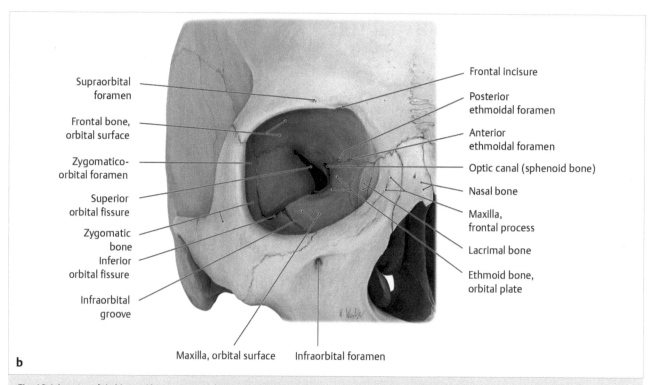

b

Fig. 18.1 (*continued*) (a,b) Facial bones. Artist's depiction of the bones forming the face, and a magnified view of the bones comprising the orbit. From Atlas of Anatomy, © Thieme 2012, Illustration by Karl Wesker.

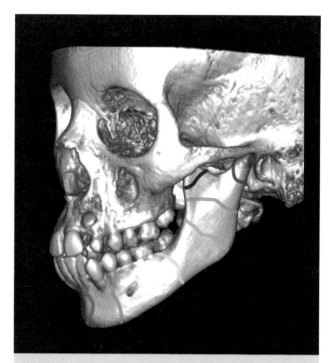

Fig. 18.2 Locations of mandibular fractures. Three-dimensional rendering of the face from a computed tomogram showing the different locations of mandibular fractures, including symphyseal (red) and parasymphyseal (orange) fractures; fractures in the body (yellow), angle (green), and ramus (blue); and condylar/subcondylar (purple) and coronoid (black) fractures.

including the maxillary, frontal, zygomatic, ethmoid, sphenoid, lacrimal, and palatine bones (▶ Fig. 18.1b). The nose is formed by the maxilla and nasal bones, and the nasal septum by the vomer and ethmoid bones, along with cartilage. The forehead is predominantly supported by the frontal bone and the squamous portions of the temporal bones. The cheek is supported largely by the zygoma, a very important bone, which rigidly articulates with the maxillary, temporal, frontal, and sphenoid bones. The cranium is composed of flat bones creating the cranial cap (calvarium) and by a set of bones creating the cranial base. The anatomy of the skull, orbits, and oral cavity is discussed in further detail in Chapters 15, 21, and 23, respectively.

18.3 Facial Trauma

Facial trauma in children has patterns similar to those in adults, but identifying abnormalities in the setting of developing bones may be more complex than in mature bones. Additionally, it is important to attempt to use the most radiation-optimized diagnostic algorithm when imaging children.

Because mandibular fractures typically do not occur in isolation, it is important to follow the identification of such a fracture with an investigation for an occult secondary fracture. Alternatively, the disruption/displacement of the temporomandibular joint may serve as a second point of pressure release, instead of a second fracture being present (▶ Fig. 18.2). Mandibular fractures are also often seen in conjunction with fractures of the spine. Additionally, greenstick-type bowing fractures can occur in the face in children just as they do in the extremities.

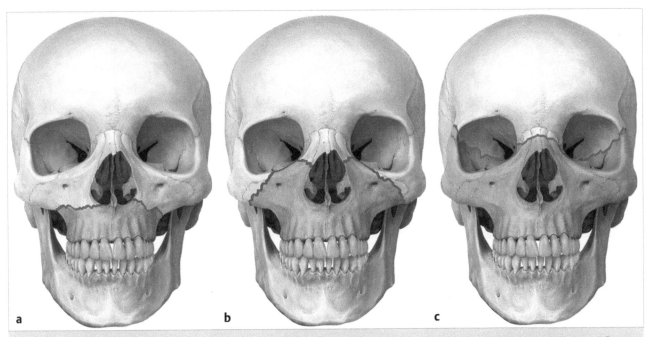

Fig. 18.3 Le Fort fractures. (a) Le Fort type I—Horizontally oriented fractures through the maxilla, and the pterygoid plates, resulting in a "floating palate." (b) Le Fort type II—angled fractures through the maxilla and inferior orbital rims, crossing the midline, as well as involvement of the pterygoid plates. (c) Le Fort type III—Horizontally oriented fracture through the zygomatic arches, lateral orbital wall, and across the midline through the ethmoid sinuses, also involving the pterygoid plates. This results in craniofacial dissociation ("floating face"). From Atlas of Anatomy, © Thieme 2012, Illustration by Karl Wesker.

Complex maxillofacial trauma is sometimes described with the Le Fort classification system, which describes common patterns of facial skeletal trauma and can provide useful descriptors to surgeons. Because all subtypes of fracture in the Le Fort system involve fractures of the pterygoid plates, the finding of such a fracture should raise a degree of high suspicion for a Le Fort fracture. Fractures at other sites determine the type of Le Fort fracture. Thus, for example, a Le Fort I fracture extends through the piriform rim and posterolaterally through the maxillary sinuses and zygomaticomaxillary buttress to the lower aspect of the pterygoid plates. With respect to a frontal view of the face, Le Fort I fractures are said to follow the distribution of a moustache. A Le Fort II fracture involves the nasal bridge and extends laterally through the orbit, down through the inferior orbital rim, and posteriorly through the zygomaticomaxillary buttress to the pterygoid plates. With respect to a frontal view of the face, Le Fort II fractures follow the distribution of the nasal bridge of a pair of eyeglasses. A Le Fort III fracture also involves the nasal bridge and extends from the nasal bones laterally through the orbit, but continues through the lateral orbital wall and inferiorly involves the zygomatic arch and pterygoid plate. With respect to a frontal view of the face, Le Fort III fractures follow the orientation of a pair of eyeglasses (▸ Fig. 18.3).

Classically, Le Fort fractures are bilateral; the term *hemi-Le Fort* can be used for a fracture that is unilateral. In summary, all types of Le Fort fracture involve the pterygoid plates. Fractures classified uniquely by type in the Le Fort system include those involving the piriform rim (type I), inferior orbital rim (type II), and lateral orbital wall along with the zygomatic arch (type III).[1]

Another important fracture pattern is one that involves the zygomaticomaxillary complex (ZMC), sometimes called a "tripod" fracture, although this is a misnomer because the pattern of injury in such a fracture has more than three components. As mentioned, the zygoma articulates with four other facial bones. In the setting of direct trauma, fracture can occur at the sites of any of these four sutures, which are: (1) the zygomaticofrontal (lateral orbit), (2) zygomaticosphenoid (orbital floor), (3) zygomaticotemporal (arch), and (4) zygomaticomaxillary (maxillary sinus and inferior orbital rim) sutures. If this fracture pattern is seen, a ZMC fracture can be documented, with additional information provided about the degree of displacement and adjacent tissue injury at each suture site.

Orbital trauma, including fractures of the orbital floor and medial orbital wall, is further discussed in Chapter 21.

18.4 Craniofacial Syndromes

Congenital syndromes of craniofacial development have characteristic osseous and soft tissue features. The class of disorders known as hemifacial (or craniofacial) microsomia is marked by unilateral hypoplasia of structures arising from the first and second branchial apparati. Goldenhar syndrome is a type of hemifacial microsomia with associated vertebral anomalies. Involved structures include the mandible, maxilla, orbit, external ear, facial soft tissues, and cranial nerve VII (▸ Fig. 18.4). The inner ear, which arises from the otic placode, will typically be normal in Goldenhar syndrome. The acronym OMENS, representing the first letters of "orbit," "mandible," "ear," "nerve" (CN VII), and "soft tissue," is the basis for a surgical scoring system used to describe the abnormalities in hemifacial microsomia (▸ Table 18.1).

Treacher–Collins syndrome (TCS) is a developmental condition in which mandibular and zygomatic hypoplasia is accompanied by abnormalities of the external and middle ear.

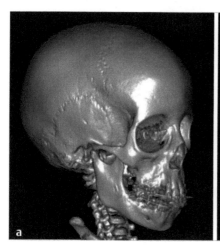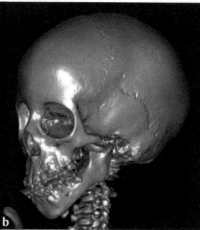

Fig. 18.4 Hemifacial microsomia. Three-dimensional computed tomographic images from (a) right and (b) left frontal oblique projections, showing hypoplasia of the left mandible.

Table 18.1 OMENS surgical scoring system for abnormalities in hemifacial microsomia[a]

Orbit		
O0		Normal orbital size, position
O1		Abnormal orbital size
O2		Abnormal orbital position
O3		Abnormal orbital size, position
Mandible		
M0		Normal mandible
M1		Small mandible and glenoid fossa with short ramus
M2		Ramus short and abnormally shaped
	2A	Glenoid fossa in anatomically acceptable position
	2B	Temporomandibular joint inferiorly, medially, and anteriorly displaced, with severely hypoplastic condyle
M3		Complete absence of ramus, glenoid fossa, and temporomandibular joint
Ear		
E0		Normal ear
E1		Minor hypoplasia and cupping with all structures present
E2		Absence of external auditory canal with variable hypoplasia of the auricle
E3		Malposition of the lobule with absent auricle, lobular remnant usually inferior anteriorly displaced
Facial nerve		
N0		No facial-nerve involvement
N1		Upper facial-nerve involvement (temporal or zygomatic branches)
N2		Lower facial-nerve involvement (buccal, mandibular, or cervical)
N3		All branches affected
Soft tissue		
S0		No soft tissue or muscle deficiency
S1		Minimal tissue or muscle deficiency
S2		Moderate tissue or muscle deficiency
S3		Severe tissue or muscle deficiency

[a]OMENS: orbit, mandible, ear, nerve (CN VII), soft tissue.
Used with permission from Vento AR, et al., The O.M.E.N.S classification of hemifacial microsomia, 1991, Cleft Palate Craniofac, J 28, p. 68–76.

The developmental abnormalities of the ear in this condition commonly result in a conductive hearing loss, and there is also an increased incidence of cleft palate. The function of the facial nerve (CN VII) is intact in TCS, differentiating it from bilateral hemifacial microsomia. The facial deformities of TCS are also remarkably symmetric, further distinguishing this syndrome from bilateral hemifacial microsomia.

The Pierre Robin sequence (PRS) is a series of developmental malformations that include cleft palate, micrognathia, and glossoptosis (▶ Fig. 18.5). The sequence is thought to be primarily related to micrognathia, which results in glossoptosis, which in turn prevents the hard palate from forming. The condition is referred to as a sequence (and sometimes simply as the Robin sequence) because these events happen in a sequential manner, and can result from mandibular hypoplasia of differing etiologies.

Midface hypoplasia is a feature of achondroplasia, together with other features, including frontal bossing, stenosis of the foramen magnum and jugular foramen, and lumbar spinal stenosis.

Recent genetic work has allowed the classification of many skeletal dysplasias related to abnormalities of the fibroblast growth factor receptor (FGFR), including Pfeiffer syndrome, Apert syndrome, Crouzon syndrome, and achondroplasia (▶ Fig. 18.6). Several craniofacial syndromes related to abnormalities in the FGFR are listed in ▶ Table 18.2, but many additional syndromes exist. Description of the key features of these syndromes on imaging, including abnormalities in development of the mandible, maxilla, orbits, and temporal bone, in conjunction with a radiographic skeletal survey for additional musculoskeletal manifestations, can help in clinically categorizing a particular syndrome.

Many abnormalities of craniofacial development result in atypical positioning of the orbits, which can be either too closely spaced (hypotelorism) or too widely spaced (hypertelorism). As an approximation, a distance between the medial walls of the orbits that is approximately equal to the width of the globe of the eye is considered to represent normal spacing. However, considerable variation exists in the spacing of the orbits, and ultimately this is a facial feature that is more evident clinically than upon imaging, for which reason imaging should not be the primary means of diagnosis of an abnormality in craniofacial development.

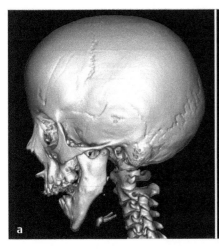
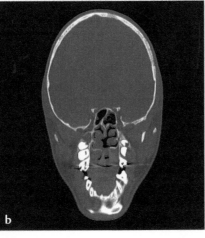

Fig. 18.5 Pierre Robin sequence. (a) Lateral projection from a three-dimensional computed tomographic rendering of the head of an 11-year-old boy with Pierre Robin sequence shows mandibular hypoplasia with an associated underbite. (b) Coronal bone algorithm computed tomographic image shows a midline cleft in the hard palate (*red arrowheads*).

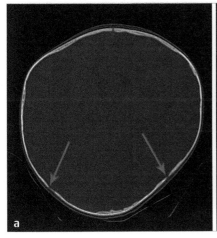
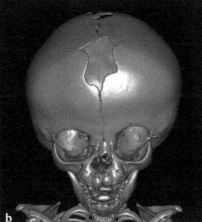

Fig. 18.6 Bilateral coronal craniosynostosis. (a) Axial computed tomographic image of the head of a 10-month-old girl with Crouzon syndrome shows patency of the lambdoid sutures bilaterally (*red arrows*) and of the metopic suture; however, the coronal sutures are not identified. (b) Three-dimensional rendering of a frontal projection of the same patient's head shows subtle bony ridges/angulations corresponding with the expected locations of closed coronal sutures. The metopic suture is patent, and the anterior fontanelle remains widely patent.

Table 18.2 Select syndromes affecting craniofacial development

Name of syndrome	Findings	Genetics/associations
Pfeiffer	Craniosynostosis, developmental abnormalities of the hands and feet	FGFR1 and FGFR2
Apert	Developmental abnormalities of the skull and face (first and second branchial apparati), hands, and feet (acrocephalosyndactyly)	FGFR2
Crouzon	Craniofacial developmental abnormalities, cleft palate, typically normal hands and feet	FGFR2
Achondroplasia	Retarded growth of long bones	FGFR3
Goldenhar	Developmental abnormalities of the skull and face (first and second branchial apparati), abnormalities of the soft palate and lip, vertebral anomalies, subtype of hemifacial microsomia	
Treacher–Collins	Craniofacial abnormalities, including micrognathia and aural atresia, intact facial nerve (cranial nerve VII)	TCOF1

18.5 Clefts

A number of facial clefts have been described. Most commonly, cleft lip with or without cleft palate will be encountered. Isolated cleft palate, without cleft lip, is considered a separate entity with different implications about the genetic syndromes in which it can occur and about the abnormalities associated with it. Cleft lip can be unilateral or bilateral and complete or incomplete. A complete cleft involves the maxillary alveolus and upper lip, extending through the nasal floor.[2]

Additional osseous and soft tissue clefts of the face exist, characterized by the Tessier classification system, however these are very rare and are beyond the scope of this chapter.

18.6 Suggested Reading

[1] Som PM, Naidich TP. Illustrated review of the embryology and development of the facial region, Part 1: Early face and lateral nasal cavities. AJNR Am J Neuroradiol 2013; 34(12):2233–2240

[2] Som PM, Naidich TP. Illustrated review of the embryology and development of the facial region, Part 2: Late development of the fetal face and changes in the face from the newborn to adulthood. AJNR Am J Neuroradiol 2014; 35(1): 10–18

[3] Som PM, Streit A, Naidich TP. Illustrated review of the embryology and development of the facial region, Part 3: An overview of the molecular interactions responsible for facial development. AJNR Am J Neuroradiol 2014; 35(2):223–229

[4] Johnson JM, Moonis G, Green GE, Carmody R, Burbank HN. Syndromes of the first and second branchial arches, Part 1: Embryology and characteristic defects. AJNR Am J Neuroradiol 2011; 32(1):14–19

[5] Johnson JM, Moonis G, Green GE, Carmody R, Burbank HN. Syndromes of the first and second branchial arches, Part 2: Syndromes. AJNR Am J Neuroradiol 2011; 32(2):230–237

[6] Alcalá-Galiano A, Arribas-García IJ, Martín-Pérez MA, Romance A, Montalvo-Moreno JJ, Juncos JMM. Pediatric facial fractures: Children are not just small adults. Radiographics 2008; 28(2):441–461, quiz 618

[7] Winegar BA, Murillo H, Tantiwongkosi B. Spectrum of critical imaging findings in complex facial skeletal trauma. Radiographics 2013; 33(1):3–19

References

[1] Rhea JT, Novelline RA. How to simplify the CT diagnosis of Le Fort fractures. AJR Am J Roentgenol 2005; 184(5):1700–1705

[2] Abramson ZR, Peacock ZS, Cohen HL, Choudhri AF. Radiology of cleft lip and palate: Imaging for the prenatal period and throughout life. Radiographics 2015; 35:2053–2063 Published online 10.1148/rg.2015150050

19 Vascular Abnormalities of the Head and Neck

19.1 Introduction

Multiple vascular malformations and vascular neoplasms of the neck are relatively unique to the pediatric population and merit clinical familiarity. The terminology used to describe these vascular malformations and neoplasms can initially be confusing, but they differ in age of onset, features on imaging, and treatment, and the correct terminology for describing them is therefore important. Additionally, traumatic and infectious complications can affect the major arterial and venous structures of the neck and must be recognized and characterized.

19.2 Anatomy

The major arterial structures of the neck are the bilateral carotid and vertebral arteries (▶ Fig. 19.1). The common carotid arteries branch in the midneck to give rise to the internal and external carotid arteries. The internal carotid arteries predominantly supply the intracranial contents, while the external carotid arteries supply the face and neck. The vertebral arteries predominantly supply the posterior cranial fossa, including the brainstem and cerebellum, as well as the thalami and occipital lobes, and contribute to the blood supply of the cervical spinal cord.

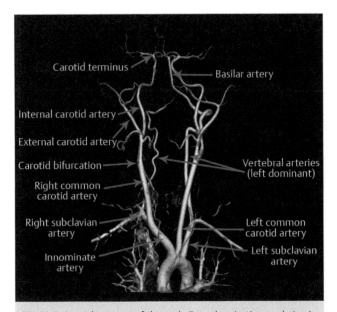

Fig. 19.1 Arterial anatomy of the neck. Frontal-projection rendering in three dimensions of a computed tomographic angiogram showing a three-vessel branching pattern from the aortic arch, giving rise to the innominate, left common carotid, and left subclavian arteries. The innominate artery branches into the right subclavian and right common carotid arteries. Each of the two common carotid arteries branches in the midneck into the internal and external carotid arteries. The two subclavian arteries give rise to the vertebral arteries.

19.3 Hemangiomas of Infancy

Vascular malformations of the head and neck are commonly encountered in children, including malformations identified after symptomatic presentation and those found incidentally in the course of examinations for other reasons. These lesions may present as swellings or through mass effect on another structure, sometimes with skin discoloration. A majority, however, are small capillary hemangiomas identified on clinical examination and do not require imaging evaluation.

Rather than being classified as a vascular malformation, the lesions known as capillary hemangiomas are in actuality vascular neoplasms. They differ from "cavernous hemangiomas," which can, for example, be seen in the adult orbit and are venous malformations rather than vascular neoplasms (and are therefore not hemangiomas, and accordingly the term "cavernous hemangioma" should be avoided), and the prefix "capillary" should be used to describe these lesions to differentiate them from other entities described as hemangiomas.

Capillary hemangiomas have several patterns of presentation. An infantile hemangioma, sometimes called a "strawberry mark," is a capillary hemangioma that is not present at birth, but grows during the first 6 to 12 months of life (proliferative phase), after which it shows a variable period of stability (plateau phase), and eventually involutes (involution phase). Capillary hemangiomas have a characteristic hyperintense appearance on T2 W images, may have internal flow voids, and demonstrate diffuse enhancement (▶ Fig. 19.2). On dynamic imaging the enhancement tends to be in the arterial phase of blood flow through the lesion. The lesions show diffuse vascularity on Doppler ultrasonography.

Although capillary hemangiomas eventually involute spontaneously, the process of involution can be accelerated by beta blocker (propranolol) therapy. The decision to use propranolol is based on several possible indications. One such indication may be large size and/or rapid growth of a hemangioma, and/or mass effect on important structures, such as the airway or major vascular structures. Even small lesions that impair eye movement or eyelid opening may be treated to prevent amblyopia. In some instances, the decision to treat a hemangioma is based on cosmetic rather than clinical concerns.

Magnetic resonance imaging (MRI) and ultrasonography serve a complementary role in evaluating capillary hemangiomas. Computed tomography is typically not needed, given that the information required for identifying and treating these lesions can be obtained by other means, without the use of ionizing radiation.

In addition to infantile hemangiomas, the category of vascular lesions known as capillary hemangiomas includes the lesions known as congenital hemangiomas. In contrast to infantile hemangiomas, congenital hemangiomas are present at birth. Congenital hemangiomas fall into two categories; those that spontaneously involute, and those that do not. These are respectively named rapidly involuting congenital hemangiomas (RICH) and noninvoluting congenital hemangiomas (NICH). However, it may not be possible, without follow-up, to know whether a particular hemangioma belongs in the first or second of these two categories.

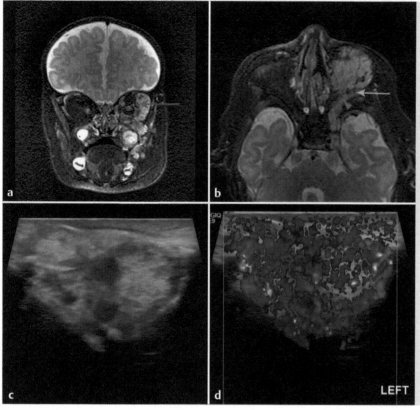

Fig. 19.2 Capillary hemangioma as seen with magnetic resonance imaging and ultrasonography. (a) Axial T2 W fat-saturated (FS) image of the head of a 1-month-old girl shows a hyperintense lesion in the orbit (*red arrow*), with extension into the masticator space (*red arrowhead*). (b) Axial T2 W FS image shows posterior extension that fills the pterygopalatine fossa (*red arrowhead*) and extends through foramen rotundum to the cavernous sinus (*red arrow*), and of the lateral extension of the pterygopalatine fossa through the pterygomaxillary fissure (*green arrow*). (c) Gray-scale and (d) Doppler ultrasonographic images of the infraorbital portion of the lesion show a heterogeneous mass with diffuse internal vascularity. This represents a capillary (infantile) hemangioma.

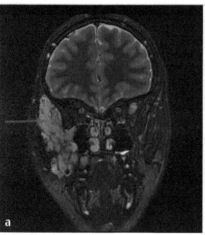
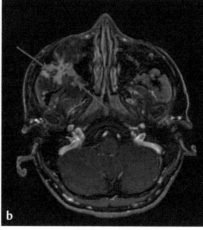

Fig. 19.3 Venous malformation. (a) Coronal T2 W fat-saturated (FS) image of the head of a 17-year-old boy with a history of facial swelling shows a multilobulated right facial mass (*red arrow*), with a focal area of hypointensity (*red arrowhead*) representing a phlebolith. (b) Axial T1 W FS plus contrast image shows heterogeneous enhancement within the lesion (*red arrows*). This represents a venous malformation.

19.4 Venous Malformations

A venous malformation is a vascular malformation with very slow blood flow and that tends to have internal enhancement, particularly on delayed images. Like capillary hemangiomas, venous malformations tend to be hyperintense on T2 W images (▶ Fig. 19.3), but have a more lobulated external contour. They may have internal phleboliths, and they have previously been described as "cavernous hemangiomas," although they are not hemangiomas. Venous malformations are more likely than capillary hemangiomas to present in late childhood or adolescence than in the infantile period. They can be treated with percutaneous sclerotherapy, using agents like ethanol and sodium tetradecyl sulfate, as well as by surgical excision and by a multimodal approach.

Some venous malformations, commonly referred to as venolymphatic malformations, have areas that resemble lymphatic malformations and additional, internally enhancing areas that resemble venous malformations. Among venolymphatic malformations are some that are predominantly venous and others that are predominantly lymphatic, with still others having greater or lesser degrees of each of these two characteristics. Therefore, when describing these lesions, it is important, for their appropriate management, to discuss their different

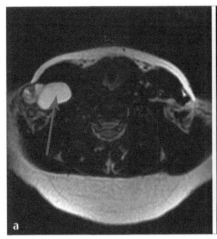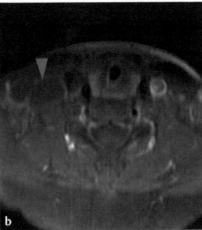

Fig. 19.4 Lymphatic malformation. (a) Axial T2 W image of the neck of a 10-year-old boy with neck swelling shows a cystic-appearing right supra-clavicular mass (*red arrow*). (b) Axial T1 W fat-saturated (FS) plus contrast image shows a peripheral rim of enhancement (*red arrowhead*) but no internal enhancement. This represents a lymphatic malformation.

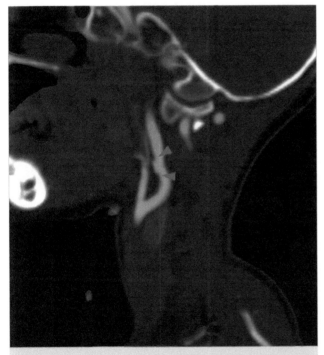

Fig. 19.5 Arterial dissection/dissecting aneurysm. Sagittal image made with computed tomographic angiography of the head and neck of a 6-year-old boy with trauma to the neck shows a focal contour irregularity along the anterior wall of the internal carotid artery (*red arrowheads*), representing a dissecting aneurysm ("pseudoaneurysm").

lesion can have macroscopic or microscopic cystic areas. Because of spontaneous hemorrhage, the macrocystic lymphatic components of a lymphatic malformation may have layering hematocrit levels (▶ Fig. 19.4). A lymphatic malformation may have weak enhancement of its periphery or of internal septations, but it will not have solid, mass-like enhancement. The management of lymphatic malformations may involve observation; sclerotherapy with agents like ethanol, bleomycin, doxycycline, and OK-432; surgical excision; or a combination of these modalities.

19.6 Traumatic Vascular Injury

Trauma, and particularly penetrating trauma, can result in injury to the arteries of the neck. Blunt trauma to the neck is less likely to result in vascular injury in children than in adults.[1] Trauma can result in a focal arterial dissection (▶ Fig. 19.5), which predisposes to embolus formation and stroke. Penetrating trauma predisposes to the formation of a dissecting aneurysm, also referred to as a pseudoaneurysm (▶ Fig. 19.5). Traumatic arterial dissection from an acceleration–deceleration injury can occur at the entry to the carotid canal, a location in the skull base where the internal carotid artery enters the petrous temporal bone.

Besides causing injury to the carotid artery, trauma can result in vertebral dissection. Vertebral fractures that extend to the foramen transversarium have an association with vertebral dissection, but the exact incremental risk of such dissection with such fractures is debated. Vertebral dissections can also result from violent movements of the head, from a tic in the setting of Tourette syndrome, from chiropractic manipulation, from cracking one's neck, and even from a violent sneeze. Vertebral dissection can result in stroke within the posterior circulation, including a stroke from injury to the posterior inferior cerebellar artery that can result in Wallenberg syndrome. Also known as lateral medullary syndrome, Wallenberg syndrome results in ipsilateral ataxia (through injury to the dorsal column and inferior cerebellar peduncle), an ipsilaterally decreased gag reflex/dysphagia (nucleus ambiguus), and decreased pain and temperature sensation in the ipsilateral face (spinal trigeminal nucleus) and contralateral body. There is also often vertigo and other nonspecific brainstem symptoms.[2]

components and to specify which portions are venous and which are cystic/lymphatic. The nonenhancing areas of some venolymphatic malformations may fill upon delayed imaging, suggesting very slow blood flow in these areas, and some such lesions may actually be entirely venous malformations, without a discrete lymphatic component.

19.5 Lymphatic Malformations

Another type of vascular malformation in children is the lymphatic malformation. The lymphatic component of this type of

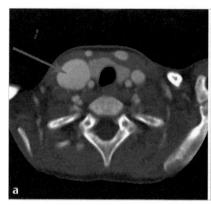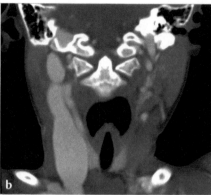

Fig. 19.6 Phlebectasia. (a) Axial and (b) coronal postcontrast computed tomographic images of the neck of a 6-year-old boy with painless, afebrile swelling of the lower neck, showing no mass, but marked enlargement of the internal jugular vein (*red arrow*), without identification of a stenosis. Clinically, the enlargement further increased with the Valsalva maneuver and represented idiopathic internal jugular phlebectasia that was presumably without pathologic significance.

19.7 Venous Abnormalities of the Neck

Pharyngeal infections can result in a septic thrombophlebitis of the internal jugular veins (▶ Fig. 17.7), a condition known as Lemierre's syndrome. This condition is frequently associated with infection by *Fusobacterium necrophorum*, a gram-negative anaerobic bacillus, which can result in septic emboli to the lungs.

The internal jugular vein can sometimes become focally dilated, typically caudally, in the condition known as phlebectasia (▶ Fig. 19.6). This idiopathic dilation is exacerbated by the Valsalva maneuver, and in the absence of other signs of venous congestion is likely to be asymptomatic.

19.8 Suggested Reading

[1] Tekes A, Koshy J, Kalayci TO et al. S.E. Mitchell vascular anomalies flow chart (SEMVAFC): A visual pathway combining clinical and imaging findings for classification of soft-tissue vascular anomalies. Clin Radiol 2014; 69(5):443–457

[2] Bonekamp D, Huisman TAGM, Bosemani T et al. Gadofosveset trisodium and TWIST for the evaluation of pediatric head and neck soft tissue vascular anomalies. Neurographics 2013; 3(1):33–40

[3] Griauzde J, Srinivasan A. Imaging of vascular lesions of the head and neck. Radiol Clin North Am 2015; 53(1):197–213

[4] Puttgen KB, Pearl M, Tekes A, Mitchell SE. Update on pediatric extracranial vascular anomalies of the head and neck. 2010;10;26(10):1417–1433. Available from: http://link.springer.com/10.1007/s00381–010–1202–2

[5] Lowe LH, Marchant TC, Rivard DC, Scherbel AJ. Vascular malformations: Classification and terminology the radiologist needs to know. Semin Roentgenol 2012; 47(2):106–117

References

[1] Desai NK, Kang J, Chokshi FH. Screening CT angiography for pediatric blunt cerebrovascular injury with emphasis on the cervical "seatbelt sign." AJNR Am J Neuroradiol 2014; 35(9):1836–1840

[2] Kim JS. Pure lateral medullary infarction: Clinical-radiological correlation of 130 acute, consecutive patients. Brain 2003; 126(Pt 8):1864–1872

20 Sinuses

20.1 Nasal Cavity and Paranasal Sinuses

The paranasal sinuses are aerated cavities within the facial bones that serve a variety of roles, including the humidification of inhaled air, contributing to immunologic defenses, and decreasing the weight of the skull. A variety of infectious, inflammatory, and neoplastic entities can occur within the paranasal sinuses throughout childhood and adolescence, largely mirroring pathologic conditions in adults. Additionally, there are a variety congenital abnormalities of the paranasal sinuses, and variants of these abnormalities, that require awareness.

20.2 Anatomy

There are four pairs of paranasal sinuses, within different facial bones (▶ Fig. 20.1). The largest are the maxillary sinuses, which are lateral to the nasal cavity, below the orbits and above the

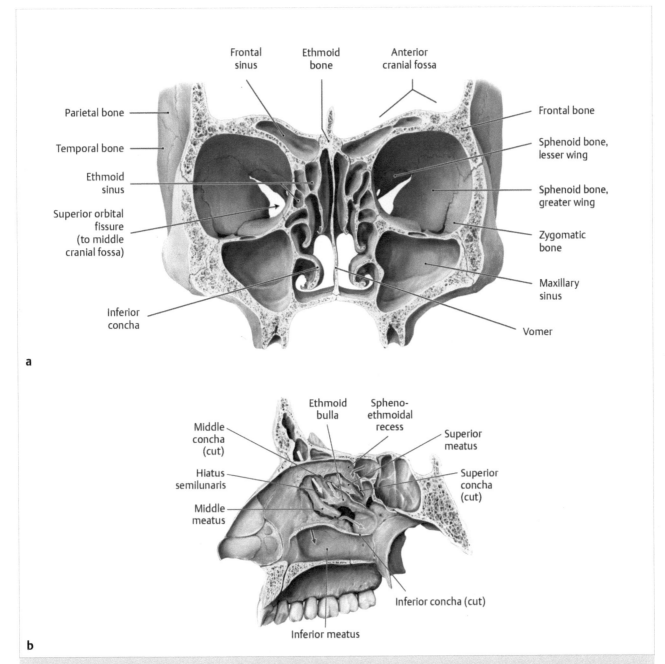

Fig. 20.1 Anatomy of paranasal sinuses. (a) Diagram of a coronal section through the frontal, ethmoid, and maxillary sinuses showing the osseous boundaries of the sinuses and their relationship to the nasal cavity and orbits. (b) Diagram of a sagittal section through the nasal cavity, showing drainage pathways of the paranasal sinuses as they relate to the hiatus semilunaris and nasal turbinates. From Atlas of Anatomy, © Thieme 2012, Illustration by Karl Wesker.

Table 20.1 Nasal passages into which the paranasal sinuses empty

Sinuses/Duct		Nasal passage	Pathway
Sphenoid sinus		Sphenoethmoidal recess	Direct
Ethmoid sinus	Posterior cells	Superior meatus	Direct
	Anterior and middle cells	Middle meatus	Ethmoid bulla
Frontal sinus		Middle meatus	Frontonasal duct into hiatus semilunaris
Maxillary sinus		Middle meatus	Hiatus semilunaris
Nasolacrimal duct		Inferior meatus	Direct

Used with permission from Gilroy A, MacPherson B, Ross L. Head & Neck: Nasal Cavity and Nose. In: Gilroy A, MacPherson B, Ross L, eds. Atlas of Anatomy. 2nd ed. New York, NY: Thieme;2012:552.

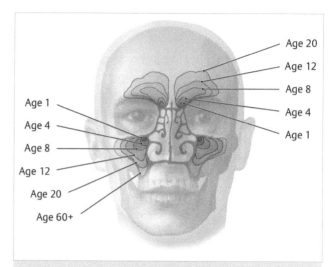

Fig. 20.2 Sinus development. Diagram showing the pattern of sinus development for the frontal and maxillary sinuses. Note that there is a great degree of variability on an individual basis. From Atlas of Anatomy, © Thieme 2012, Illustration by Karl Wesker.

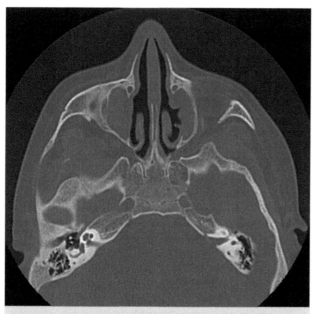

Fig. 20.3 Arrested pneumatization. Axial computed tomographic image of the head of a 12-year-old girl shows a somewhat lytic lesion in the sphenoid bone (*red arrow*), with a thin, circumscribed, sclerotic margin and heterogeneous internal matrix, in the expected location of a developing sphenoid sinus. These findings are consistent with arrested pneumatization of the sphenoid sinus, which is a variant of normal development.

posterior maxillary alveolus. The maxillary sinuses communicate with the nasal cavity through the osteomeatal complex, and drain near the hiatus semilunaris. The ethmoid sinuses are a multiseptated series of air cells located above the nasal cavity and medial to the orbit. The ethmoid sinuses are separated from the orbit by the lamina papyracea. Superiorly, the ethmoid sinuses are separated from the anterior cranial fossa by the cribriform plate medially and the fovea ethmoidalis laterally.

The frontal sinuses, in the frontal bones superior to the anterior aspect of the orbits, drain through a frontoethmoidal recess that extends toward the hiatus semilunaris. Posterior to the ethmoid bones are the sphenoid sinuses, which develop within the basisphenoid. The sphenoid sinuses drain into the posterior ethmoid sinuses through the sphenoethmoidal recess (▶ Table 20.1).

The sinuses develop over the course of childhood. The ethmoid sinuses are present at birth, as are the maxillary sinuses in their rudimentary form. The maxillary sinuses develop over the first decade of life, followed by the sphenoid sinuses and, variably, the frontal sinuses (▶ Fig. 20.2). The sphenoid sinuses develop within the basisphenoid, and at times there is lateral pneumatization of pterygoid recesses extending into the pterygoid process of the sphenoid bone. In some children, the development of the sphenoid sinus is arrested, typically in an asymmetric manner (▶ Fig. 20.3). It is important to be aware of this entity because it can be mistaken for a lesion of the skull base.

20.3 Sinonasal Infections

Sinonasal infections are common throughout childhood. Mucosal thickening along the margins of the paranasal sinuses does not necessarily represent an acute bacterial sinusitis. Focal globular thickening usually represents a mucous retention cyst (▶ Fig. 20.4) rather than a polyp. Discrete polyps are typically not visible on cross-sectional imaging. The presence of fluid levels or bubbly secretions may be indicative of acute sinusitis, but fluid levels alone are nonspecific, and can be seen after swimming. The drainage pathways to a sinus can become obstructed, preventing the drainage of infectious debris and possibly exacerbating symptoms of sinusitis (▶ Fig. 20.5). Acute sinusitis can result in bony erosion.

Three complications of acute sinusitis require awareness. The first is erosion through the lamina papyracea, which can result in orbital cellulitis (▶ Fig. 20.6). The other two,

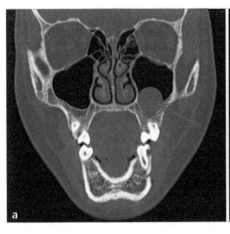 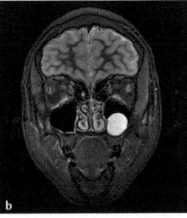

Fig. 20.4 Mucous retention cyst. (a) Coronal bone algorithm computed tomographic image shows a homogeneous, circumscribed, soft tissue lesion in the inferior aspect of the left maxillary sinus (*red arrow*). (b) Coronal short tau inversion recovery image shows the lesion to be diffusely hyperintense. This represents a mucous retention cyst.

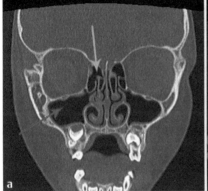 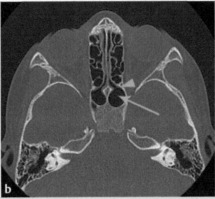 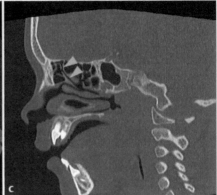

Fig. 20.5 Sinus anatomy and drainage pathways. (a) Coronal computed tomographic image of the sinuses in a 6-year-old girl shows the maxillary sinus (*red arrow*), which drains through the osteomeatal complex (*red arrowhead*) to the middle meatus, adjacent to the drainage of a middle ethmoid air cell (*green arrow*). (b) Axial image shows the sphenoid sinus (*green arrow*) draining through the sphenoethmoidal recess (*green arrowhead*). (c) Sagittal computed tomographic image shows drainage of the frontal recess (*green arrowheads*), also to the middle meatus; however, the frontal sinuses themselves have not yet developed in this patient.

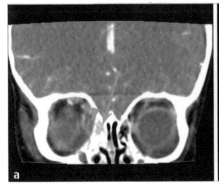 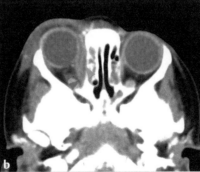

Fig. 20.6 Orbital abscess/cellulitis. (a) Coronal contrast-enhanced computed tomographic image of the head of a 21-month-old girl shows mucosal disease of the right maxillary sinus (*blue arrow*) and a fluid collection in the medial extraconal space of the right orbit (*blue arrowhead*). (b) Axial computed tomographic image shows the fluid collection (*blue arrowhead*), which is probably a subperiosteal abscess along the orbital margin of the lamina papyracea, and lateral deviation of the right medial rectus muscle (*red arrowheads*).

Pott's puffy tumor and epidural/subdural empyema, originate from the frontal sinuses, and can extend through the anterior wall into the subcutaneous soft tissues of the forehead, resulting in the swelling known as Pott's puffy tumor (▸ Fig. 10.2) (which despite its name is a non-neoplastic condition). The extension of an infectious process in the frontal sinus through the posterior wall can result in its further intracranial extension and an epidural and/or subdural empyema (▸ Fig. 10.2), which is a surgical emergency.

Chronic infection can result in thickening and sclerosis of the osseous margins of the paranasal sinuses (▸ Fig. 20.7).

A subtype of chronic sinusitis is allergic fungal sinusitis (▸ Fig. 20.8). The characteristic appearance of this on imaging is that of high-density matter within the paranasal sinuses. The high density represents noninvasive fungal hyphae, with the density possibly also related to the presence of metalloproteases. The chronic space-filling process in this sinusitis can result in expansion of the sinuses and even in hypertelorism

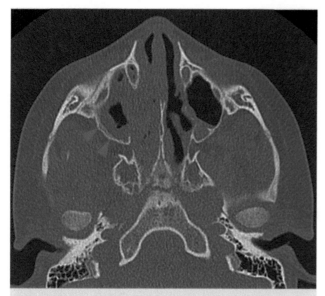

Fig. 20.7 Chronic sinusitis. Axial bone algorithm computed tomographic image of the head of a 10-year-old boy shows nearly complete opacification of the right maxillary sinus. There is thickening of the bony margins of the posterior wall of the maxillary sinus (*red arrowheads*), representing the osteitis of chronic sinusitis.

(▶ Fig. 20.8). When suggesting this diagnosis, it is important to specifically state that the diagnosis is allergic fungal sinusitis, which is a chronic process. This is in contradistinction to invasive fungal sinusitis, an acute aggressive process seen most commonly in immunocompromised patients and which represents a surgical emergency.

A partial obstruction of the osteomeatal complex of the maxillary sinuses can effectively create a one-way valve. If this allows air to move out of the sinus more easily than it can move into the sinus, it will result in a chronic vacuum effect within the sinus, causing the sinus to become smaller over the course of time. An asymmetrically smaller, or atelectatic, maxillary sinus is a sequela of this chronic sinus problem that may be clinically asymptomatic, yielding the name "silent sinus syndrome" (▶ Fig. 20.9). This is important to recognize because the syndrome can eventually result in lowering of the floor of the orbit, creating visual symptoms, such as double vision.

20.4 Masses and Neoplasms

Sinonasal neoplasms are much more rare in children than in adults, but they can occur in the pediatric population. An important tumor with which to be familiar is juvenile nasal angiofibroma (JNA). A JNA is a highly vascular tumor that arises at the sphenopalatine foramen, which connects the pterygopalatine fossa and the nasal cavity (▶ Fig. 20.10). The tumor is supplied by branches of the internal maxillary artery, and preoperative endovascular embolization is commonly done before its surgical excision. This lesion clinically presents with recurrent unilateral epistaxis, most commonly in an adolescent and always in a male. The diagnosis of JNA in a female should prompt either review of the pathology or genetic karyotyping of the patient.

An additional entity of which to be aware is an antrochoanal polyp (▶ Fig. 20.11), which is a polyp that arises from the maxillary sinus, protrudes through the maxillary sinus, and extends posteriorly into the nasopharynx. Because an antrochoanal polyp is a polyp and not a solid neoplastic mass, it does not enhance centrally on imaging. The characteristic location and appearance on imaging of an antrochoanal polyp help to differentiate it from a neoplastic entity.

Obstruction of the drainage to a sinus can result in a chronic buildup of secretions. This results in complete filling of the sinus and eventually in the expansion of its walls, and is known as a mucocele (▶ Fig. 20.12). A mucocele will have a homogeneous low density and will have no central enhancement on magnetic resonance imaging (MRI).

20.5 Congenital and Developmental Conditions

Newborn children occasionally undergo computed tomographic examination of the sinuses, typically for one of two indications. One of these is concern for a sinonasal developmental abnormality prompted by a failed attempt at passage of a nasogastric tube. There is also concern for a sinonasal developmental abnormality in children who have respiratory distress during feeding, suggesting that they are reliant on mouth breathing. The most common entity of concern in newborn children is choanal atresia or stenosis (▶ Fig. 20.13), which represents hypoplasia of the posterior nasal cavity and can be unilateral or bilateral. This condition is caused by thickening of the vomer

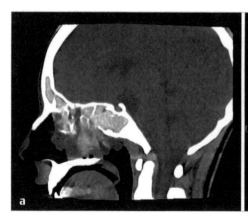
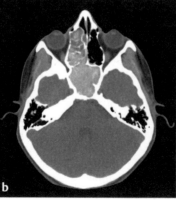

Fig. 20.8 Allergic fungal sinusitis with hypertelorism. (a) Sagittal computed tomographic image of the head of a 14-year-old boy with headaches shows high-density contents in the right frontal, ethmoid, and sphenoid sinuses. (b) Axial soft tissue algorithm computed tomographic image shows that the sinuses are filled and somewhat expanded in this patient with polyposis and allergic fungal sinusitis.

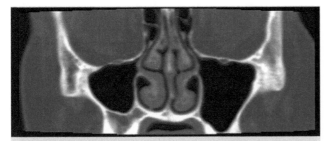

Fig. 20.9 Silent sinus syndrome. Coronal computed tomographic image of the head of a 13-year-old girl with headache but no history of sinusitis shows an asymmetrically smaller right than left maxillary sinus, with patent osteomeatal complexes bilaterally. Maxillary hypoplasia can be related to silent sinus syndrome.

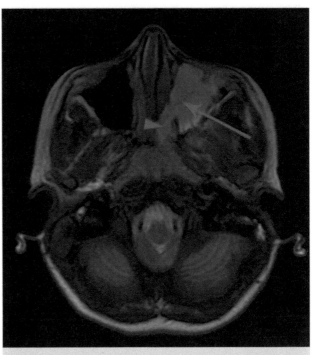

Fig. 20.11 Antrochoanal polyp. Axial T2 W image of the head of a 15-year-old girl shows filling of the left maxillary sinus (*red arrow*), with extension into the nasal cavity and toward the nasopharynx (*red arrowhead*), representing an antrochoanal polyp.

and medialization of the pterygoid plates and lateral nasal walls, resulting in narrowing of the transverse diameter of the posterior nasal cavity to less than approximately 3.5 mm. It is possible for there to be complete osseous atresia, or more commonly osseous stenosis, of the choana. Osseous stenosis of the choana can be associated with membranous atresia, which is more amenable to surgical correction than is osseous atresia. In performing a computed tomographic scan for detecting these conditions, it is important to suction the nasal cavity immediately before the scan, because it can be difficult (or impossible) for a scan to differentiate a membranous atresia of the nasal cavity from an osseous stenosis with retained fluid/secretions opacifying a narrowed but patent nasal cavity.

In the absence of signs of choanal atresia in a newborn infant, attention must be given to the remainder of the nasal cavity, and to the entire passage from the nares to the hypopharynx. In particular, the anterior nasal cavity may have the narrowing known as piriform aperture stenosis (▸ Fig. 20.14). This diagnosis is suspected if the transverse measurement of the anterior piriform opening is less than 10 mm, and if it is less than 8 mm, it is probably confirmatory of stenosis. When the piriform aperture is stenotic, the presence of other midline anomalies must be suspected, including holoprosencephaly spectrum disorders, pituitary abnormalities, and a single central incisor.

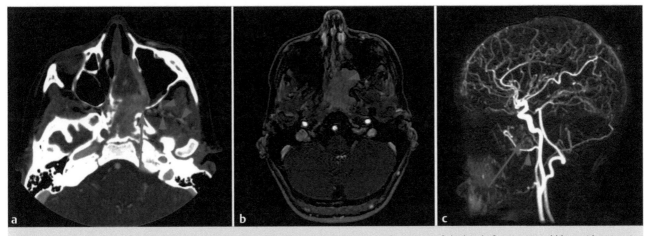

Fig. 20.10 Juvenile nasal angiofibroma (JNA). (a) Axial computed tomographic image with contrast of the head of an 11-year-old boy with epistaxis shows an enhancing soft tissue mass in the posterior nasal cavity arising from the left sphenopalatine foramen (*red arrow*). There is ipsilateral prominence of branches of the internal maxillary artery (*red arrowheads*). (b) Axial T1 W plus contrast fat-saturated image shows that the mass (*red arrowhead*) demonstrates homogeneous enhancement. (c) Sagittal maximum-intensity projection from dynamic contrast-enhanced magnetic resonance angiogram in the arterial phase shows serpentine vessels within the mass (*red arrow*) and a prominent ipsilateral internal maxillary artery (*red arrowhead*).

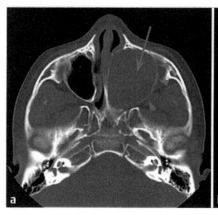
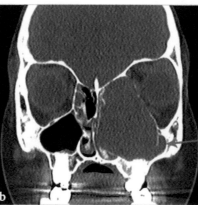

Fig. 20.12 Mucocele. (a) Axial computed tomographic image of the head of a 9-year-old girl with diplopia demonstrates a homogeneously opacified pranasal sinus (*red arrow*), with expansion/remodeling of the walls (*red arrowheads*), representing a mucocele.
(b) Coronal computed tomographic image shows that the mucocele has remodeled the lamina papyracea and effaces the maxillary sinus (*red arrow*), indicating that it originates from an ethmoid air cell.

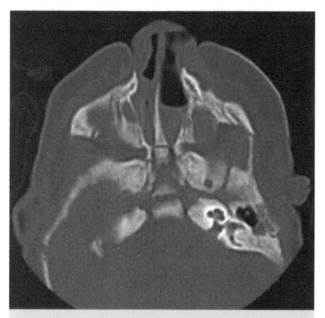

Fig. 20.13 Choanal atresia. Axial computed tomographic image of the head of a 10-day-old girl with respiratory difficulty shows a thickened vomer (*red line*, transverse dimension 4 mm), with medialization of the pterygoid processes of the sphenoid bone and resulting atresia of the right posterior choana and osseous stenosis (with membranous atresia) of the left posterior choana. Note the fluid level in the left nasal cavity (*red arrowhead*).

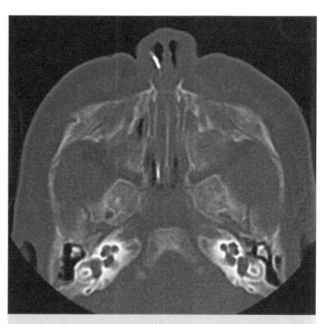

Fig. 20.14 Piriform aperture stenosis. Axial computed tomographic image of the head of a 2-week-old boy with difficulty breathing shows a narrowed piriform aperture (*red line*), with a medial position of the maxillary bones and lateral flaring of the frontal processes of the maxilla. This is piriform aperture stenosis.

20.6 Suggested Reading

[1] Daniels DL, Mafee MF, Smith MM et al. The frontal sinus drainage pathway and related structures. AJNR Am J Neuroradiol 2003; 24(8):1618–1627

[2] Som PM, Naidich TP. Illustrated review of the embryology and development of the facial region, Part 1: Early face and lateral nasal cavities. AJNR Am J Neuroradiol 2013; 34(12):2233–2240

[3] Hanna M, Batra PS, Pride GL Jr. Juvenile nasopharyngeal angiofibroma: Review of imaging findings and endovascular preoperative embolization strategies. Neurographics 2014; 4(1):20–32

21 Orbits

21.1 Imaging Techniques

The orbits are osseous cavities in the anterior skull that contain the globe of the eye ("eyeball") and serve as the source of vision. Imaging of the orbits plays a critical role in the diagnosis and management of various acute, chronic, and congenital conditions of the eye, orbit, and brain. In such imaging, computed tomography (CT) is superior for osseous detail and is rapidly available, whereas magnetic resonance imaging (MRI) is superior for revealing anatomic features and soft tissue characterization.

Computed tomography is typically the mainstay of acute orbital imaging for trauma and infection. In imaging for trauma, no intravenous contrast material is needed; however, postcontrast imaging is helpful for identifying abscesses in the setting of infection. Because of the dose of radiation needed, it is not appropriate to perform imaging both before and after the administration of contrast material, and if contrast is needed, the osseous structures of the orbit and surrounding areas can still be evaluated without dedicated unenhanced imaging.

Magnetic resonance imaging is very helpful in the examination of inflammatory conditions and both neoplastic and non-neoplastic masses affecting the orbit, and it is also helpful in characterizing congenital abnormalities of the eyes. Imaging both without and with contrast is typically indicated in MRI of the orbits, and for many indications it is important to also perform a dedicated MRI of the brain.

21.2 Anatomy

The globe of the eye has several substructures that can be identified through careful analysis of imaging. Along the anterior aspect of the globe is the lens, and anterior to this is the anterior chamber of the eye (▶ Fig. 21.1 and ▶ Fig. 21.2). The movement of the globe is controlled by six extraocular muscles, five of which extend posteriorly to the orbital apex in a conelike configuration (▶ Fig. 21.1 and ▶ Fig. 21.2), while the inferior rectus muscle attaches to the anterior floor of the orbit. The virtual cone created by the extraocular muscles is used to describe the location of structures in and around the orbit, with the optic nerve, superior ophthalmic vein, and intraconal retrobulbar fat in the intraconal space, and with the extraconal space predominantly containing fat as well as the lacrimal gland (▶ Fig. 21.1 and ▶ Fig. 21.2).

21.3 Size and Position of the Globe

The size of the globe can be measured from the anterior aspect of the cornea to the position of the insertion of the optic nerve (▶ Fig. 21.1a and ▶ Fig. 21.2), a measurement known as the axial length of the globe. The globe increases in size during infancy. In the setting of microcephaly, the appearance of the globes in relation to that of the head can suggest enlargement of the globes, and exact measurements can therefore help determine whether they are of appropriate size. The axial length of globe is approximately 18 mm in infancy, and reaches an adult size of approximately 24 mm over the first decade of life.

A measurement from the anterior aspect of the cornea to the lens provides the depth of the anterior chamber of the eye. This measurement can be inexact, especially because of slight obliquity of the lens, but typically ranges from 2 to 3.5 mm. A depth of the anterior chamber that exceeds 4 mm can be suggestive of glaucoma (▶ Fig. 21.3). A shallow anterior chamber can be seen after a corneal laceration, and in some patients may be the only sign, on imaging, of an open globe (▶ Fig. 21.4).

The midpole of the globe should be at, or slightly posterior to, a line connecting the medial and lateral points on the orbital rim (▶ Fig. 21.5). Projection of the globe anterior to this line represents proptosis, which can be seen with a retrobulbar space-occupying lesion, including a tumor, hematoma, or muscle hypertrophy in thyroid eye disease.

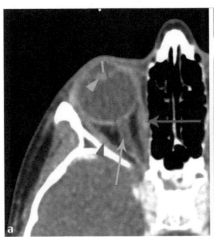
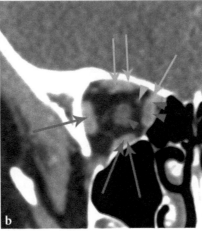

Fig. 21.1 Anatomy of the globe and orbit. (a) Axial computed tomographic image of the right orbit shows the depth of the anterior chamber (*green line*) measured to the anterior margin of the lens (*green arrowhead*), and the axial length of the globe (*red line*). The medial rectus (*red arrow*) and lateral rectus (*red arrowhead*) muscles are seen, as is the optic nerve (*green arrow*). (b) Coronal computed tomographic image shows the optic nerve in the center of the orbit (*red arrowhead*), and above it the superior ophthalmic vein (*green arrowhead*). The image shows the medial rectus (*double red arrowheads*) and lateral rectus muscles (*red arrow*), inferior rectus muscle (*double red arrows*), and superior rectus/levator muscle complex (*double green arrows*). The superior oblique muscle is also seen (*green arrow*), but the inferior oblique muscle is seen only at the anterior aspect of the orbit because it does not extend posteriorly to the apex.

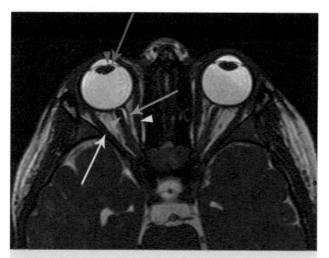

Fig. 21.2 Magnetic resonance image of orbital anatomy. Axial image made with fast imaging employing steady-state acquisition shows the iris (*red arrow*), which forms the margins of the pupil (*red arrowhead*) along the anterior aspect of the lens (*green arrowhead*). Along the posterior retina, the head of the optic nerve (*green arrow*) is seen at the insertion of the optic nerve (*blue arrowhead*). The optic nerve is surrounded by cerebrospinal fluid and bounded by a layer of dura known as the optic nerve sheath (*blue arrow*). The medial (*white arrowhead*) and lateral (*white arrow*) rectus muscles are seen.

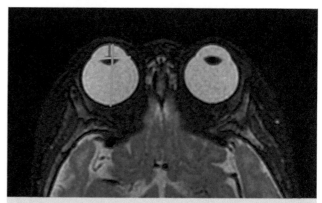

Fig. 21.3 Glaucoma. Axial T2 fat-saturated image of the anterior head of a 5-month-old female with congenital glaucoma shows a markedly increased depth of the anterior chamber (4.5 mm, *red line*), an increased axial length of the globe (23 mm, *blue line*), and a large width of the cornea (14 mm, *green line*).

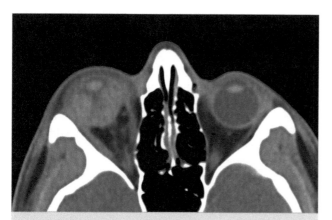

Fig. 21.4 Vitreous hemorrhage. Axial computed tomographic image of the anterior head of a 16-year-old boy with orbital trauma shows vitreous hemorrhage and a shallow anterior chamber. The shallow anterior chamber is an indicator of an open globe injury.

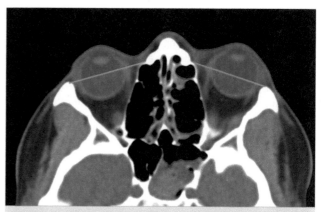

Fig. 21.5 Proptosis/retrobulbar hematoma. Axial computed tomographic image of the anterior head of a 13-year-old girl after trauma shows left-sided proptosis, with the midglobe extending beyond a line drawn from the medial to the lateral orbital rim (*blue line*).

The posterior contour of the globe should conform to that of a circle. Any outward deviation raises concern about a possible coloboma or morning glory disc anomaly (MGDA), which is discussed below (▶ Fig. 21.6). Inward projection along the posterior globe is suggestive of papilledema, and warrants funduscopic examination and a workup for possible causes of increased intracranial pressures (▶ Fig. 21.7).

21.4 Orbital Region Infections

Infections in the region of the orbit typically originate in two locations, either the facial soft tissues or the ethmoid sinuses.

Ethmoid sinus disease has the potential for extending through the lamina papyracea and into the medial extraconal fat. This is often accompanied by dehiscence/demineralization of the lamina papyracea, but it can be unclear whether the extension of the disease to the orbit is due to such demineralization or occurred through venous channels and then secondarily resulted in dehiscence. In either case, the infection can threaten vision after it reaches the orbit, and an abscess in the orbit represents a surgical emergency. Because this constitutes an infection within the orbit, it is referred to as an orbital infection, in the form of either orbital cellulitis or an orbital abscess. The anterior orbit has a fibrous septum that extends from the globe to the margins of the orbit, and any infection posterior to this septum is referred to as a postseptal process. Because of this, orbital cellulitis and postseptal cellulitis are synonymous terms for the same condition.

A preseptal cellulitis is one that involves the face and periorbital region (and is therefore also known as periorbital cellulitis), without extension posterior to the septum (▶ Fig. 21.8).

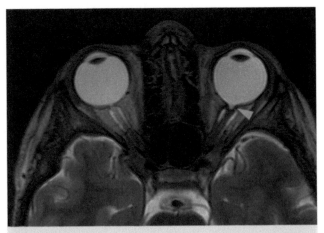

Fig. 21.6 Morning glory disc anomaly (MGDA). Axial T2 W image of the anterior head of an 8-year-old girl shows a focal protrusion (*blue arrowhead*) of the left globe at the location of the insertion of the head of the optic nerve, consistent with an MGDA.

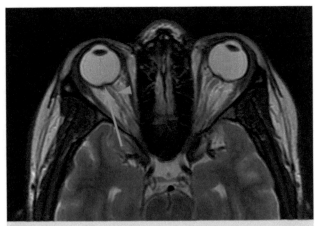

Fig. 21.7 Papilledema. Axial T2 W image of the anterior head of a 16-year-old girl with severe headaches and pseudotumor cerebri shows elevation of the optic nerve head (*blue arrow*), representing the correlate on magnetic resonance imaging of elevation/papilledema of the head of the optic nerve. There is also prominence of cerebrospinal fluid within the optic nerve sheaths (*blue arrowhead*), which with papilledema is suggestive of elevated intracranial pressure.

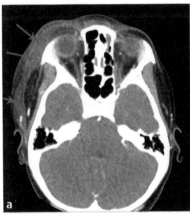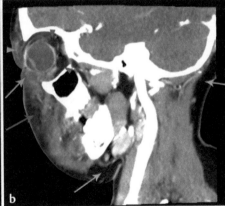

Fig. 21.8 Preseptal cellulitis. (a) Axial postcontrast computed tomographic image of the head of a 10-year-old boy with periorbital erythema and swelling shows subcutaneous stranding (*red arrows*) but no fluid collection. (b) Sagittal post-contrast CT image shows facial subcutaneous soft tissue stranding (*red arrow*) extending to involve the lower (*blue arrow*) and upper (*blue arrowhead*) eyelids; however, there is no stranding in the postseptal fat (*red arrowheads*), which resembles subcutaneous fat in uninvolved areas of the face (*green arrows*). This represents preseptal (periorbital) cellulitis without postseptal extension and without abscess.

All infectious processes in the orbital region carry the risk of inducing a septic thrombophlebitis in the veins of the face and orbit (▶ Fig. 21.9), and accordingly it is imperative to evaluate the caliber and patency of the superior ophthalmic vein and cavernous sinus in all studies of the orbit in which there is concern about infection. Following is a checklist for infectious processes affecting the orbit:

1. Preseptal or postseptal?
2. Cellulitis or abscess?
3. Any osseous demineralization?
4. Involvement of the ethmoid sinuses?
5. Patency of the superior ophthalmic vein and/or cavernous sinus?

21.5 Orbital Trauma

The two main patterns of osseous injury in orbital trauma are a fracture of the orbital floor and a fracture of the lamina papyracea (medial orbital wall).[1] Fractures of the orbital floor are commonly associated with the layering of blood products in the maxillary sinus, which may be the initial clue to the presence of a subtle fracture of the orbital floor (▶ Fig. 21.10). Fractures of the orbital floor may also be accompanied by an associated intramuscular hematoma of the inferior rectus muscle, herniation of fat through the fracture defect, or by herniation of the muscle itself through the defect. When there is herniation through the defect, there may be impaired movement of the eye, known as entrapment. Regardless, the appearance on imaging can neither diagnose nor exclude the entrapment of an extraocular muscle, which is a clinical finding based on impaired ocular motility.

Fractures of the medial orbital wall can also be associated with intramuscular hematoma and/or herniation of the medial rectus muscle (▶ Fig. 21.11). Acute fractures will usually have associated blood products in the adjacent paranasal sinus, as well as stranding in the adjacent extraconal fat (▶ Fig. 21.11). A chronic fracture can have herniation of fat through a persistent defect, but there will be no stranding in the fat and no blood products in the paranasal sinuses (▶ Fig. 21.11).

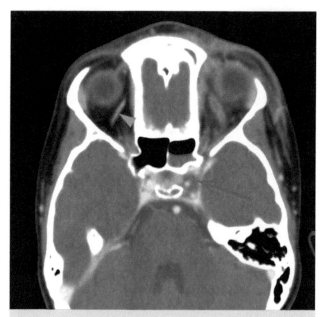

Fig. 21.9 Cavernous sinus thrombosis. Axial computed tomographic plus contrast image in an 11-year-old with eye pain and fever shows a normal right superior ophthalmic vein (*blue arrowhead*). There is an enlarged left superior ophthalmic vein (*red arrowhead*) that shows no central enhancement, and there is relative non-enhancement of the left cavernous sinus (*red arrow*). This represents left cavernous sinus and superior ophthalmic vein thrombosis.

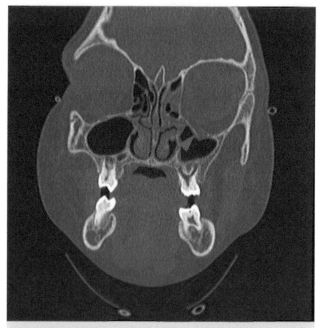

Fig. 21.10 Fracture of the orbital floor. Coronal bone algorithm computed tomographic image of the head of a 6-year-old girl with trauma shows a discontinuity (*red arrowhead*) in the floor of the left orbit, consistent with a fracture of the orbital floor.

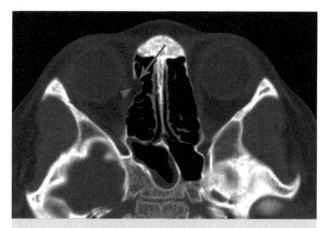

Fig. 21.11 Chronic orbital fracture. Axial computed tomographic image of the anterior head of an 8-year-old boy with headache but no history of recent trauma shows a defect in the right lamina papyracea (*red arrow*); however, there is a homogeneous appearance to the medial extraconal fat that extends into the defect (*red arrowhead*), consistent with an old fracture of the lamina papyracea.

Trauma may cause a retrobulbar hematoma, which can result in proptosis. The retrobulbar hematoma may be an amorphous hematoma in the intraconal fat, presenting only as stranding, or a lentiform subperiosteal hematoma along the orbital roof (▶ Fig. 6.8). Accordingly, it is critical to evaluate the orbits with both bone and soft tissue settings when evaluating posttraumatic imaging.

A normal size and shape of the globe do not exclude an open globe; this can only be excluded on physical examination.

A corneal laceration causes an open globe that may lack any detectable abnormality on imaging. Therefore, description of ocular findings on imaging should never state that the globes are intact, but only that they have a normal shape. Only a small percentage of open globes will have a "squished-grape" appearance. Evaluation for orbital foreign bodies is important, particularly if there is a history of penetrating trauma. It is also important to note that wood has a very porous structure and can resemble air on computed tomographic scans, and that a wooden foreign body, such as a stick, toothpick, or pencil fragment, can be missed without careful examination of such a scan.[2]

21.6 Masses and Neoplasms

Congenital inclusion cysts can occur in the region of the orbit, most commonly adjacent to the frontozygomatic suture (▶ Fig. 21.12). Histologically these may be dermoid or epidermoid cysts, and although the presence of macroscopic fat or calcium suggests a dermoid cyst, the two types of cyst can be difficult to differentiate on imaging. Congenital inclusion cysts will be circumscribed lesions, and can be evaluated with CT, MRI, or ultrasonography. A key concern when evaluating these lesions is their size, relationship to the globe of the eye and other structures, and whether there are signs of any underlying osseous defect that could suggest intracranial extension. If there are signs of possible intracranial extension of a congenital inclusion cyst, MRI is needed before surgical excision, to exclude the possibility of an encephalocele or other developmental lesion with a sinus tract that could predispose to meningitis, a CSF leak, or both.

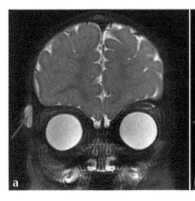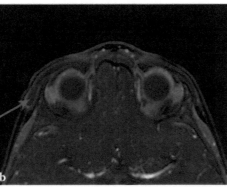

Fig. 21.12 Orbital dermoid cyst. (a) Coronal T2 W fat-saturated (FS) image of the orbits in a 1-year-old boy shows a circumscribed ovoid lesion along the lateral margin of the zygomaticofrontal suture (*red arrow*). (b) Axial T1 W FS plus contrast image shows no central enhancement within this lesion (*red arrow*), which represents a dermoid cyst.

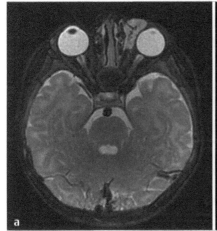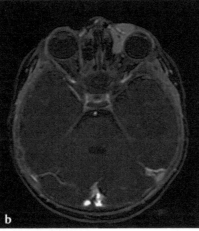

Fig. 21.13 Capillary hemangioma of orbit. (a) Axial T2 W fat-saturated (FS) image of the orbits in a 2-month-old male shows a circumscribed hyperintense mass in the anterior aspect of the medial extraconal space of the left orbit. (b) Axial T1 W FS plus contrast image shows postcontrast enhancement of the lesion, which represents a capillary (infantile) hemangioma. The lesion results in lateral deviation of the left globe, but the lack of an abnormality in the contour of the globe indicates that the lesion has low internal pressures.

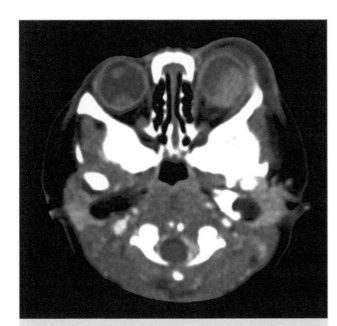

Fig. 21.14 Retinoblastoma. Axial computed tomographic image of the head of a 2-month-old girl shows a large mass in the left globe, with left-sided proptosis and periorbital swelling. A smaller mass is seen in the right globe. This represents bilateral retinoblastoma, probably related to a germline mutation in the *Rb* gene on chromosome 13.

A capillary hemangioma (▶ Fig. 21.13) is a vascular neoplasm that is characteristically not visible at birth but grows over the first 6 to 12 months of life (proliferative phase), at which time it stops growing (plateau phase), possibly for several years, and then tends to spontaneously involute (involution phase). Capillary hemangiomas are discussed in further detail in Chapter 19; however, it is important to be aware that the reason for treating hemangiomas and other lesions in the orbital region is to prevent amblyopia. Even without any intrinsic problem in the visual pathway, anything that impairs binocular vision, including a hemangioma or other lesion that prevents full eyelid opening or impairs ocular movement, results in understimulation of the visual cortex during early development, and can induce amblyopia.

Retinoblastoma is the most common malignant tumor of the eye in children, typically presenting before 6 years of age (▶ Fig. 21.14). Retinoblastoma occurs when there are two copies of a defective *Rb* tumor-suppressor gene within a given cell. In some patients one copy of the *Rb* gene, on chromosome 13, will be defective, and any mutation of the paired, functioning *Rb* gene may result in retinoblastoma, giving a high risk of multifocal disease, including bilateral disease, the occurrence of more than a single tumor within one eye, or both.

On imaging, a retinoblastoma will typically be an enhancing mass, often with calcifications. Conversely, calcifications within an orbital mass are strongly suggestive of retinoblastoma, and

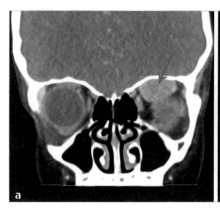
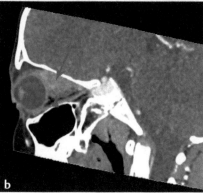

Fig. 21.15 Rhabdomyosarcoma. (a) Coronal and (b) sagittal oblique computed tomographic images, following the administration of a contrast agent, of the head of a 7-year-old boy with a short history of painless proptosis show mass-like thickening of the superior rectus muscle (*red arrows*) with inferior deflection of the optic nerve (*red arrowhead*). This represents orbital rhabdomyosarcoma.

are better depicted on CT than on MRI; however, CT should not be done solely to detect calcifications. If retinoblastoma is known or suspected, MRI should be the imaging modality of choice and CT should be avoided unless absolutely necessary. Patients who have an inherited form of retinoblastoma are highly radiosensitive and subjecting them to scanning increases the risk of inducing additional retinoblastomas.[3]

The most common primary orbital tumor (but not primary ocular tumor) of infancy is rhabdomyosarcoma, for which the median age at presentation is approximately 8 years and which has a slight male predominance. The typical presentation of a rhabdomyosarcoma will be painless proptosis in a patient without signs of an infectious process. This tumor is most commonly seen in the superior half of the orbit, and can invade or possibly arise from within an extraocular muscle, although the tumor mass may be circumscribed (▶ Fig. 21.15).[4]

21.7 Neurocutaneous Manifestations

Many neurocutaneous disorders have characteristic ocular manifestations. These conditions are discussed in greater detail in Chapter 7. Although their ocular manifestations are not seen in all patients, ophthalmologic examination is important in anyone with any of these conditions. Some ocular findings of neurocutaneous disorders may be visible only on cross-sectional imaging, despite normal findings in an ophthalmologic examination (▶ Table 21.1).

Table 21.1 Optic findings in neurocutaneous syndromes

Neurocutaneous syndrome	Optic and orbital findings
Neurofibromatosis type 1	Optic pathway glioma, plexiform neurofibromas, buphthalmos, sphenoid-wing hypoplasia
Neurofibromatosis type 2	Juvenile posterior subcapsular/lenticular cataract, cortical cataract
von Hippel–Lindau disease	Retinal hemangioblastoma
Tuberous sclerosis complex	Astrocytic hamartoma
Sturge–Weber syndrome	Retinal angioma, glaucoma, nevus of Ota

21.8 Congenital and Developmental Conditions

Leukocoria is a term that means "white pupil," and it describes the absence of a red reflex of the eye. Although leukocoria can have a variety of causes, the primary concern in its causation is retinoblastoma. The causes of leukocoria are:

- Retinoblastoma (typically in children under 3 years, and nearly always under 6 years, of age)
- Persistent hyperplastic primary vitreous (PHPV)
- Coats' disease
- Sequelae of toxoplasmosis, other, rubella, cytomegalovirus, and herpes (TORCH) infection
- Retinopathy of prematurity (ROP) (seen only in patients with a history of prematurity)
- Cataract
- Coloboma

Persistent hyperplastic primary vitreous, also known as persistent fetal vasculature, is a condition in which the embryologic arterial supply to the hyaloid canal does not appropriately involute, leading to a small eye (microphthalmos) (▶ Fig. 21.16). This can be associated with retinal detachment and proteinaceous fluid within the eye, as detected by incomplete suppression on fluid-attenuated inversion recovery (FLAIR) images.

A coloboma is a malshaped eye related to a developmental defect, and can be associated with a variety of genetic conditions. A specific type of abnormality of eye contour is one in which there is focal protrusion at the location of the insertion of the optic nerve; this is known as a morning glory disk anomaly (MGDA) on the basis of the similarity of its funduscopic appearance to that of a morning glory flower (▶ Fig. 21.6).[5] At times, MGDA has been considered a form of coloboma and at others a discrete entity.

Coats' disease is a developmental retinal abnormality that can present with leukocoria. The globe in Coats' disease is usually small, and on funduscopic examination abnormal tortuous vessels will be found within the retina. There should not be any solid enhancement within the globe in Coats' disease; enhancement raises concern for retinoblastoma.

Retinopathy of prematurity (ROP) is a condition in which there is abnormal retinal development because of stresses associated with prematurity, including altered oxygen tension

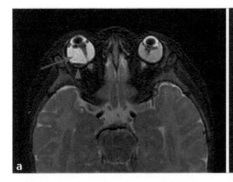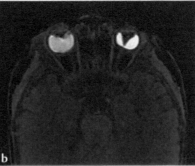

Fig. 21.16 Persistent hyperplastic primary vitreous (PHPV). (a) Axial T2 fat-saturated (FS) image in a 4-month-old male shows bilateral retinal/choroidal detachments (*red arrow*) and a fluid level in the right globe (*red arrowhead*). (b) Axial T1 W FS image shows hyperintense signal within the subretinal/subchoroidal effusions in both globes, consistent with proteinaceous/hemorrhagic material. In the setting of microphthalmia, these findings are consistent with bilateral PHPV in Norrie syndrome.

21.9 Inflammatory Conditions of the Orbit

Magnetic resonance imaging is the mainstay modality for detecting and characterizing noninfectious inflammatory conditions of the orbit. Perhaps the most commonly encountered such entity is optic neuritis, an inflammatory process chiefly seen in demyelinating disorders, such as multiple sclerosis, acute disseminated encephalomyelitis (ADEM), and Devic's disease (▶ Fig. 21.18). This results in an edematous appearance of the optic nerve with enhancement in the clinical setting of blurred vision and eye pain. While the nerve may be minimally larger due to the edema, it does not have a mass-like appearance.

Inflammatory orbital pseudotumor is an idiopathic inflammatory process. It results from orbital inflammation that can mimic either an infectious process or a tumor (hence the name pseudotumor). Inflammatory orbital pseudotumor is an entirely distinct process from pseudotumor cerebri (i.e., idiopathic intracranial hypertension), and will usually respond to steroid therapy. A prospective diagnosis of inflammatory orbital pseudotumor can be difficult to make; however, there will typically be no signs of infection.

21.10 Miscellaneous Conditions

Pseudotumor cerebri, also known as idiopathic intracranial hypertension, is a condition that results in increased intracranial pressure. This increased pressure is transmitted into the CSF of the optic nerve sheaths, which become distended, and can result in papilledema (▶ Fig. 21.7). Pseudotumor cerebri is further discussed in Chapter 12 (12.4.14).

Another condition is a hypoplastic optic nerve, which can be a developmental finding (▶ Fig. 21.19) or can be related to sequelae of prior optic neuritis. Bilateral optic nerve hypoplasia may be seen in septo-optic dysplasia (SOD) (▶ Fig. 3.17), and attention to the presence of the septum pellucidum and the morphology of the pituitary gland is warranted, as these can be involved in SOD.

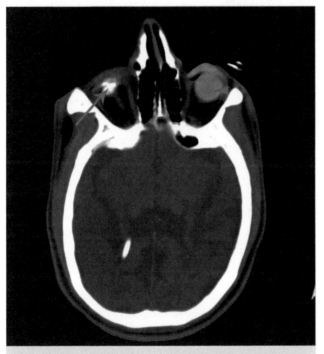

Fig. 21.17 Retinopathy of prematurity/phthisis bulbi. Axial computed tomographic image of the head of an infant who was born prematurely shows a shrunken calcified right globe (*red arrow*), consistent with phthisis bulbi. A prosthesis is present in the left globe as the result of prior enucleation of the left eye (*red arrowhead*). The image provides partial visualization of intracranial findings of shunted posthemorrhagic hydrocephalus and white-matter disease of prematurity.

and resulting alterations in the drive for vascular proliferation. The acute manifestations of ROP are characterized by funduscopic examination, but children with this disorder often undergo lifelong brain imaging for other purposes, and the consequences of ROP will be encountered. Mild ROP may be undetectable, or may be associated with microphthalmia, but more severe ROP can result in chronic retinal detachment. The most severe cases of ROP may result in phthisis bulbi, in which the eye is shrunken and nonfunctional, and often contains calcifications. Phthisis bulbi can result from any form of severe eye injury or infection. (▶ Fig. 21.17).

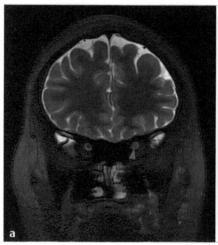
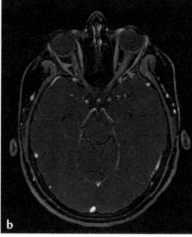

Fig. 21.18 Optic neuritis. (a) Coronal T2 W fat-saturated (FS) image of the head of a 17-year-old girl with eye pain shows an ill-defined and hyperintense appearance of the orbital segment of the left optic nerve (*red arrowhead*). (b) An axial T1 W FS plus contrast image shows enhancement of the orbital segments of the optic nerves bilaterally, greater for the left than for the right nerve (*red arrowheads*), indicating that the optic neuritis in this patient is a bilateral process.

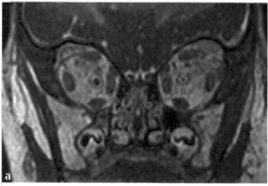
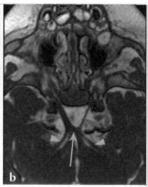

Fig. 21.19 Optic nerve hypoplasia. (a) Coronal image made with fast imaging employing steady-state acquisition (FIESTA) of the head of a 1-year-old boy shows an asymmetrically decreased volume of the orbital segment of the left optic nerve (*red arrowhead*), representing optic nerve hypoplasia. (b) Axial oblique FIESTA image of the optic chiasm confirms a diminutive caliber of the left optic nerve (*red arrowhead*) and a normal caliber of the right optic nerve (*red arrow*). Posterior to the chiasm (*green arrow*), there is a symmetrically smaller-than-expected volume of the optic tracts (*green arrowheads*). No etiology was identified for the hypoplasia in this patient.

21.11 Suggested Reading

[1] Jacquemin C, Bosley TM, Svedberg H. Orbit deformities in craniofacial neurofibromatosis type 1. AJNR Am J Neuroradiol 2003; 24(8):1678–1682

References

[1] Sung EK, Nadgir RN, Fujita A et al. Injuries of the globe: What can the radiologist offer? Radiographics 2014; 34(3):764–776

[2] Shelsta HN, Bilyk JR, Rubin PAD, Penne RB, Carrasco JR. Wooden intraorbital foreign body injuries: Clinical characteristics and outcomes of 23 patients. Ophthal Plast Reconstr Surg 2010; 26(4):238–244

[3] Razek AAKA, Elkhamary S. MRI of retinoblastoma. Br J Radiol 2011; 84 (1005):775–784

[4] Chung EM, Smirniotopoulos JG, Specht CS, Schroeder JW, Cube R. From the archives of the AFIP: Pediatric orbit tumors and tumorlike lesions: Nonosseous lesions of the extraocular orbit. Radiographics 2007; 27(6):1777–1799

[5] Ellika S, Robson CD, Heidary G, Paldino MJ. Morning glory disc anomaly: Characteristic MR imaging findings. AJNR Am J Neuroradiol 2013; 34(10): 2010–2014

22 Temporal Bone

22.1 Introduction

The temporal bone has a complex anatomy and varied functions, and its cross-sectional imaging tends to be an intimidating endeavor. It is to be hoped that a basic understanding of the anatomy of the temporal bone, and a systematic approach to the various pathologic entities that can affect it, can reduce the anxiety associated with, and improve the diagnostic yield of, its imaging.

Imaging of the temporal bone in children is done for several reasons. First and foremost is hearing loss. Additional reasons for imaging the temporal bone include infection, trauma, and facial nerve pathology. The mainstay modalities for imaging the temporal bone are computed tomography (CT) and magnetic resonance imaging (MRI).

22.2 Anatomy

The temporal bone is a bone of complex anatomy located within the skull base. Its main parts include its petrous portion, tympanic portion, and mastoid portion, all of which are parts of the skull base, and its squamous and zygomatic portions (▶ Fig. 22.1). The tympanic portion of the temporal bone

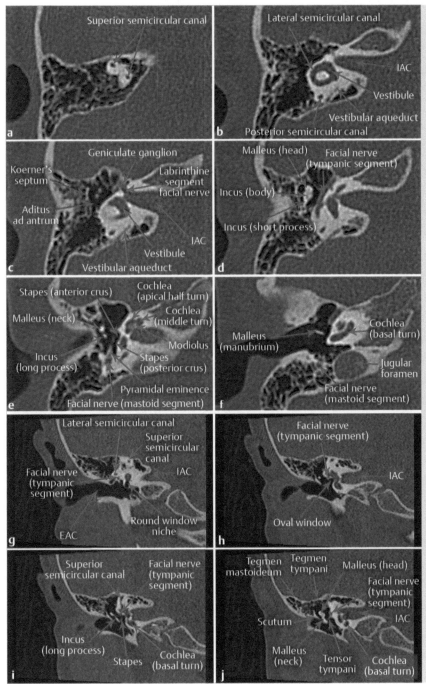

Fig. 22.1 Temporal bone anatomy. Axial bone algorithm computed tomographic images of the right temporal bone, from superior to inferior. (a) Axial computed tomographic image shows the mastoid air cells and the anterior and posterior crura of the superior semicircular canal. (b) Axial computed tomographic image at a slightly lower level than in (a) shows the internal auditory canal (IAC), vestibule, and lateral semi-circular canal (with its internal "bony island"). (c) Axial computed tomographic image at a slightly lower level than in (b) begins to show the osseous course of the facial nerve (labyrinthine segment and geniculate ganglion). (d) Axial computed tomographic image at a lower level than in (c) begins to show the ossicles, including the head of the malleus overlying the body of the incus. The triangular body and short process of the incus have been referred to as resembling an ice-cream cone, with the head of the malleus representing the ice cream. (e) Axial computed tomographic image at a slightly lower level than in (d) demonstrates the crura of the stapes, which extend to the oval window, and the cochlea. Between the modiolus and IAC is the cochlear aperture. (f) Axial computed tomographic image showing the basal turn of the cochlea, the manubrium of the malleus, and the jugular bulb/foramen. Four separate coronal bone algorithm computed tomographic images of the right temporal bone from posterior to anterior, include (g) a coronal bone algorithm computed tomographic image showing the vertically oriented round window niche and the location of the tympanic segment of the facial nerve relative to the tympanic cavity; (h) a coronal bone algorithm image anterior to that in (g), showing the relationship of the tympanic segment of the facial nerve to the oval window; (i) a coronal bone algorithm image anterior to that in (h) shows the relationship of the inferiorly directed long process of the incus to the superomedially directed stapes (which extends toward the oval window); (j) a coronal computed tomographic image showing the relationship of the neck and head of the malleus to the scutum, with the intervening lateral epitympanic space. (*continued*)

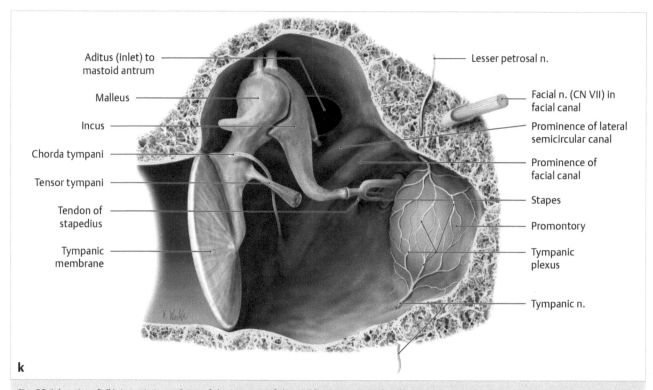

Aditus (inlet) to mastoid antrum

Malleus

Incus

Chorda tympani

Tensor tympani

Tendon of stapedius

Tympanic membrane

Lesser petrosal n.

Facial n. (CN VII) in facial canal

Prominence of lateral semicircular canal

Prominence of facial canal

Stapes

Promontory

Tympanic plexus

Tympanic n.

k

Fig. 22.1 (*continued*) (k) An artist's rendition of the anatomy of the middle ear cavity within the temporal bone. "k" From Atlas of Anatomy, © Thieme 2012, Illustration by Karl Wesker.

contains the middle ear cavity, also known as the tympanic cavity. The petrous temporal bone can be subdivided into the labyrinthine portion and the petrous apex (pathologic processes involving the petrous apex are further discussed in Chapter 16). The external auditory canal leads to the middle ear, which is separated from the outer ear by the tympanic membrane.

Within the middle ear are three ossicles: the malleus, incus, and stapes (▶ Fig. 22.1d,e,f,i,j), which span from the tympanic membrane to the oval window. The structures of the inner ear include the cochlea, vestibule, and three semicircular canals (▶ Fig. 22.1e,f). The cochlea has approximately from two-and-a-quarter to two-and-a-half turns, and at its center is a small osseous structure known as the modiolus, which contains the spiral ganglion, or ganglion for the cochlear nerve. The cochlear nerve passes through the cochlear aperture, traverses the internal auditory canal (IAC) and cerebellopontine angle cistern (CPA), and projects to the brainstem.

The IAC and CPA also contain the facial nerve and two vestibular nerves (▶ Fig. 16.13b). The facial nerve travels between the cochlea and vestibule of the inner ear (labyrinthine segment), with nearly all of its fibers synapsing in the geniculate ganglion. The fibers then course along the superior aspect of the middle ear (tympanic segment) and descend between the middle ear and mastoid air cells (mastoid segment) before exiting the stylomastoid foramen.

The main portion of the middle ear cavity is the mesotympanum, above which is the epitympanum (▶ Fig. 22.1b,c,h,i,j). The epitympanum communicates with the mastoid air cells through the aditus ad antrum, an opening bounded laterally by Koerner's septum

(▶ Fig. 22.1c), and which communicates posteriorly with the mastoid antrum and air cells and anteriorly with the nasopharynx through the eustachian tube. The lateral aspect of the epitympanum contains a sub-area sometimes referred to as Prussak's space, which is bounded laterally by the scutum (▶ Fig. 22.1h,i,j).

22.3 Embryology Basics

The middle and external ear arise from the first and second branchial (pharyngeal) apparati. Accordingly, an abnormality in one of these areas has a high degree of association with abnormalities in these two parts of the ear. Thus, for instance, abnormalities of the external ear tend to be associated with ossicular malformation.

22.4 Hearing Loss

Hearing loss is one of the most common indications for dedicated temporal bone imaging in children. Hearing loss is characterized audiologically and otologically as being conductive, sensorineural, or mixed. Knowledge of the type and duration of hearing loss and side of the head on which it occurs is important, and for acquired hearing loss it is important to know whether the loss was abrupt or progressive and if there were associated symptoms, such as infection or cranial neuropathy. This information helps in determining the ideal modality for imaging the ear in a case of hearing loss, and whether to use intravenous contrast material in such imaging.

Conductive hearing loss is typically related to problems affecting the external auditory canal or middle ear, including

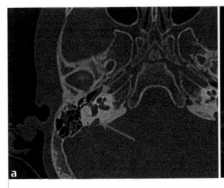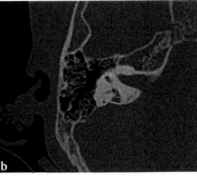

Fig. 22.2 Incomplete partitioning, type II (Mondini dysplasia). (a) Axial computed tomographic image of the right side of the head of a child with right-sided sensorineural hearing loss shows a bulbous appearance of the middle and apical turns of the cochlea (*red arrowhead*), and an enlarged vestibular aqueduct (*red arrow*), consistent with incomplete partition type II. (b) Axial computed tomographic image showing measurements of the vestibular aqueduct, which can be a transverse measurement at the mid-aqueduct (*red line*) or at the operculum (*green line*).

the ossicular chain. Computed tomography is the gold standard for evaluating conductive hearing loss, with an estimated sensitivity for detecting a pathologic cause of such loss of approximately 90%. Accordingly, rescrutinization of images is warranted before concluding that a computed tomographic examination done for conductive hearing loss is normal. (n.b. this is for true, audiology confirmed conductive hearing loss. Conductive hearing loss identified by physical examination with a tuning fork will have a lower incidence of pathologic findings on CT).

22.4.1 Sensorineural Hearing Loss

Although adult-onset sensorineural hearing loss (SNHL) is best evaluated with contrast-enhanced MRI for seeking tumors like vestibular schwannoma, both CT and MRI can be effective techniques for evaluating congenital sensorineural hearing loss. Computed tomography can provide excellent bony detail about developmental abnormalities of the inner ear. Although CT has a high diagnostic yield for conductive hearing loss, both CT and MRI may be normal in patients with SNHL. This is the case in approximately 50% of cases, and pediatric SNHL is often idiopathic without an identifiable cause.

The labyrinthine structures can fail to develop completely, with effects ranging from complete labyrinthine aplasia (i.e., Michel aplasia) to incomplete partition of the middle and apical turns of the cochlea with an enlarged vestibular aqueduct (incomplete partition type II, originally described as the Mondini malformation) (▶ Fig. 22.2).[1,2]

The gradation between the most severe and milder forms of cochlear and vestibular dysplasia includes multiple additional abnormalities with characteristic features, which are described in ▶ Table 22.1 and are covered in greater detail in dedicated articles on this topic.[3]

The mildest abnormality seen, if any is present, is an enlarged vestibular aqueduct (▶ Fig. 22.2), which is thought to transmit pressure from cerebrospinal fluid pulsations from the subarachnoid space into the inner ear. Accordingly, an enlarged vestibular aqueduct in a patient without hearing loss is felt to be a factor that increases the risk of eventual development of SNHL, which in turn is often instigated by a traumatic event. For this reason, an enlarged vestibular aqueduct is sometimes considered to be a contraindication to contact sports.

Some patients have absence or hypoplasia of the cochlear nerve. This will result in a narrow cochlear aperture (cochlear aperture stenosis), of typically less than 1 mm diameter (▶ Fig. 22.3). When this finding is made, MRI should be suggested, to permit differentiation between cochlear nerve aplasia and hypoplasia. A patient with cochlear nerve aplasia is typically not a candidate for an ipsilateral cochlear implant device.

Table 22.1 Ear dysplasias in congenital sensorineural hearing loss

Malformation	Gestational age of occurrence of developmental abnormality	Findings
Labyrinthine aplasia (Michel deformity)	Third week	Agenesis of the cochlea, vestibule, and semicircular canals
Cochlear aplasia	Third to fourth week	Agenesis of the cochlea. Vestibule present; semicircular canals likely to be dysplastic
Common cavity deformity	Fourth week	Confluent cystic cavity, without separation or differentiation of structures, rather than normal cochlea and vestibule
Cystic cochleovestibular anomaly (incomplete partition type I)	Fifth week	Cystic cochlea without modiolus or appreciable internal partitioning. Cystic vestibule without semicircular canals of normal appearance
Cochlear hypoplasia	Sixth week	Cochlea and vestibule are distinctly formed but hypoplastic
Incomplete partition type II (Mondini malformation)	Seventh week	There is a bulbous appearance of the middle and apical turns of the cochlea due to incomplete partitioning, resulting in 1.5 turns. Vestibular aqueduct typically enlarged. Vestibule and semicircular canals may be normal.
Enlarged vestibular aqueduct	Unclear	Enlargement of the vestibular aqueduct in the absence of definable abnormality in the cochlea, vestibule, or semicircular canals

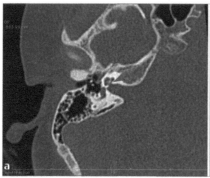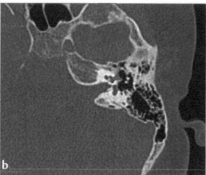

Fig. 22.3 Stenosis of the cochlear aperture. (a) Axial computed tomographic image of the right temporal bone shows a normal cochlear aperture (*red arrowhead*). (b) Axial computed tomographic image of the left temporal bone shows a diminutive left cochlear aperture (*red arrowhead*), consistent with stenosis of the cochlear aperture in the setting of aplasia of the left cochlear nerve.

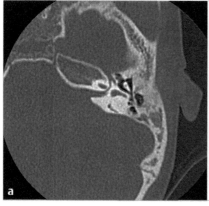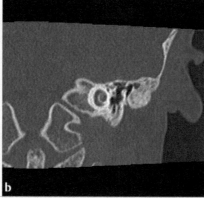

Fig. 22.4 Aural atresia. (a) Axial computed tomographic image of the head of a patient with left microtia shows soft tissue and osseous atresia of the external auditory canal. (b) Coronal image shows that the neck and manubrium of the malleus are in continuity with a thick osseous atresia plate.

22.5 Conductive Hearing Loss

Abnormalities of the external and middle ear can result in a conductive hearing loss, which can be of a congenital or acquired etiology. Congenital conductive hearing loss is seen in abnormalities of the first and second branchial apparati, which often have associated ossicular and middle ear developmental abnormalities. A dysplastic external ear serves as a clue to the presence of middle ear dysplasia.

The external auditory canal may be atretic, and imaging is critical to determine whether the atresia is osseous or simply soft tissue atresia. In a case of osseous atresia, it is critical to report to the otolaryngologist the thickness of the atresia plate (▶ Fig. 22.4), to help in determining whether and how the EAC can be reconstructed. Otolaryngologists sometimes use a 10-point scale to determine the complexity of aural atresia and help predict the likelihood of success in its surgical treatment (▶ Table 22.2). In this 10-point scale, scores lower than 5 or 6 indicate atresia that is typically not amenable to surgery, although other factors also enter into the decision, such as whether the atresia is unilateral or bilateral.

A congenital conductive hearing loss can result from dysplastic ossicles. An acquired conductive hearing loss can result from osseous erosion, either by chronic infection or cholesteatoma (▶ Fig. 22.5), and with traumatic injury to the ossicles.

22.5.1 Mixed Hearing Loss

Some types of hearing loss are found on audiologic examination to have components of both conductive and sensorineural hearing loss. This is known as mixed hearing loss. One entity that can result in mixed hearing loss is atresia of the oval window, in which the oval window is absent and the stapes is dysplastic (▶ Fig. 22.6).

22.6 Temporal Bone Infection

Infections of the middle ear are common throughout childhood, and typically do not require imaging. When imaging is done, it will often reveal fluid in the tympanic cavity and mastoid air cells. A common treatment for persistent middle ear infection

Table 22.2 Jahrsdoerfer grading scale score for congenital aural atresia

Structure	Points
Stapes bone	2
Oval window open	1
Middle-ear space	1
Facial nerve	1
Malleus–incus complex	1
Mastoid pneumatization	1
Incus–stapes connection	1
Round window	1
External ear	1
Total possible score	10

Used with permission from Jahrsdoerfer RA, Yeakley JW, Aguilar EA, Cole RR, Gray LC. Grading system for the selection of patients with congenital aural atresia. Am J Otol. 1992;13(1): 6–12.

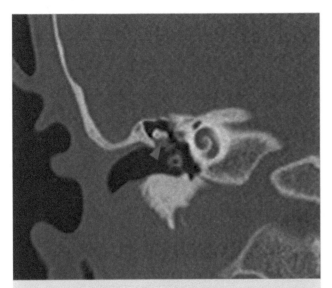

Fig. 22.5 Cholesteatoma. Coronal computed tomographic image of the right temporal bone of a patient with a history of ear infections and presenting with conductive hearing loss shows a soft tissue lesion in the lateral epitympanic space, between the scutum and neck of the malleus (*red arrowhead*), consistent with a cholesteatoma. This was reported on otoscopy to be a white retrotympanic lesion.

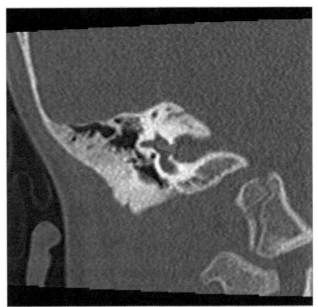

Fig. 22.6 Oval window atresia. Coronal bone algorithm computed tomographic image of the right temporal bone of a patient with congenital mixed hearing loss shows absence of the oval window (*red arrowhead*), consistent with atresia of the oval window.

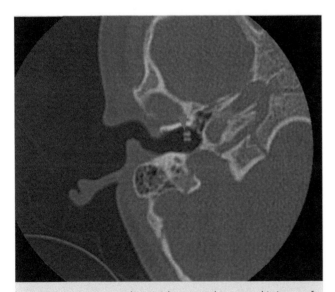

Fig. 22.7 Myringotomy tubes. Axial computed tomographic image of the right temporal bone shows parallel lines of myringotomy (a.k.a., tympanostomy, or pressure-equalization) tubes (*red arrowhead*).

is the insertion of tympanostomy (or myringotomy) tubes, which can be seen on CT (▶ Fig. 22.7). Chronic infection can result in osseous destruction, which, if it occurs in the mastoid air cells, is referred to as coalescent mastoiditis (▶ Fig. 22.8). It is important to be aware that infection can spread from the mastoid air cells via several routes. One of these is posteromedial extension through the sigmoid plate (▶ Fig. 22.8a), which can result in a septic thrombophlebitis of the sigmoid sinus. Extension can also occur superiorly, through the tegmen tympani and tegmen mastoideum (▶ Fig. 22.8b), which can result in

an epidural empyema along the floor of the middle cranial fossa, and possibly also in infectious involvement of the inferior temporal lobe. Infection in the mastoid bones can also spread outward into the postauricular soft tissues (▶ Fig. 22.8; ▶ Fig. 22.9), and if this infection extends extracranially and caudally into the sternocleidomastoid muscle, it can result in an intramuscular abscess (Bezold abscess).

In some patients, hearing loss will begin after an episode of bacterial meningitis. This is probably related to the extension of infection into the membranous labyrinth (cochlea, vestibule, and semicircular canals). Infection in these structures can result in the inflammation known as labyrinthitis and can be seen on postcontrast MRI. On CT there may be postinfectious dystrophic mineralization of the labyrinth, known as labyrinthitis ossificans (▶ Fig. 22.10). This can be subtle on early imaging, but can lead to irreversible hearing loss. When detected early, patients with this condition may be candidates for emergent cochlear implantation.

Infections of the labyrinth do not have to be bacterial, and viral labyrinthitis is a common cause of acute vertigo. Viral labyrinthitis will typically yield a normal appearance on imaging, but there may be incomplete suppression of the labyrinthine signal on fluid-attenuation inversion recovery (FLAIR) images, without postcontrast enhancement (▶ Fig. 22.11).

Bell's palsy is a viral infectious process involving the facial nerve, and is further described in Chapter 16.

22.7 Cholesteatoma

In the setting of recurrent infection, it is possible for the tympanic membrane to retract and trap epithelial cells at the superior insertion of the membrane. This leads to an accumulation of keratin from desquamation, with the keratin forming a mass

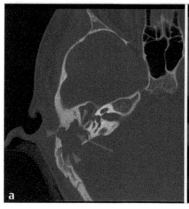
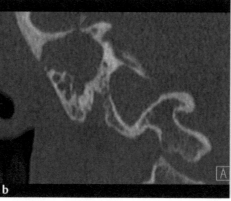

Fig. 22.8 Coalescent mastoiditis with osseous dehiscence. (a) Axial bone algorithm computed tomographic image of the right side of the head of a patient with recurrent right mastoiditis shows demineralization of the mastoid air cells (*red arrow*), with dehiscence through the outer mastoid cortex (*red arrowhead*) and through the sigmoid plate (*double red arrowheads*). (b) Coronal bone algorithm computed tomographic image shows an additional area of focal dehiscence through the mastoideum (*red arrowhead*).

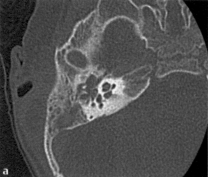
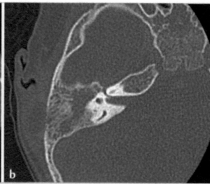
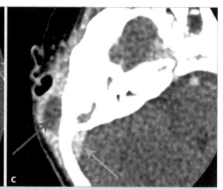

Fig. 22.9 External extension of mastoid bone infection. (a) Axial computed tomographic image of the right side of the head of a patient with fever and right postauricular swelling shows opacification of the right mastoid air cells and focal dehiscence of the sigmoid plate (*red arrowhead*). (b) An axial computed tomographic image at a slightly lower level than in (a) shows demineralization of the outer mastoid cortex (*red arrowheads*). (c) Axial soft tissue algorithm image at this level in a postcontrast computed tomographic study shows a postauricular abscess (*red arrow*) overlying the area of demineralization. While there is dehiscence of the sigmoid plate, the sigmoid sinus remains patent (*green arrow*).

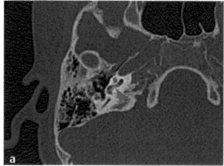
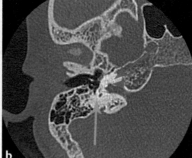

Fig. 22.10 Labyrinthitis ossificans. (a) Axial computed tomographic image of the inner ear of a patient with new sensorineural hearing loss shortly after an episode of meningitis shows an area of subtly increased density along the basal turn of the cochlea (*red arrowhead*), representing early labyrinthitis ossificans. At this stage, cochlear implantation may still be possible. (b) Severe labyrinthitis ossificans. Axial computed tomographic image of the right temporal bone of a patient with a history of sensorineural hearing loss after an episode of meningitis shows a cochlear aperture (*red arrowhead*), confirming that the cochlea was once present, but there is now complete ossification of the cochlea (*red arrow*) and vestibule (*blue arrow*).

known as a cholesteatoma. A cholesteatoma is histologically identical to an epidermoid cyst, can enlarge, and results in erosions in adjacent osseous structures. The most common location for an acquired cholesteatoma is in the lateral epitympanic space, or Prussak's space, and the first structures to be demineralized are the scutum and the neck and head of the malleus (▶ Fig. 22.5). Because it is histologically an epidermoid cyst, a cholesteatoma will restrict diffusion on diffusion-weighted imaging (DWI), but because of susceptibility to artifact from the air and bone adjacent to the cyst, a non-echo-planar diffusion-weighted technique should be used to diagnose a cholesteatoma. Non-echo-planar techniques, such as spin-echo diffusion-weighted imaging, are more resistant than echo-planar MRI to artifacts at the skull base. In addition to aiding the primary diagnosis of a cholesteatoma, a non-echo-planar technique can be used after surgical resection to identify a

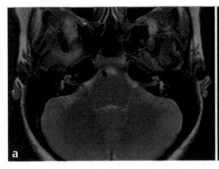
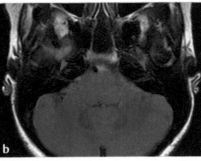

Fig. 22.11 Viral labyrinthitis. (a) Axial T2 W image of the head of a 4-year-old girl with vertigo shows a normal appearance of the inner ear structures. (b) Axial fluid attenuation inversion recovery (FLAIR) image shows incomplete FLAIR suppression of signal in the cochlea (*red arrowheads*), vestibule, and semicircular canals, indicative of proteinaceous fluid. In the setting of vertigo, without postcontrast enhancement, this is likely to represent viral labyrinthitis.

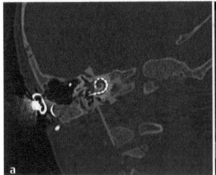
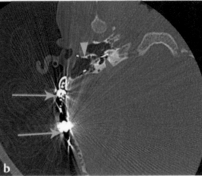

Fig. 22.12 Cochlear implant. (a) Coronal oblique computed tomographic image of the right side of the head of a patient with a cochlear implant shows the implant lead traversing the round window (*red arrow*) and making approximately one turn within the cochlea (*red arrowheads*). The proximal-most lead of the implant is at the level of the round window. (b) Axial computed tomographic image shows the extracranial implant device (*green arrows*). The lead is seen entering the round window niche (*red arrowhead*). The anterior margin of the mastoidectomy, which is the posterior wall of the internal auditory canal (*green arrowhead*), remains intact in this canal-wall-up mastoidectomy.

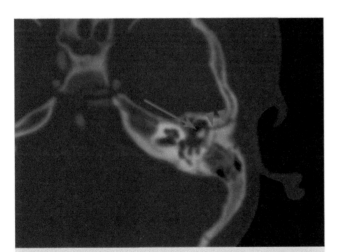

Fig. 22.13 Oblique temporal bone fracture/ossicular dissociation. Axial computed tomographic image of the left temporal bone of a patient with high-velocity trauma shows an oblique fracture through the temporal bone (*red arrowheads*), with the malleus head out of its expected location anterior to the body of the incus (*red arrow*).

recurrent cholesteatoma. Recurrent cholesteatoma will restrict diffusion but does not enhance, in contrast to granulation tissue, which enhances but does not restrict diffusion, and retained fluid, which will neither enhance nor restrict diffusion.[4]

22.8 Cochlear Implants

Cochlear implant devices can be used in patients with congenital or acquired sensorineural hearing loss. The lead from the implant traverses a mastoidectomy cavity, enters the round window to enter the inner ear, and makes approximately one to one-and-a-half turns within the cochlea (▶ Fig. 22.12). Presurgical planning for the insertion of a cochlear implant requires a description of anatomic variants in the ear, head, and neck, and particularly aberrant courses of the internal carotid artery, a high-riding jugular bulb, and a dehiscent facial nerve.[5,6]

22.9 Trauma

Fractures of the temporal bone can result in hearing loss, including conductive hearing loss when there is dissociation of the ossicular chain and sensorineural hearing loss when there is violation of the otic capsule.[7] Fractures of the temporal bone have traditionally been classified as longitudinal or transverse, but many fractures of the bone will be oblique (▶ Fig. 22.13). When evaluating a fracture, features to seek and describe include:

1. Extension to the carotid canal, which may be associated with dissection of the petrous segment of the internal carotid artery.
2. Extension into the otic capsule (the dense bone around the cochlea, vestibule, and semicircular canal), which has a high likelihood of causing permanent hearing loss. If no such fracture is identified, pneumolabyrinth (or air within the labyrinth) suggests an occult fracture of the otic capsule.
3. Ossicular dissociation. Disruption of the normal articulation between the malleus and incus (best seen on axial images) (▶ Fig. 22.13) or the incus and stapes (often best seen on coronal images).

4. Pneumocephalus, which indicates the likelihood of a fracture extending from the mastoid bone, tympanic cavity, or paranasal sinuses into the intracranial compartment. This puts the patient at high risk for meningitis, and also carries the risk of a subsequent leak of CSF.

5. Any intra-articular extension of the fracture to the glenoid fossa, and whether there is asymmetry of the temporomandibular joint, which may indicate a joint-space hematoma and may be associated with dental malocclusion.

References

[1] Mondini C. Minor works of Carlo Mondini: The anatomical section of a boy born deaf. Am J Otol 1997; 18(3):288–293

[2] Sennaroglu L, Saatci I. A new classification for cochleovestibular malformations. Laryngoscope 2002; 112(12):2230–2241

[3] Huang BY, Zdanski C, Castillo M. Pediatric sensorineural hearing loss, Part 1: Practical aspects for neuroradiologists. AJNR Am J Neuroradiol 2012;33:2117

[4] Baráth K, Huber AM, Stämpfli P, Varga Z, Kollias S. Neuroradiology of cholesteatomas. AJNR Am J Neuroradiol 2011; 32(2):221–229

[5] Young JY, Ryan ME, Young NM. Preoperative imaging of sensorineural hearing loss in pediatric candidates for cochlear implantation. Radiographics 2014; 34(5):E133–E149

[6] Fishman AJ. Imaging and anatomy for cochlear implants. Otolaryngol Clin North Am 2012; 45(1):1–24

[7] Zayas JO, Feliciano YZ, Hadley CR, Gomez AA, Vidal JA. Temporal bone trauma and the role of multidetector CT in the emergency department. Radiographics 2011; 31(6):1741–1755

23 Oral Cavity

23.1 Oral Cavity, Salivary Glands, and Pharynx

The oral cavity is the gateway for food into the body and is involved with breathing and verbal communication, and consequently it may serve as the point of entry into the body for infectious agents. Against this, physical barriers (the tongue, glottis, etc.) and immunologic barriers (Waldeyer's ring of lymphatic tissue) serve to protect the airway and the body from unwanted intruders. The salivary glands provide lubrication, pH buffering, and antibacterial substances to help maintain normal functions and prevent infection. Lesions of the oral cavity and pharynx in children are of infectious etiology much more often than in adults, in whom neoplastic lesions of these structures are the primary concern. However, just as adults can get infections, neoplasms can develop in children.

23.2 Anatomy

The oral cavity is bounded anteriorly by the lips, inferiorly by the tongue and floor of the mouth, superiorly by the hard and soft palates and dental arches, and laterally by the buccal mucosa, and communicates posteriorly with the oropharynx (▶ Fig. 23.1). The posterior portion of the oral cavity is bounded laterally by the palatine tonsils and palatal and pharyngeal folds (▶ Fig. 23.2). Posteriorly, the oral cavity communicates with the oropharynx, which is inferior to the nasopharynx and superior to the hypopharynx.

The parotid glands are superficial to the masticator space and anteromedial to the sternocleidomastoid muscle. The submandibular glands are located in the submandibular triangle beneath the inferior border of the mandible, and wrap around the posterior edge of the mylohyoid muscle to enter the floor of

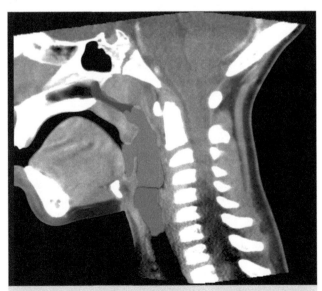

Fig. 23.1 Oropharynx/hypopharynx. Midsagittal soft tissue algorithm computed tomographic image showing the nasopharynx (red), oropharynx (green), and hypopharynx (blue).

the mouth. The sublingual glands are adjacent to the base of the tongue in the floor of the mouth. Additionally, the oral cavity contains thousands of minor salivary gland ducts.

A brief mention of the location of the salivary gland ducts is important because they are the sites of certain pathologies. The parotid duct (Stensen's duct) pierces the buccinator muscle and empties into the oral cavity through the buccal mucosa just lateral to the maxillary second molar. The submandibular duct (Wharton's duct) empties next to the frenulum in the floor of the mouth. The sublingual glands excrete their saliva into many ducts and their number and size are variable, but all empty into the floor of the mouth.

It is worth noting the various definitions and descriptions of the parapharyngeal space (▶ Fig. 23.3). The parapharyngeal space is relatively large, extending from the angle of the mandible inferiorly to the skull base superiorly, bounded laterally by the masticator space, and bounded medially by the pharynx. Some textbooks refer to a fascial ligament from the styloid process to the tensor veli palatini, dividing the parapharyngeal space into the prestyloid (lateral) and poststyloid (posteromedial) spaces. The terms parotid space and carotid space are often used and essentially represent the prestyloid and poststyloid spaces, respectively.

A source of confusion is that neither the prestyloid nor poststyloid space contains the submucosal connective tissue and parapharyngeal fat pads. The submucosal space that contains these structures is also called the parapharyngeal space in some texts concerning the head and neck, and is also called this by oral and maxillofacial surgeons, and one can argue that this space is more deserving of the term "parapharyngeal space" because it surrounds the pharynx. However, given that this space is not included in the parapharyngeal spaces described above, these areas are referred to as the "pharyngeal submucosal space." This submucosal space is very important for two reasons: (1) displacement of the fat in this space (seen on computed tomography [CT] and magnetic resonance imaging [MRI]) by lesions in the other parapharyngeal spaces can help determine the location and diagnostic identification of these lesions; and (2) this space is a pathway for the downward spread of odontogenic infections from the oral cavity into the neck and mediastinum.

Lesions in the prestyloid space are typically of salivary gland (parotid gland) origin. A small portion of the parotid gland often extends medially between the posterior border of the mandible and the styloid ligament (a space referred to the stylomandibular tunnel), and sometimes extends all the way up to the parapharyngeal fat. Lesions in the prestyloid space will displace the parapharyngeal fat pad anteromedially and the carotid artery posteriorly.

Lesions in the poststyloid space (carotid space) are often vascular lesions, paragangliomas, or neural lesions. Most neural lesions in the poststyloid space involve the vagus nerve, which is typically located posterior to the carotid artery. A lesion that displaces the carotid artery anteriorly or one that is located posterior to the styloid process and extends laterally and enters the poststyloid space narrows the differential diagnosis to lesions arising in the poststyloid space.

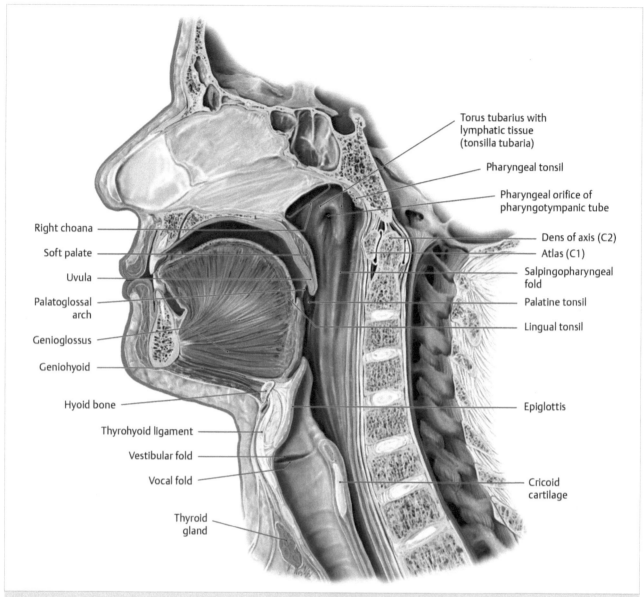

Fig. 23.2 Oral cavity. Artist's drawing of a midsagittal section of the oral cavity and pharynx. From Atlas of Anatomy, © Thieme 2012, Illustration by Karl Wesker.

The retropharyngeal space (part of the submucosal pharyngeal space) lies between the prevertebral fascia and the visceral fascia of the neck (see Chapter 17) and extends inferiorly into the mediastinum, serving as a pathway through which oropharyngeal infections can spread and cause mediastinitis.

23.3 Salivary Glands

Primary neoplasms of the salivary glands are rare in children, although capillary hemangiomas of infancy can be associated with the parotid gland. Infection adjacent to a salivary gland can lead to secondary inflammation. Stones within the ducts of the salivary glands (sialoliths) increase the risk of sialadenitis.

The ducts of the sublingual gland can become damaged and leak salivary fluid into the submucosa. A leaking salivary duct eventually becomes walled off by connective tissue, forming a pseudocyst termed a mucocele. When this occurs in the floor of the mouth, the mucocele is known as a ranula, and will be hyperintense on T2 W imaging, show no central enhancement, and have a thin peripheral wall without focal nodularity. A ranula can be confined to the sublingual space or can have cervical extension by coursing posterior to the mylohyoid muscle (or through a congenital defect in the mylohyoid); this is known as a plunging (or diving) ranula, and will nearly always be located lateral to the midline.[1] A midline cystic lesion in the floor of the mouth, typically in the posterior base of the tongue, is more likely to be a thyroglossal duct cyst (▶ Fig. 17.4), which is discussed in Chapter 17.[2]

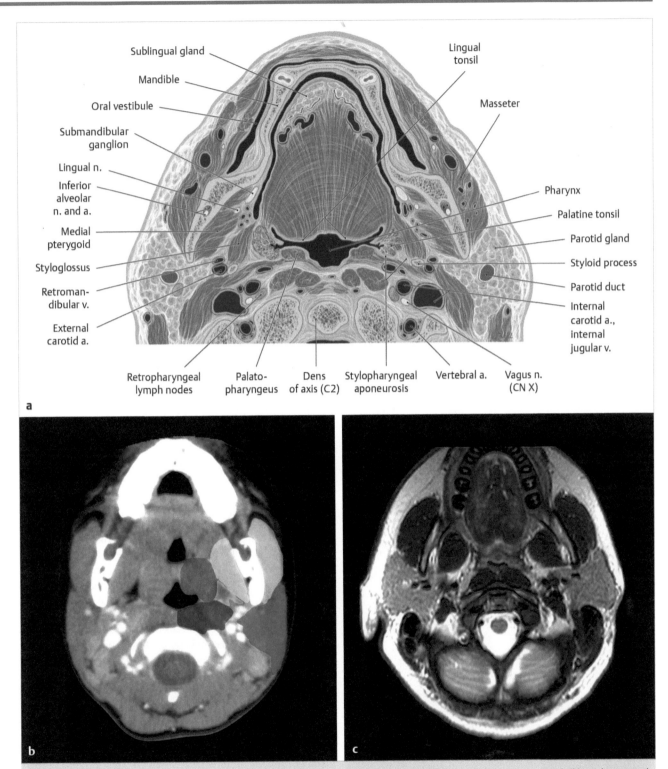

Fig. 23.3 Neck spaces, (a) Artist's drawing of an axial section through the suprahyoid neck with anatomic structures annotated. (b) Axial computed tomographic image of the suprahyoid neck showing the palatine tonsils (*red overlay*), retropharyngeal tissues, including the longus colli muscles (*black overlay*), parapharyngeal fat pad (*green overlay*), masticator space, including the masseter and lateral pterygoid muscles (*yellow overlay*), and parotid space containing the parotid gland (*purple/blue overlay*). (c) Axial T2 W magnetic resonance image at a level similar to that in (b) demonstrates the appearance of these same structures on magnetic resonance imaging. "a" From Atlas of Anatomy, © Thieme 2012, Illustration by Karl Wesker.

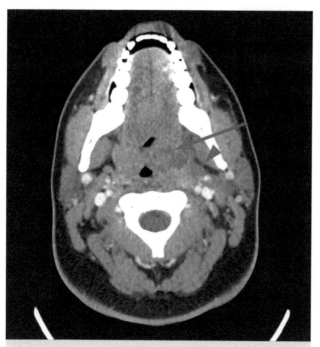

Fig. 23.4 Tonsillar phlegmon. Axial computed tomographic image of the head of a 17-year-old girl shows enlarged palatine tonsils bilaterally, with the enlargement of the left tonsil greater than that of the right tonsil. There is heterogeneous enhancement of the left palatine tonsil, without a discrete fluid collection (*red arrow*), representing a tonsillar phlegmon. Stranding is seen in the adjacent parapharyngeal fat (*red arrowhead*).

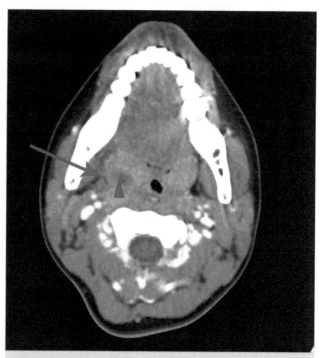

Fig. 23.5 Tonsillar abscess. Axial computed tomographic post contrast image of the head of a 12-year-old girl with throat pain shows a focal hypodense area within the depth of the right palatine tonsil (*red arrowhead*), representing a tonsillar abscess. There is stranding in the adjacent parapharyngeal fat (*red arrow*).

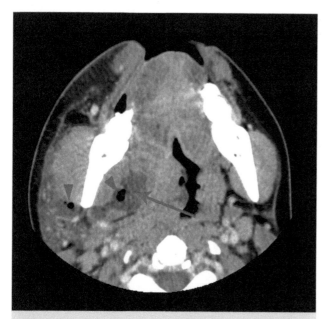

Fig. 23.6 Parapharyngeal abscess involving the neck and face. Axial computed tomographic plus contrast image of the head of a 15-year-old girl with throat pain and fever shows a parapharyngeal fluid collection (*red arrow*) with foci of air (*red arrowheads*). The inflammatory process extends to the masticator space. These findings represent a parapharyngeal abscess in the setting of necrotizing fasciitis.

23.4 Tonsils

The palatine tonsils are paired lymphatic structures at the lateral aspect of the posterior oral cavity. The palatine tonsils can become infected, resulting in the clinical diagnosis of tonsillitis. On imaging, this has a spectrum of appearances ranging from glandular swelling and hyperemia, through heterogeneous enhancement with fluidlike areas (tonsillar phlegmon) (▶ Fig. 23.4), to a discrete tonsillar abscess (▶ Fig. 23.5). In examining for tonsillar infections, it is important to look for involvement of the adjacent parapharyngeal fat.

An abscess centered in the parapharyngeal fat is sometimes called a "peritonsillar" abscess, and is a distinct entity from a tonsillar abscess. A tonsillar abscess will often spontaneously drain/decompress into the oral cavity, and if it does not do this spontaneously, can be drained through a transoral route. A parapharyngeal abscess is an abscess in the deep neck space that cannot typically be directly accessed through a transoral route and requires either open surgical drainage or image-guided drainage (▶ Fig. 23.6). Differentiating a parapharyngeal from a tonsillar abscess is important, as is use of the appropriate terminology for each condition to prevent confusion. Communication with local otolaryngologists and oral-maxillofacial surgeons is helpful to minimize confusion in the terminology for these abscesses.

Following the diagnosis of a tonsillar infection, typically on contrast-enhanced computed tomography (CT), it is important to evaluate the adjacent vasculature of the neck. The infection

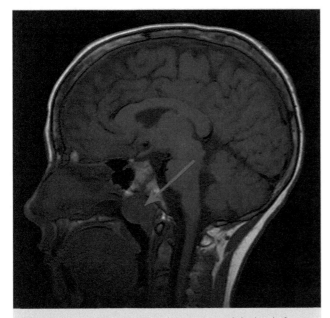

Fig. 23.7 Normal adenoids. Sagittal T1 W image of the head of a 9-year-old female with a history of headaches demonstrates prominence of the adenoids (*red arrow*). The patient had no symptoms of acute infection, and the findings in this case are felt to be normal findings in a child of this age. In an adult, these findings warrant direct visualization and possible biopsy.

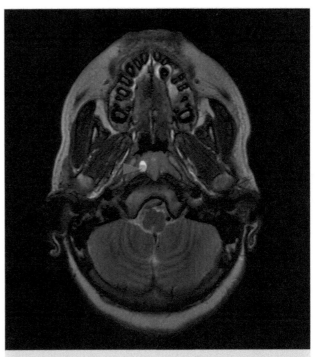

Fig. 23.8 Adenoid mucous retention cyst. Axial T2 W image of the head shows a mucous retention cyst (*red arrowhead*) within the right lateral aspect of the adenoids. Because this is not a midline lesion it does not represent a Tornwaldt cyst. In an adult, the findings shown here would raise concern about a neoplasm.

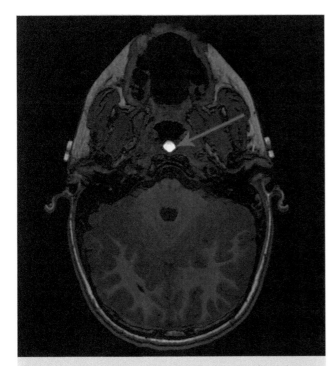

Fig. 23.9 Axial T1 W image of the head of a 10-year-old boy shows a circumscribed, T1 hyperintense, cystic-appearing structure in the midline and along the anterior aspect of the clivus at the level of the sphenooccipital synchondrosis, representing a Tornwaldt cyst (*red arrow*).

can result in vasospasm of the internal carotid artery, and infections in the neck can result in septic thrombophlebitis of the internal jugular vein (▶ Fig. 17.7).

Apart from the palatine tonsils is a ring of lymphoid tissue surrounding the oropharynx and posterior nasopharynx. This tissue includes the lingual and adenoid tonsils, collectively known as Waldeyer's ring. Adenoidal soft tissue prominence can be normal in children (▶ Fig. 23.7), particularly during the seasons when head and chest colds are common, and mucous retention cysts can be found within the adenoids in children (▶ Fig. 23.8). In contrast, soft tissue prominence in the adenoidal region in adults should raise concern about possible nasopharyngeal carcinoma. In an adult, any cystic change within the adenoidal region that is not a midline Tornwaldt cyst (a remnant of the notochord) (▶ Fig. 23.9) must raise concern for nasopharyngeal carcinoma.

23.5 Hypopharynx and Larynx

The hypopharynx and larynx play roles in the transit of food, protection of the airway, and phonation. Infection of the epiglottis can lead to the process known as epiglottitis (▶ Fig. 23.10). The incidence of infectious epiglottitis has diminished significantly as a result of vaccination against *Haemophilus influenzae* type B, but when encountered is an acute airway emergency. When imaging identifies epiglottitis in a child, the airway should not be examined and the child should not be agitated until definitive airway protection has been established through intubation under direct visualization. This is typically

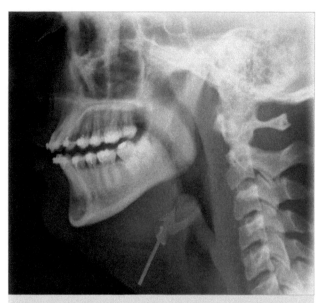

Fig. 23.10 Lateral radiograph of the neck showing thickening of the epiglottis (*red arrow*), an appearance suggestive of epiglottitis.

done in the operating room by an otolaryngologist and/or anesthesiologist, with the immediate availability of tracheostomy should it be needed. The lateral radiographic appearance of epiglottitis has been referred to as the "thumb sign" because it gives the epiglottis an appearance similar to a hitchhiker's thumb.

23.6 Teeth

The teeth reside in the maxillary and mandibular arches. Each arch is bilaterally symmetric, with the right and left half of each arch called a quadrant and housing a specific set and order of teeth. In adult humans, each quadrant, beginning from the midline and moving posterolaterally, contains two incisors (central and lateral), a canine tooth, two premolars (first and second), and three molars (first, second, and third), resulting in 8 teeth per quadrant, 16 per arch, and 32 in total. The primary dentition, consisting of deciduous teeth, consists of no premolars and only two molars, resulting in 5 teeth per quadrant, 10 per arch, and 20 in total.

The most common naming convention for the teeth involves their numbering from 1 through 32, beginning from the most posterior right maxillary tooth (third molar) and progressing along the dental arch to the left maxillary third molar, followed by the most posterior left mandibular tooth (third molar), and again progressing along the arch to the right mandibular third molar. On the basis of this numbering system, the four "wisdom" teeth are numbers 1, 16, 17, and 32; the central maxillary incisors are numbers 8 and 9 (right and left, respectively); and the central mandibular incisors are numbers 24 and 25 (left and right, respectively). Exact numbering of the teeth can be difficult if there are missing teeth and/or mixed dentition (some permanent and some primary teeth present). The 20 primary teeth are assigned the letters A through T (▸ Fig. 23.11).

Dental infection can result in decay/loss of the enamel of the teeth (caries). When an infection extends to the pulp of the tooth causing pulpal necrosis, the periapical inflammation commonly leads to abscess or granuloma formation, with each of these lesions appearing as a lucency on radiographs and CT (▸ Fig. 23.12), and occasionally leads to reactive bone formation with a sclerotic appearance on imaging. A localized periapical infection can extend through the cortex of the bone to cause a subperiosteal odontogenic abscess with surrounding soft tissue swelling. The abscess will centrally have the appearance of complex fluid and have an enhancing rim, and the surrounding cellulitis will appear as amorphous soft tissue stranding (▸ Fig. 23.13). It is important to note that in a dental abscess, unlike abscesses in other areas of the body, the absence of an organized fluid collection does not preclude surgical drainage.

The exposure of infected tissue to oxygen is thought to alter the course of dental infection and may prevent the spread of anaerobic infection and/or abscess formation. In addition, oral mucosal tissue heals remarkably well, with minimal scar formation, making the benefit of drainage of a dental infection typically outweigh its risks. Therefore, the finding on imaging of a dental infection of a phlegmon and fat stranding should be noted. The imaging report should not state that there is no drainable collection, which may mistakenly lead to the inappropriate discharge of a patient from an emergency department without an oral surgery consultation. This should be confirmed with local emergency physicians and oral surgeons to learn their practice patterns.

At times, a cystic lesion is seen surrounding an unerupted tooth. This can be a normal finding of an enlarged follicle, depending on the age of the patient and size of the cyst. When

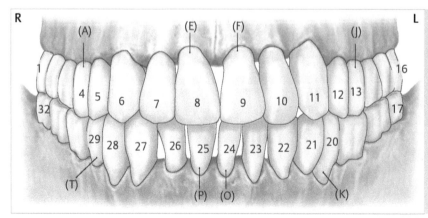

Fig. 23.11 Dental arch. Image showing the numbering of the permanent teeth (1 through 32), as well as schematic labeling showing the location of the primary teeth (A through T). From Atlas of Anatomy, © Thieme 2012, Illustration by Karl Wesker.

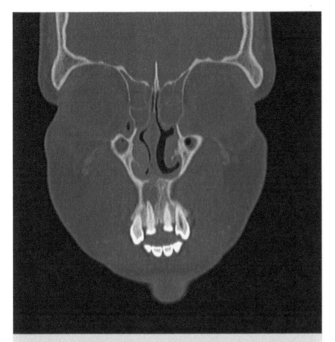

Fig. 23.12 Periapical lucency. Coronal bone algorithm computed tomographic image shows a lucency (*red arrowhead*) around the right central maxillary incisor (tooth number 8), representing demineralization from a dental infection.

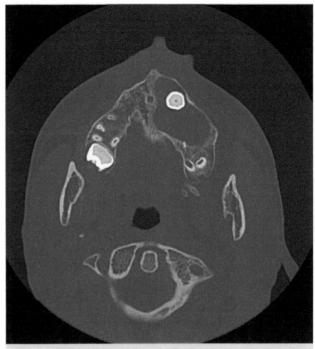

Fig. 23.14 Axial bone algorithm computed tomographic image of the maxilla shows a cystic lesion within the left maxillary bone, with an internal tooth, representing a dentigerous cyst.

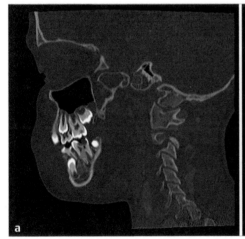

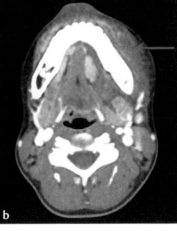

Fig. 23.13 Odontogenic abscess. (a) Sagittal bone algorithm computed tomographic image shows a focal area of enamel loss in a left mandibular molar tooth (*red arrowhead*), representing a dental cavity. (b) Axial soft tissue algorithm computed tomographic image shows soft tissue swelling and stranding along the superficial margin of the gingiva (*red arrow*), as well as along the medial margin, reprenseting an odontogenic cellulitis with a focal abscess.

such a cyst becomes larger than 2 cm, the likelihood of the tooth eventually erupting becomes very low (▶ Fig. 23.14). Known as dentigerous cysts, cysts surrounding unerupted teeth can occur in both the maxilla and mandible, and should not be mistaken for lytic neoplastic lesions.

Lytic mandibular or maxillary lesions that do not contain tooth material must be further evaluated. The differential diagnosis for lytic lesions in the mandible includes neoplastic entities, such as keratocystic odontogenic tumor (KOT, previously referred to as an odontogenic keratocyst), ameloblastoma (previously referred to as adamantinoma), aneurysmal bone cysts, and central giant-cell granuloma, and non-neoplastic entities, such as intraosseous vascular malformations and simple bone cysts. KOT is seen with increased frequency in patients with

Gorlin syndrome, which is a risk factor for developing medulloblastoma.

There is also an entity known as a mandibular salivary gland defect that appears as a well-corticated radiolucency on panoramic radiography but actually represents a bony indentation of a submandibular gland. This is a normal variant and does not require biopsy. It can be distinguished from a pathologic entity by its well-defined cortical borders and its location below the inferior alveolar nerve (IAN) canal, in the region of the submandibular gland. The vast majority of odontogenic lesions will be found or centered above the IAN canal. Sclerotic lesions in the mandible can include reactive changes from prior infection and fibrous dysplasia, among other entities.[3]

23.7 Suggested Reading

[1] Chapman MN, Nadgir RN, Akman AS et al. Periapical lucency around the tooth: Radiologic evaluation and differential diagnosis. Radiographics 2013; 33(1):E15–E32

[2] Dunfee BL, Sakai O, Pistey R, Gohel A. Radiologic and pathologic characteristics of benign and malignant lesions of the mandible. Radiographics 2006; 26 (6):1751–1768

[3] Capps EF, Kinsella JJ, Gupta M, Bhatki AM, Opatowsky MJ. Emergency imaging assessment of acute, nontraumatic conditions of the head and neck. Radiographics 2010; 30(5):1335–1352

[4] Meuwly J-Y, Lepori D, Theumann N et al. Multimodality imaging evaluation of the pediatric neck: Techniques and spectrum of findings. Radiographics 2005; 25(4):931–948

[5] Ludwig BJ, Foster BR, Saito N, Nadgir RN, Castro-Aragon I, Sakai O. Diagnostic imaging in nontraumatic pediatric head and neck emergencies. Radiographics 2010; 30(3):781–799

[6] Hoang JK, Eastwood JD, Branstetter BF, IV et al. Masses in the retropharyngeal space: Key concepts on multiplanar CT and MR imaging. Neurographics 2011; 1:49–55

References

[1] La'porte SJ, Juttla JK, Lingam RK. Imaging the floor of the mouth and the sublingual space. Radiographics 2011; 31(5):1215–1230

[2] Zander DA, Smoker WRK. Imaging of ectopic thyroid tissue and thyroglossal duct cysts. Radiographics 2014; 34(1):37–50

[3] Curé JK, Vattoth S, Shah R. Radiopaque jaw lesions: An approach to the differential diagnosis. Radiographics 2012; 32(7):1909–1925

Part 4

Spine Imaging

24 Anatomy and Craniocervical Junction

24.1 Spine Anatomy

The vertebral column is the central supportive structure of the body, linking the skull base to the pelvis, with the ribs and extremities connected directly to the periphery of the column or connected indirectly to it through other bones, such as the shoulder or pelvic girdle. The vertebral column also serves to protect the spinal cord, and is a defining anatomic feature of higher-order life forms. In addition to the structure and protection provided by the bones of the vertebral column, the fibrocartilagenous intervertebral disks provide the ability for movement.

The vertebral column consists of 24 articulating vertebrae, including 7 cervical (C1–C7), 12 thoracic (T1–T12), and 5 lumbar vertebrae (L1–L5), and 9 fused and relatively immobile vertebrae, including 5 sacral (S1–S5) and 4 coccygeal (Cx1–Cx4) segments. The morphology of the coccyx is highly variable, and there are often transitional vertebrae at the lumbosacral junction, typically a sacralized (or hemisacralized) L5 vertebra or a lumbarized (or partly lumbarized) S1 vertebra. There are also variations in the number of ribs, including occasional cervical ribs at C7, absent ribs at T12, or rudimentary ribs at L1. Throughout the articulating portions of the vertebral column, the vertebrae are separated from one another by fibrocartilagenous intervertebral disks. At each vertebral level are right and left nerve roots that emanate from the neural foramen. In the cervical spine, the C2–C3 neural foramen carries the C3 nerve root, and in the thoracic spine (as in the lumbar and sacral regions) the T1–T2 neural foramen carries the T1 nerve root. At the cervicothoracic junction is a C8 nerve root, although there is no C8 vertebra. Also, although the coccyx has four osseous segments, there is only one coccygeal nerve.

24.1.1 Typical Articulating Vertebrae

The articulating vertebrae have a vertebral body and a posterior neural arch. The posterior neural arch consists of two pedicles that extend posteriorly to the superior and inferior articulating facets. Posterior to that are medially directed laminae that come together to form the posteriorly directed spinous processes. Beneath the pedicles of the neural arch are the neural foramina, through which nerve-root sleeves project. (It is a satisfaction in pediatric neuroradiology to almost never have to describe neural foraminal stenosis, except at the apex of a severe scoliotic curvature and in several other rare situations.) The vertebrae have laterally directed transverse processes that arise anterior to the facets in the cervical and lumbar spine and posterior to the facets in the thoracic spine (▶ Fig. 24.1).

24.1.2 Special Anatomic Considerations

The first two cervical vertebrae have unique morphologic and functional characteristics. The first cervical vertebra, C1, does not contain a vertebral body, and represents a ring. The ring has an anterior and posterior neural arch, with two lateral masses. These lateral masses articulate with the occipital condyles, and because the C1 vertebra supports the cranium, it is sometimes referred to as the atlas (derived from the name of Atlas, the Greek god who supported the world on his back). The articulation of the atlas with the occipital condyles allows vertical motion of the head (e.g., nodding of the head) (▶ Fig. 24.1a,b; ▶ Fig. 24.2, ▶ Fig. 24.3, ▶ Fig. 24.4, ▶ Fig. 24.5).

The body of the C2 vertebra has a superiorly directed vertical protrusion known as the odontoid process (also known as the dens). The odontoid process serves as a post around which C1 can rotate, and by allowing such rotation of the head, C2 is also known as the axis. The posterior neural arch of C2 is similar to those of C3–C7, described above.

The vertebral bodies of C2 through C7 do not have a purely planar inferior surface, because the side edges of the vertebrae immediately below each of these vertebrae have the hook-shaped processes known as uncinate processes, which prevent C2 through C7 from sliding backward and off the surfaces of C3 through T1, respectively. This provides an additional articulation known as the uncovertebral joint. Each of the cervical vertebrae also has within its transverse processes an opening known as the foramen transversarium through which the left and right vertebral arteries pass (typically entering at approximately the C6 level) before merging within the skull to form the basilar artery. In summary:

- The thoracic vertebrae articulate with ribs.
- The lumbar vertebrae typically do not have any special features.
- The sacral vertebrae are typically fused with one another without a formed disk space between them. Instead of transverse processes, the sacral vertebrae have winglike lateral projections (alae).
- The coccyx is largely ignored when evaluating imaging of the spine.

24.1.3 Alignment

The adult cervical spine typically has a mild lordosis, with a mild kyphosis in the thoracic spine and a mild lordosis in the lumbar spine. In childhood, the cervical alignment is often straight or slightly kyphotic, which is normal (see Chapter 28 for further discussion). It is important to also be aware of an additional variant in spinal alignment in young children, which is the apparent subtle (up to approximately 3 mm) anterolisthesis of C2 with respect to C3, known as pseudosubluxation (▶ Fig. 24.6). It is normal for children under approximately 8 years of age to have a subtle alignment variant at this location, and this should not be mistaken for a fracture.

24.1.4 Ligaments

The anterior surfaces of the vertebrae are connected by a continuous anterior longitudinal ligament (ALL). The posterior margins of the vertebral bodies, which together form the anterior margin of the spinal canal, are connected by the posterior longitudinal ligament (PLL). The posterior/posterolateral margin of the spinal canal consists of the ligamenta flava, which connect the laminae of adjacent vertebrae. Between the spinous processes are interspinous ligaments, and overlying the tips of the

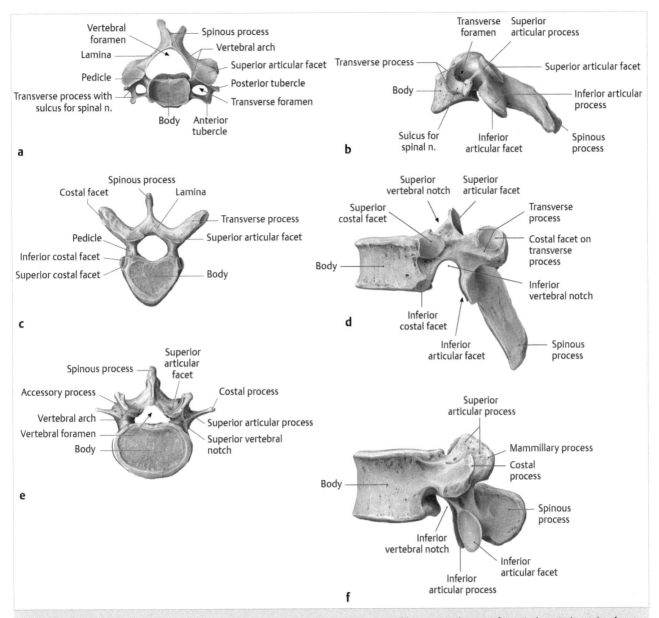

Fig. 24.1 (a) Anatomic drawing of a typical cervical vertebra from a superior projection. (b) Anatomic drawing of a typical cervical vertebra from a lateral projection (c) Anatomic drawing of a typical thoracic vertebra from a superior projection. (d) Anatomic drawing of a typical thoracic vertebra from a lateral projection. (e) Anatomic drawing of a typical lumbar vertebra from a superior projection. (f) Anatomic drawing of a typical lumbar vertebra from a lateral projection. From Atlas of Anatomy, © Thieme 2012, Illustrations by Karl Wesker. (*continued*)

spinous processes, from C7 to the sacrum, is the supraspinous ligament.

The ALL extends to the anterior surface of the clivus, at the skull base, as the anterior atlanto-occipital ligament. The PLL extends superiorly from the odontoid process as the tectorial membrane, where it becomes the dorsal dura of the clivus, and the ligamentum flavum extends superiorly to the posterior margin of the foramen magnum (opisthion) as the posterior atlanto-occipital ligament. The supraspinous ligament in the upper cervical spine does not remain adjacent to the tips of the spinous processes, and is known as the nuchal ligament, attaching to the occipital bone at the external occipital protuberance.

The tip of the odontoid process has a ligamentous connection, known as the apical ligament of the odontoid, that extends

superiorly to the basion. Two superior-oblique ligaments, the alar ligaments, extend from the odontoid process to the occipital condyles. A horizontally oriented ligament connecting both sides of the anterior neural arch of C1 and extending posterior to the odontoid process is the transverse ligament.

24.2 Embryology

The spine and spinal cord develop together, starting in the third gestational week, through a process known as neurulation. During this process, the neural plate (a special area of ectoderm) begins to fold inward, and eventually forms a hollow tube. The boundaries between the neural plate and the normal ectoderm

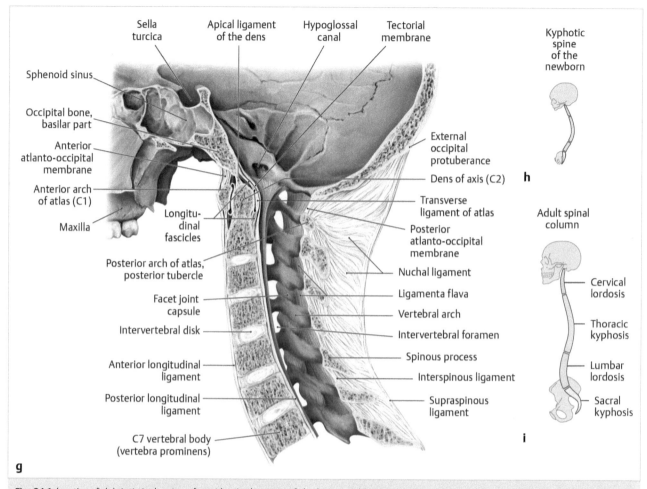

Fig. 24.1 (*continued*) (g) Artist's drawing of a midsagittal section of the bones and ligaments of the skull base, craniocervical junction, and cervical spine. Diagrams showing the differences in sagittal alignment of the vertebral column in (h) infancy and (i) in adulthood. From Atlas of Anatomy, © Thieme 2012, Illustrations by Karl Wesker.

are known as the neural folds, and converge at approximately 4 weeks of gestation to create the neural crest. The neural tube has cranial and caudal openings, known as neural pores, which close during the fourth week of gestation; cranial defects in closure of the neural tube, including anencephaly and encephalocele, are discussed in Chapters 3 and 15. Caudal defects in closure of the neural tube, resulting in conditions like myelomeningocele, are further discussed in also Chapter 5.[1,2,3,4]

Ventral to the neural tube is a linear mesodermal structure known as the notochord, which serves as the backbone for neurulation. Along the sides of the notochord develop the paired mesodermal elements, one on each side of the notochord, known as the paraxial mesoderm, which give rise to the somites. The somites, of which there are 44 pairs, differentiate into the vertebrae of the spine and into the ribs, skeletal muscle, and other structures. Associated with the development of each somite is a component known as a sclerotome, which is the lower, medioventral part of the somite, a dermatome, or area of skin supplied with afferent nerve fibers from a single spinal nerve root, and a myotome, which develops into the group of muscles supplied by a single spinal nerve root. As the somites differentiate into vertebral chondrification and ossification centers, the

notochord regresses. The nucleus pulposus of the intervertebral disk is a remnant of the notochord.

Each vertebra arises from multiple primary and secondary ossification centers. In the infant, the nonossified portions of a vertebra should not be mistaken for a fracture. It is possible for some of the ossification centers of vertebra to close incompletely, resulting in a series of congenital clefts[5] further described in the anatomic variants section of this chapter and in Chapter 26.

Most vertebrae (C3 to L5) have three primary and five secondary ossification centers. One primary ossification center gives rise to the bone of the vertebral body, and two other primary ossification centers give rise to the left half and to the right half, respectively, of the posterior elements of the spine. Two of the five secondary ossification centers of each vertebral body give rise to the two transverse processes of each vertebra. Another secondary ossification center exists at the tip of the spinous process, and two further secondary ossification centers exist as ring epiphyses at the superior and inferior endplates of the vertebral bodies (▶ Fig. 24.2, ▶ Fig. 24.3, ▶ Fig. 24.4, ▶ Fig. 24.5). The unossified ring epiphyses result in the "bullet" shape of immature vertebrae, the bodies of which become more

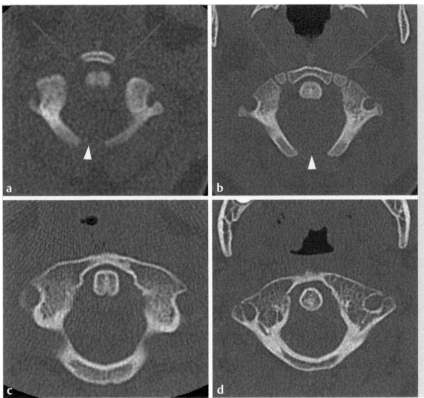

Fig. 24.2 Development of C1 and C2, axial views. Axial computed tomographic images of C1 at 4 months, 20 months, 5 years, and 9 years of age. (a) At 4 months, the anterior ossification center is in isolation (*red arrowheads*) because of the incompletely ossified neurocentral synchondroses (*red arrows*). The posterior median intraneural synchondrosis is not yet closed (*white arrowheads*). (b) At 20 months, there are ossicles forming in the neurocentral synchondroses (*red arrows*). (c) At 5 years of age and (d) 9 years of age, the C1 ring is fully ossified.

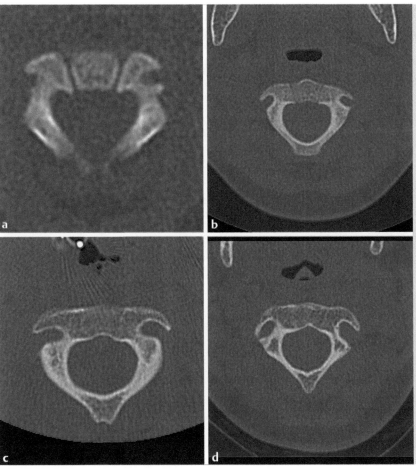

Fig. 24.3 Development of C1 and C2, axial views. Axial computed tomographic images of C2 at 4 months, 20 months, 5 years, and 9 years of age. (a) At 4 months, the neurocentral synchondroses are still present, and the posterior neural arch is not yet unified. (b) At 20 months, the neurocentral synchondroses are fusing and the posterior neural arch has closed. (c) At 5 years of age and (d) 9 years of age, the C2 ring is fully ossified.

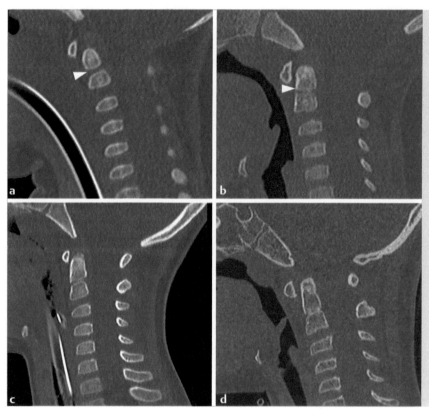

Fig. 24.4 Development of C1 and C2, sagittal views. Sagittal computed tomographic images of the craniocervical junction at 4 months, 20 months, 5 years, and 9 years of age. (a) At 4 months, the odontoid synchondrosis is patent (*white arrowhead*), and it progressively ossifies/fuses throughout childhood at (b) 20 months, (c) 5 years and (d) 9 years. The posterior neural arch of C1 is visible at 5 years and 9 years of age, corresponding to the appearance in Fig. 24.3c and Fig. 24.3d, respectively.

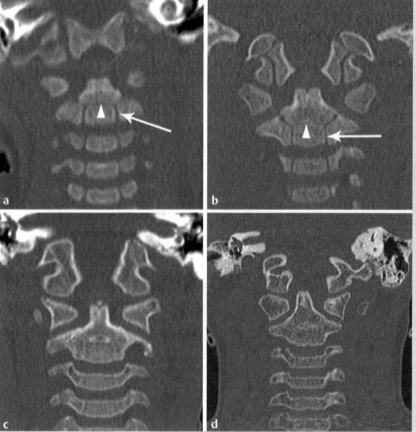

Fig. 24.5 Development of C1 and C2, coronal views. Coronal CT images of the craniocervical junction at 4 months, 20 months, 5 years, and 9 years of age. (a) At 4 months, the neurocentral (*white arrow*) and odontocentral (*white arrowhead*) synchondroses of C2 are patent. There is no apical secondary ossification (*red arrow*). (b) At 20 months, the neurocentral synchondrosis (*white arrow*) is closing and the odontocentral synchondrosis is nearly closed (*white arrowhead*). There is no apical secondary ossification (*red arrowhead*). (c) At 5 years of age, the primary ossification centers have all fused and there is partial visualization of the odontoid apical secondary ossification center, giving a "trident" appearance. (d) At 9 years of age, the odontoid apical secondary ossification center has fused with the odontoid process.

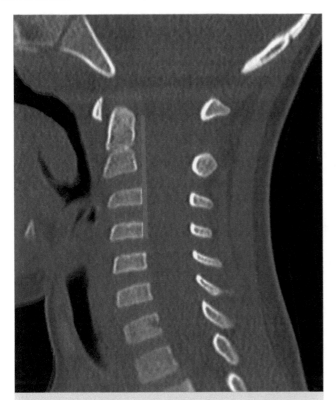

Fig. 24.6 Pseudosubluxation. Sagittal bone algorithm computed tomographic image of the cervical spine of a 4-year-old boy shows that the posterior cortex of the vertebral body of C2 does not directly line up with the posterior cortex of the vertebral bodies of C3 and C4, as shown by the *red line*. This is known as pseudosubluxation, and is a physiologic process normal in the first 6 to 8 years of life.

cylindrical as the vertebrae mature (▶ Fig. 24.7). The incompletely ossified ring epiphysis of an immature vertebra should not be mistaken for a fracture.

Some special developmental considerations apply to the first and second cervical vertebrae, C1 and C2. The odontoid process of C2 has two additional primary ossification centers beyond the three such centers for most vertebrae, as well as an odontoid apical secondary ossification center. No secondary ossification centers exist in C1. The ossification of the sacrum is complex, but without much clinical significance other than variants in segmentation. The ossification of the coccyx is simple, without much clinical significance.

24.3 Bone Marrow

Within each vertebra is trabeculated bone with bone marrow. In childhood, this is red marrow, comprising hematopoietic cells, and accordingly has intermediate signal intensity on T1 W and T2 W magnetic resonance imaging (MRI). Throughout childhood and adolescence, red marrow undergoes conversion to yellow marrow. Yellow marrow, which is fatty, has a hyperintense signal on T1 W and T2 W MRI (▶ Fig. 24.8 and ▶ Fig. 24.9).

24.4 Imaging Techniques

Plain radiographic films are less sensitive to fractures than computed tomographic scans. However, radiographs involve less radiation than CT, and the limitations are less in children than in adults. The role of plain films for the primary evaluation of fractures must be established on the basis of local practice protocols and evidence-based guidelines. Radiographs are very good for evaluating and following spinal alignment, and particularly so for conditions like scoliosis.

24.4.1 Computed Tomography

Computed tomography (CT) provides excellent bone and soft tissue detail, and is the best means of evaluating patients for fractures in the setting of trauma. It can provide additional information about congenital osseous malformations and about the status of fracture-repair hardware after bone fusion. Given that the radiation doses entailed by CT are significantly higher than those for plain films, care must be taken to find the optimum balance between a lowest useful radiation dosage (favoring plain films) and a dosage revealing more detail (favoring CT), an issue for which there is rarely a perfect answer.

24.4.2 Magnetic Resonance Imaging

Magnetic resonance imaging has several main roles in evaluation of the spine. The first of these is in evaluating the spinal cord and nerve roots of the cauda equina, which are not well seen on CT. Magnetic resonance imaging can be used to look for intradural and extradural soft tissue abnormalities, such as tumors, abscesses, or hematomas. Although inferior to CT for bone evaluation, MRI can permit better evaluation of bone marrow in examining for edema (e.g., in trauma, infection, etc). Postcontrast MRI provides additional information when there is concern about tumor, infection, or a noninfectious inflammatory process. In complicated cases, MRI and CT can be complementary and increase the diagnostic accuracy of both studies.

24.4.3 Ultrasonography

Ultrasonographic examination of the spine is typically limited to the first few months of life. When there is concern about a possibly tethered cord, such as in a patient with a sacral dimple, ultrasonography can identify the location of the conus medullaris, the thickness of the filum terminale, the presence of a dermal sinus tract, or a congenital lesion, such as a dermoid or lipoma.

24.4.4 Nuclear Imaging

Nuclear imaging, such as in bone scanning and subsequent single-photon emission computed tomography (SPECT), can help in evaluating for possible defects in the pars interarticularis and for stress fractures. Although not commonly used for children, and largely supplanted by MRI in patients without contraindications to the latter, a gallium scan can aid in the evaluation of suspected diskitis/osteomyelitis.

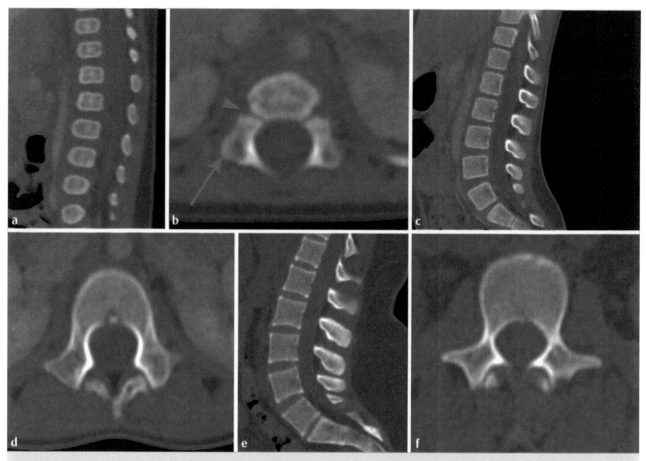

Fig. 24.7 Lumbar development. Sagittal computed tomographic images of the lumbar spine (a,c,e) and axial image of L1 (b,d,f) at various ages. (a) At 4 months of age, the disk spaces appear wide, taking up nearly 50% of the height of the adjacent vertebral body, and the endplate corners are rounded, especially anteriorly. (b) The neurocentral synchondroses remain patent (*red arrowhead*), and the transverse processes are hypoplastic (*red arrow*). The lateral cortices of the pedicles are more lateral than the lateral cortex of the vertebral body. (c) At 7 years of age, the vertebrae are more rectangular, but with slight rounding of the corners, and the disk spaces have become narrower relative to the vertebrae. (d) The neurocentral synchondroses are fused and the transverse processes are partly developed. The lateral cortices of the pedicles are at the same level as the lateral cortex of the vertebral body. (e) At 16 years of age, the vertebrae are rectangular, with well demarcated corners. (f) The transverse processes have continued to mature, and the lateral cortices of the pedicles pinch slightly inward from the vertebral body.

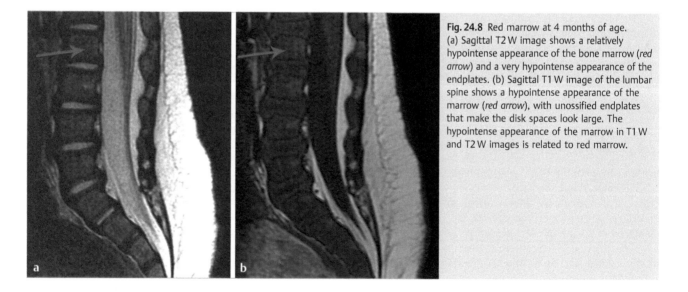

Fig. 24.8 Red marrow at 4 months of age. (a) Sagittal T2 W image shows a relatively hypointense appearance of the bone marrow (*red arrow*) and a very hypointense appearance of the endplates. (b) Sagittal T1 W image of the lumbar spine shows a hypointense appearance of the marrow (*red arrow*), with unossified endplates that make the disk spaces look large. The hypointense appearance of the marrow in T1 W and T2 W images is related to red marrow.

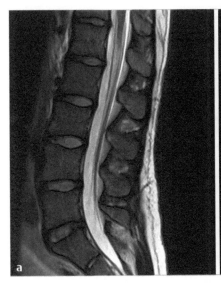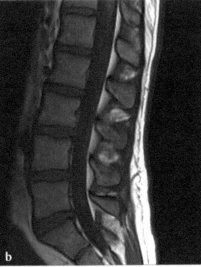

Fig. 24.9 Yellow marrow in a 17-year-old female. (a) Sagittal T2 W image shows a relatively intermediate signal character of the bone marrow. (b) Sagittal T1 W image of the lumbar spine shows an intermediate to slightly hyper-intense appearance of the marrow. The change in signal characteristics is related to increased fat content within the marrow as it converts to yellow marrow.

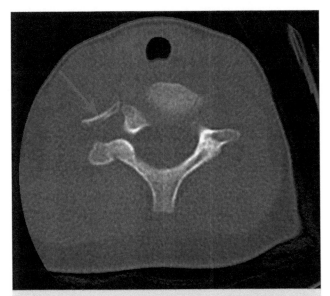

Fig. 24.10 Cervical rib. Axial CT image of C7 of the neck of a 30-month-old boy shows a rudimentary right-sided C7 cervical rib. (*red arrow*)

24.5 Variants

24.5.1 Cervical Rib

At times, there can be rudimentary ribs at C7. Although this is often a normal variant, it predisposes to neurovascular compression and symptoms of thoracic outlet syndrome, including paresthesias when the arm is raised (▶ Fig. 24.10).

24.5.2 Sacralized L5 Transverse Processes

At times, the L5 transverse processes have a sacralized appearance, which is often unilateral (hemisacralization). It is important to recognize this as involving L5 and not a partly lumbarized S1, particularly if there are plans for an image-guided surgical procedure (▶ Fig. 24.11). On CT and MRI, the ileolumbar ligaments nearly always arise from the transverse processes of L5, which helps in establishing the true identity of L5; however, this is not always the case. (▶ Fig. 24.11 a,c).

24.5.3 Persistent S1–S2 Disk Space

At times, a formed disk space exists between S1 and S2. On a sagittal CT or MRI image, or a lateral radiograph, it can be difficult to exactly identify the L5 and S1 vertebrae. When there is uncertainty, it is important to use all available information, including identification of the caudal-most rib-bearing vertebrae, to correctly identify specific lumbar and sacral vertebrae, possibly correlating this information with the findings on a prior chest radiograph if one is available, and with the location of the ileolumbar ligament, and with other information. At times, it can be difficult to confidently identify vertebral levels even with this additional information, in which case it is important to describe the areas of uncertainty. Vertebral numbering can be especially confusing if there are incompletely segmented vertebrae or hemivertebrae (▶ Fig. 24.11b).

24.6 Clefts

Several congenital clefts can occur within the vertebrae, some of which (in particular sagittal and coronal clefts of the vertebrae) are associated with skeletal dysplasia. Other clefts, including an intraspinous cleft and other clefts of the posterior neural arch, are often sporadic. These are discussed further in Chapter 26.

24.7 Anatomy and Pathology of the Craniocervical Junction

The anatomy of the craniocervical junction can be confusing, and understandably so given the inconsistent use of terminology in describing it. The normal anatomy of the craniocervical

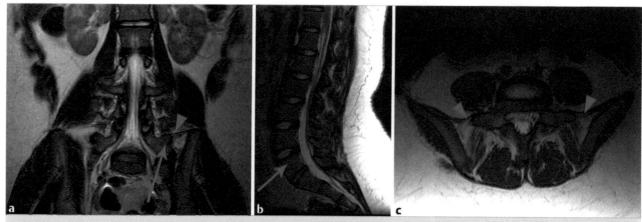

Fig. 24.11 Sacralized L5 vertebra. (a) Coronal T2 W image of the spine of a 12-year-old girl with back pain shows left hemisacralization of a transitional vertebra at the lumbosacral junction (*red arrow*). The ileolumbar ligament attaches to this transverse process (*red arrowhead*). Because there are 12 rib-bearing vertebrae (confirmed on a chest radiograph, not shown) and L5 is the fifth non-rib-bearing vertebra, this represents a partly sacralized L5 vertebra. (b) A sagittal T2 W image shows the lowest formed vertebra (*red arrow*); however, the disk space between L5 and S1 is less mature than the remainder of the imaged disk spaces. (c) Axial T2 W image of L5 shows the ileolumbar ligaments bilaterally (*red arrowheads*).

junction is reviewed in the following sections, and although the present chapter is predominantly focused on anatomy, abnormalities of the craniocervical junction are also discussed. Terms with which to be familiar in this regard include platybasia, basilar invagination, basilar impression, cranial settling, and atlantoaxial instability (▶ Table 24.1).[6,7] Rotatory subluxation and retroclival epidural hematoma are discussed in Chapter 28.

24.7.1 Anatomic Features

The clivus is comprised of the basisphenoid and basiocciput. The inferior tip of the basiocciput is the basion, which forms the anterior margin of the foramen magnum. The posterior margin of the foramen magnum is known as the opisthion, and develops embryologically from a structure known as Kerkring's ossicle, which joins the adjacent portions of the occipital bone. The margins of the foramen magnum are formed entirely by parts of the occipital bone.

24.7.2 Pathology

Platybasia

The term "platybasia" describes "flattening" of the central skull base, with an increased angle, known as the Welcker basal angle, between the dorsal aspect of the clivus and the planum sphenoidale. An angle of more than 140° is said to be diagnostic of platybasia, but this measurement was originally based on radiographic assessment (▶ Fig. 24.12).

Basilar Invagination and Basilar Impression

The term "basilar invagination" describes an abnormal relationship between the occiput and C1 as the result of a predisposing congenital abnormality. However, although the predisposing abnormality is congenital, the severity of the basilar invagination may be progressive. The relationship between C1 and C2 in patients with basilar invagination is variable, but is often normal (although some malformations of C1 may make it difficult

Table 24.1 Abnormalities of the craniocervical junction and skull base

Abnormality	O–C1 relationship	C1–C2 relationship	Acquired or congenital	Common associations
Cranial settling	Typically normal	Abnormal	Acquired	Rheumatoid arthritis (ligamentous laxity)
Basilar invagination	Abnormal	~ Normal*	Congenital,** can be progressive	Congenital abnormalities of the craniocervical junction
Basilar impression	Abnormal	Typically normal	Acquired	Trauma, bone metabolic disorders (e.g., Paget's disease)
Platybasia	Normal†	Normal†	Either	Many

*Although abnormality of the C1–C2 relationship is not a hallmark of basilar invagination, the C1 malformation often present makes it difficult in many cases to have a truly normal C1–C2 articulation.
**Although the predisposing developmental abnormality of the craniocervical junction is congenital, the severity of the basilar invagination may be progressive.
†Platybasia can be seen with basilar invagination, but the two are separate findings.

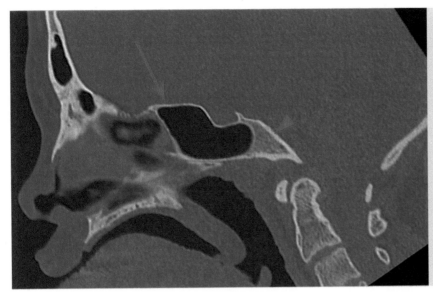

Fig. 24.12 Platybasia. Sagittal bone algorithm computed tomographic image of the skull base and craniocervical junction of a 15-year-old girl demonstrates a wide angle between the planum sphenoidale (*red arrow*) and the dorsal clivus (*red arrowhead*), known as platybasia ("flat base").

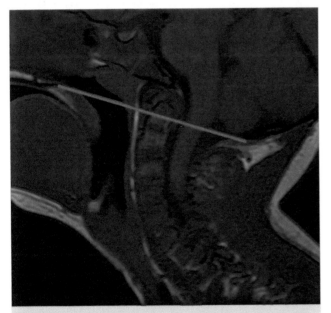

Fig. 24.13 Basilar invagination. Sagittal T1 W image of the craniocervical junction of a 6-year-old boy shows the primary ossification center of the odontoid process projecting several millimeters above the line between the posterior hard palate and the opisthion (*red line*), with the unossified secondary ossification center of the odontoid apex projecting even further above this line, representing basilar invagination. There is a somewhat sharp angle between the posterior clivus and the posterior cortex of the odontoid process, and there is borderline platybasia as well.

to have truly normal articulations). Basilar impression is an acquired form of the same abnormality as in basilar invagination, and can be seen after trauma and possibly after prior craniocervical junction surgery, such as suboccipital decompression for a Chiari type I malformation, or may result from metabolic bone disease (▶ Fig. 24.13).

The determination of basilar invagination is based on the position of the odontoid process relative to a line drawn from the posterior edge of the hard palate to the opisthion. Basilar invagination (or basilar impression, if the condition is acquired) is said to exist when the odontoid process extends above this line by more than 3 mm. If the line is drawn from the posterior edge of the hard palate to the inferior cortex of the occipital bone, a measurement of 4.5 mm above this line, rather than 3 mm, is considered to represent basilar invagination or basilar impression. Note that basilar invagination is not defined as projection of the odontoid process through the foramen magnum.

Cranial Settling

The term "cranial settling" relates to an abnormal relationship between C1 and C2 as the result of ligamentous laxity, and is most commonly seen in rheumatoid arthritis. This results in telescoping of C1 with respect to C2, as the skull and C1 "settle" onto the rest of the body. The relationship between the occiput and C1 is typically normal.

Atlantoaxial Instability

Atlantoaxial instability relates to abnormal ligamentous stability between C1 and C2 in the anterior–posterior direction. This is seen with increased frequency in children with trisomy 21, and also after traumatic injury to the transverse ligament of the atlas. Lateral radiographs of the craniocervical junction are obtained with the patient in neutral, flexed, and extended positions. A distance between the posterior cortex of the anterior neural arch of C1 and the odontoid process that exceeds approximately 5 mm in a young child (or 3 mm in an adult) is considered abnormal. Movement between flexion and extension is also considered abnormal (▶ Fig. 24.14). When this is found in patients with trisomy 21, extra attention must be given to head positioning for endotracheal intubation to prevent abnormal head movement. Accordingly, flexion-extension radiographs of the neck of such patients are often requested before the patient undergoes a surgical procedure. The relationship between the occiput and C1 in atlantoaxial instability is typically normal.

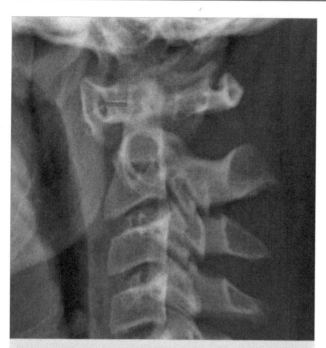

Fig. 24.14 Atlantoaxial instability. Lateral radiograph at the C1–C2 level of a 12-year-old male with trisomy 21 shows a 4 mm distance between the anterior cortex of the odontoid process and the posterior cortex of the anterior neural arch of C1 (*red line*). A distance between C1 and C2 of more than 3 mm in adults and more than 5 mm in children is considered abnormal, as is subluxation between flexion and extension of the neck.

24.8 Suggested Reading

[1] Junewick JJ. Pediatric craniocervical junction injuries. AJR Am J Roentgenol 2011; 196(5):1003–1010

[2] Junewick JJ, Chin MS, Meesa IR, Ghori S, Boynton SJ, Luttenton CR. Ossification patterns of the atlas vertebra. AJR Am J Roentgenol 2011; 197(5):1229–1234

[3] Karwacki GM, Schneider JF. Normal ossification patterns of atlas and axis: A CT study. AJNR Am J Neuroradiol 2012; 33(10):1882–1887

References

[1] Rufener SL, Ibrahim M, Raybaud CA, Parmar HA. Congenital spine and spinal cord malformations—Pictorial review. AJR Am J Roentgenol 2010; 194(3) Suppl:S26–S37

[2] Kaplan KM, Spivak JM, Bendo JA. Embryology of the spine and associated congenital abnormalities. Spine J 2005; 5(5):564–576

[3] Unsinn KM, Geley T, Freund MC, Gassner I. US of the spinal cord in newborns: Spectrum of normal findings, variants, congenital anomalies, and acquired diseases. Radiographics 2000; 20(4):923–938

[4] Pang D, Thompson DNP. Embryology and bony malformations of the craniovertebral junction. Childs Nerv Syst 2011; 27(4):523–564

[5] Johansen JG, McCarty DJ, Haughton VM. Retrosomatic clefts: Computed tomographic appearance. Radiology 1983; 148(2):447–448

[6] Lustrin ES, Karakas SP, Ortiz AO et al. Pediatric cervical spine: Normal anatomy, variants, and trauma. Radiographics 2003; 23(3):539–560

[7] Smoker WR. Craniovertebral junction: Normal anatomy, craniometry, and congenital anomalies. Radiographics 1994; 14(2):255–277

25 Infection and Inflammatory Conditions

25.1 Spinal Infections and Inflammatory Conditions

The spinal cord is a part of the central nervous system (CNS), and as such is surrounded by cerebrospinal fluid (CSF), has a dural covering, and is myelinated by oligodendrocytes. Accordingly, many of the inflammatory conditions that influence the brain, of both infectious and noninfectious origin, can affect the spinal cord. The appearance of these entities on imaging overlaps that of neoplastic entities.

The spinal cord is supported and protected by a dural layer within the scaffolding of the vertebral column. Nerves of the peripheral nervous system leave this protective dural covering to provide motor, sensory, and autonomic innervation to the body. This creates several compartments within which infectious and inflammatory conditions can occur. Appropriate recognition and characterization of these conditions, as well as the differentiation of infectious and inflammatory processes from one another and from potentially neoplastic conditions, can help in the planning of treatment for all of these disease entities.

The involvement by an inflammatory process of the spinal cord (a myelitis) can result in neurologic deficits that can be localized to a specific sensory level, to the point at which a horizontally oriented (transverse) line can be drawn that demarcates symptomatic from asymptomatic levels. Clinically, the inflammatory process in which this can be done is known as a transverse myelitis, and can result from infection, acute disseminated encephalomyelitis (ADEM), neuromyelitis optica (NMO), multiple sclerosis (MS), lupus, vasculitis, trauma, spinal cord infarctions, tumors, and other conditions. Accordingly, transverse myelitis is a clinical finding and not a specific disease process, for which reason transverse myelitis cannot and should not be diagnosed based upon imaging. However, transverse myelitis is often an indication for magnetic resonance imaging (MRI) of the spine, in order to identify which of the entities named above may be present. Because a clinical instance of transverse myelitis can sometimes be idiopathic, there is a clinical entity known as idiopathic transverse myelitis, which in many cases is likely to be related to an immune-mediated process, such as ADEM.

25.2 Spinal Infections

25.2.1 Extradural Infections

Extradural infections are those that involve the epidural space, the paraspinal space, and the intervertebral disk space, as well as the bone of the spine itself. Osteomyelitis of the spine often originates as diskitis. The intervertebral disk space is highly vascular in young children and may be susceptible to the hematogenous spread of infection. It is important to keep in mind that in young children a spinal infection such as diskitis/osteomyelitis may present as limping, hip pain, or a refusal to bear weight. The first signs of diskitis may be narrowing of the joint space on radiographs (▶ Fig. 25.1). On MRI, there will be fluid within the disk space and heterogeneous enhancement in the disk and adjacent soft tissues. Diskitis may result in osteomyelitis of the adjacent vertebra, or the infection causing it may extend into the paraspinous soft tissues with the development of an abscess, such as in the psoas muscles (▶ Fig. 25.2). This may be amenable to computed tomography (CT)–guided drain placement, particularly if the infection does not respond to intravenous (IV) antibiotics. An extradural infection that extends into the epidural space can result in an epidural abscess that may narrow the thecal sac and is typically a neurosurgical emergency (▶ Fig. 25.3).

25.2.2 Intradural Infections

Spinal meningitis is an intradural, extramedullary infection of the meninges and CSF that involves the spinal column and is usually diagnosed by lumbar puncture. Uncomplicated meningitis typically lacks any specific features on imaging. Intradural

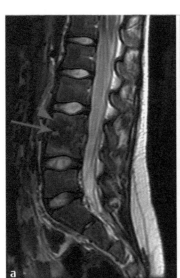
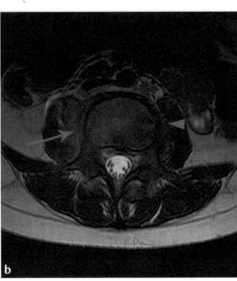

Fig. 25.1 Diskitis. (a) Sagittal T2W image of the spine of a 6-year-old girl with back pain shows nonvisualization of the L3–L4 disk space (*red arrow*) and a heterogeneous marrow signal in the adjacent vertebra (*red arrowhead*). (b) Axial T2W image shows edema in the right (*red arrow*) and to a lesser extent the left (*red arrowhead*) psoas muscles. This represents L3–L4 diskitis with adjacent osteomyelitis and psoas myositis.

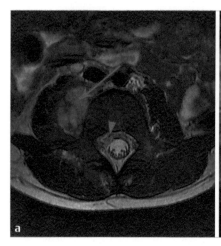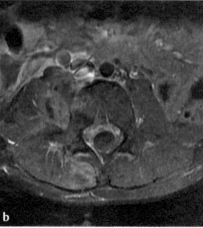

Fig. 25.2 Psoas abscess. (a) Axial T2 W image at the L4 level in a 3-year-old girl with fever and back pain shows heterogeneous edema and fluid in the right psoas muscle (*red arrow*) and asymmetric thickening of the right ventrolateral epidural space (*red arrowhead*). (b) Axial T1 W plus contrast image with fat saturation shows enhancement of the edematous areas, consistent with myositis, with focal hypoenhancing areas (*red arrows*) representing psoas abscess. There is solid enhancement of the thickened right ventrolateral epidural space (*red arrowhead*), representing an epidural phlegmon.

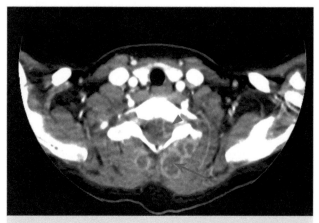

Fig. 25.3 Epidural abscess. Axial computed tomographic image at the C7 level in a 9-year-old boy with fever and neck pain shows a multiloculated abscess in the paraspinous musculature (*red arrow*). There is an epidural component along the left aspect of the central canal that has a peripheral rim of enhancement and central hypoenhancement, representing an epidural abscess (*red arrowhead*).

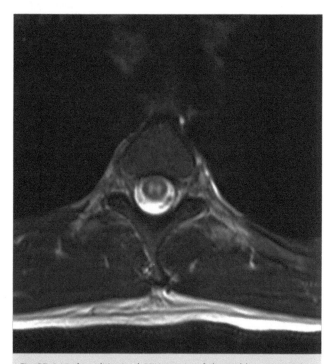

Fig. 25.4 Viral myelitis. Axial T2 W image of the midthoracic spinal cord in a 16-year-old girl with upper- and lower-extremity weakness shows a hyperintense signal in the central cord. There was no abnormal enhancement or diffusion abnormality, and this represented viral myelitis.

intramedullary infections are more commonly visible on imaging. Intramedullary bacterial infections are usually devastating. More common are viral infections of the spinal cord, or viral myelitis. Viral myelitis tends to be based within the central gray matter of the spinal cord, resulting in a T2 hyperintense signal often without abnormal postcontrast enhancement (▶ Fig. 25.4). Poliomyelitis, which reached epidemic proportions in the mid-twentieth century, is a viral myelitis that results in atrophy of the anterior horn cells of the spinal cord. In children and adolescents, an exacerbation of asthma may result in a rare condition where the patient experiences paralysis, and there are signal abnormalities in the spinal cord. This is known as Hopkins syndrome and is believed to be related to a viral myelitis that results in a poliomyelitis-like injury to the anterior horn cells of the cord. The virus is thought to be an opportunistic infection that has the impact that it does because of the immunocompromised state brought on by an exacerbation of asthma and its treatment with steroids. The exact viral etiology of Hopkins syndrome has not been determined, and may not involve a single viral agent. It is likely that a pathophysiology

similar to that in Hopkins syndrome was involved in the enterovirus D68 outbreak that occurred in the United States in 2014, which had a clinical presentation and features on imaging that resembled those of Hopkins syndrome (▶ Fig. 25.5).[1]

25.3 Noninfectious Inflammatory Conditions

Noninfectious inflammatory conditions involving the spinal cord and intradural nerve roots in children are predominantly immune mediated.

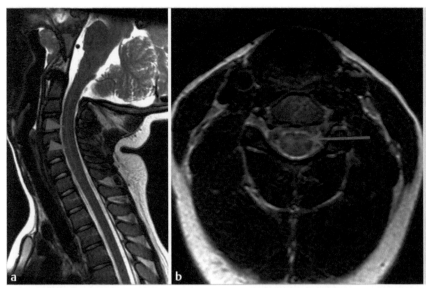

Fig. 25.5 Hopkins syndrome. (a) Sagittal T2 W image of the spine of a 7-year-old boy with upper-extremity weakness after a severe exacerbation of asthma shows a subtle linear area of hyperintense signal (*red arrowheads*). (b) Axial T2 W image shows a hyperintense signal in the central cervical cord, corresponding to the "butterfly" distribution of the cord gray matter. This represents viral myelitis in the setting of Hopkins syndrome.

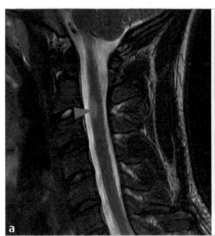
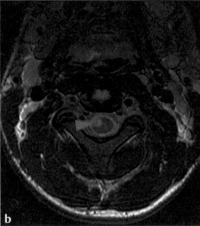

Fig. 25.6 Manifestations of multiple sclerosis (MS) in the spine. (a) Sagittal T2 W image of the cervical spine of a 17-year-old boy with right-sided weakness shows a focal (short-segment) hyperintense lesion in the ventral aspect of the cord at the C2–C3 level (*red arrowhead*). (b) Axial T2 W image shows that the area of signal abnormality (*red arrowhead*) is in the periphery of the cord and is nonexpansile. This patient was confirmed to have MS.

Multiple sclerosis is a demyelinating condition that can involve all parts of the CNS (▶ Fig. 25.6). Involvement of the spinal cord by MS is most commonly manifested in the form of patchy areas of nonexpansile, T2 hyperintense signaling within the cord. It is important to note that fluid-attenuated inversion recovery (FLAIR) imaging does not work well in the spine, and that conventional T2 W imaging is used to look for these abnormalities. Areas of active demyelination will commonly enhance after the administration of a contrast agent. Depending on the location of the lesions of MS within the spinal cord, patients may present with motor (anterior and lateral involvement) and/or sensory (posterior involvement) symptoms.

As noted earlier, ADEM can involve the spinal cord. The lesions of ADEM in the cord tend to be expansile and involve long segments (more than two or three vertebral segments in a craniocaudal orientation), and often occur as a single spinal lesion, which is in contrast to the short-segment, nonexpansile, and often multifocal lesions in MS (▶ Fig. 10.6). Acute disseminated encephalomyelitis is an immune-mediated process that follows an immunoreactive process. The latter is most commonly a recent viral infection, although ADEM can occasionally result from vaccinations and bacterial infections. Additionally, although ADEM is usually a monophasic process, it can occasionally be multiphasic.

Neuromyelitis optica is an immune-mediated condition that can result in expansile lesions of the spinal cord resembling those of ADEM (▶ Fig. 10.6). Also known as Devic's disease, NMO is caused by autoantibodies to the aquaporin-4 protein of the transmembrane water channels of cells. Spinal cord lesions and optic neuritis are the most common presentations of NMO. Although there is typically relative sparing of the brain in NMO, and intracranial involvement is rarely the predominating feature of this inflammatory condition, the presence of intracranial demyelinating lesions does not exclude the diagnosis of NMO. The antibody to aquaporin-4 is easier to detect in CSF than in serum, and the assay for it may give negative results early in the disease process.[2,3]

Awareness of the expansile nature and often heterogeneous enhancement of the spinal cord lesions in ADEM and NMO is important, and these findings should raise the consideration of these conditions as possibilities in addition to that of an intramedullary neoplasm of the cord. When such a lesion is encountered, CSF inflammatory markers should be evaluated, and

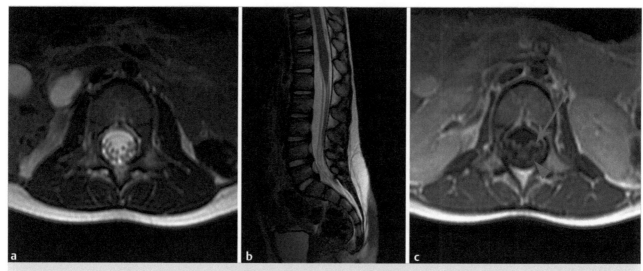

Fig. 25.7 Guillain–Barré syndrome. (a) Axial and (b) sagittal T2 W image of the lumbar spine of a 30-month-old girl with lower-extremity weakness shows thickened nerve roots of the cauda equina. (c) Axial T1 W image of the cauda equina shows preferential enhancement of the ventral nerve roots (*red arrow*) as compared with the dorsal nerve roots (*red arrowhead*). This represents Guillain–Barré syndrome.

reimaging after a trial with corticosteroids should be considered prior to considering a biopsy.

25.4 Guillain–Barré Syndrome

Although all of the conditions described above involve abnormalities of the spinal cord, Guillain–Barré syndrome (GBS), also known as acute demyelinating polyradiculoneuritis, is a postinfectious, immune-mediated inflammatory condition that specifically affects the nerve roots of the cauda equina (▶ Fig. 25.7). This syndrome presents with a polyneuropathy that includes bilateral weakness of the lower extremities. The infection that precedes GBS is most commonly a gastrointestinal infection with *Campylobacter jejuni*. The imaging manifestations of GBS include enhancement and thickening of the nerve roots of the cauda equina, with preferential involvement of the ventral nerve roots (▶ Fig. 25.7). In the late stage of the syndrome, dorsal nerve roots may also be involved. Immunomodulatory therapy with intravenous immunoglobulins (IVIg) is the primary treatment for GBS, which, unlike most inflammatory conditions, is not typically helped by steroids (which may even delay the recovery from it).

25.5 Suggested Reading

[1] Sorte DE, Poretti A, Newsome SD, Boltshauser E, Huisman TAGM, Izbudak I. Longitudinally extensive myelopathy in children. Pediatr Radiol 2015; 45(2): 244–257, quiz 241–243

[2] O'Mahony J, Shroff M, Banwell B. Mimics and rare presentations of pediatric demyelination. Neuroimaging Clin N Am 2013; 23(2):321–336

[3] Go JL, Rothman S, Prosper A, Silbergleit R, Lerner A. Spine infections. Neuroimaging Clin N Am 2012; 22(4):755–772

References

[1] Maloney JA, Mirsky DM, Messacar K, Dominguez SR, Schreiner T, Stence NV. MRI findings in children with acute flaccid paralysis and cranial nerve dysfunction occurring during the 2014 enterovirus D68 outbreak. AJNR Am J Neuroradiol 2015; 36(2):245–250

[2] Makhani N, Bigi S, Banwell B, Shroff M. Diagnosing neuromyelitis optica. Neuroimaging Clin N Am 2013; 23(2):279–291

[3] Thomas T, Branson HM. Childhood transverse myelitis and its mimics. Neuroimaging Clin N Am 2013; 23(2):267–278

26 Congenital/Developmental Spine Abnormalities

26.1 Congenital and Developmental Spinal Abnormalities

The evaluation of nontraumatic structural abnormalities is probably the aspect in which imaging of the pediatric spine differs the most from that of adults. The evaluation and study of trauma, neoplasms, and infectious/inflammatory processes of the pediatric spine have many more similarities to those of adult imaging. Ultimately, understanding many of these pediatric conditions requires familiarity with embryology. However, because familiarity does not mean mastery, it should not be a cause of fear in addressing congenital disorders of the pediatric spine.

26.2 Anomalies of Segmentation and Clefts of the Vertebral Bodies

Because the vertebral column develops from the same neural tube that segments to give rise to the vertebrae, the failure of two vertebrae to separate, leaving them instead in continuity, is referred to as incomplete segmentation. This is in contradistinction to the term "fused," which is more properly applied to an acquired fusion of two vertebrae that had already segmented in the normal manner. During segmentation, additional variants can occur in vertebral morphology, including persistent sagittal clefts between vertebrae ("butterfly vertebrae") (▶ Fig. 26.1), hemivertebrae, and mutlilevel incomplete segmentation blocks. The more complex anomalies of vertebral segmentation are often associated with congenital scoliosis. Although sagittal clefts are the most common anomalies of vertebral development, some skeletal dysplasias (e.g., Kniest dysplasia) can be associated with coronal clefts (▶ Fig. 26.2).

Anomalies of vertebral segmentation can create a challenge in numbering the vertebrae for the purposes of reporting findings in their imaging. If any atypical features of vertebral segmentation exist, the system used for vertebral numbering must be described in the report. When there are atypical features, every possible attempt should be made to determine a numbering system that allows for the appropriate number of vertebrae. Theoretical vertebrae, such as T13 and L6, do not exist, particularly because there is no T13 or L6 nerve root, dermatome, or sclerotome. Nearly all cases of anomaly in vertebral segmentation can be analyzed to determine a numbering system that accounts for the appropriate number of nerve roots and dermatomes.

26.3 Clefts of the Posterior Neural Arch

There are several characteristic locations for osseous clefts within or at the junction of the ossification centers of the posterior neural arch (▶ Fig. 26.3). Additional osseous abnormalities can occur within a given vertebral level in the joining of the different ossification centers of the vertebra and posterior neural arch at that level. Perhaps the most commonly encountered osseous cleft is midline incomplete closure of the posterior neural arch without the protrusion of meninges or neural elements (▶ Fig. 26.4). Classically this has been described as "spina bifida occulta," but this term raises concern on behalf of patients, referring physicians, and (potentially) insurance companies, and a midline incomplete closure of the posterior neural arch without the protrusion of meninges or neural elements can instead be described with the statement that "incidental note is made of focal congenital nonunion of the posterior neural arch of (vertebral level)," if this condition is to be described at all. Such incomplete closure is most commonly encountered at C1 and S1, and personally I tend to mention it in the body of a report for C1, particularly for studies performed for cervical spinal trauma, and rarely mention it when it is present in S1 because it rarely has pathologic significance at that level of the spine. Referring in a report to incomplete closure of the posterior neural arch as spina bifida occulta introduces unneeded anxiety; the clefts resulting from such incomplete closure have no clinically relevant relationship to spina bifida, which is

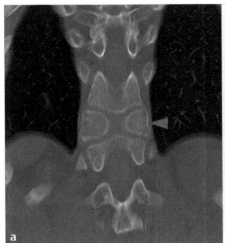
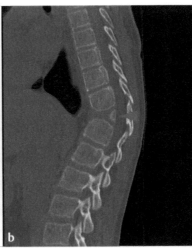

Fig. 26.1 Butterfly vertebra/sagittal cleft. (a) Coronal bone algorithm computed tomographic image of the spine of a 12-year-old boy shows a T11 "butterfly vertebra" (*red arrowhead*) related to a sagittal cleft. (b) Sagittal computed tomographic image shows a focal kyphosis (*red arrowhead*) at this level.

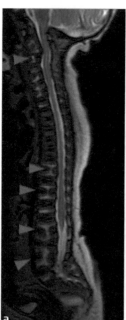 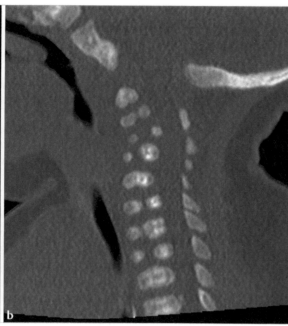

Fig. 26.2 Coronal cleft. (a) Sagittal T2 W magnetic resonance image of the spine of a 1-month-old boy shows coronal clefts within multiple vertebrae (*red arrowheads*). (b) Sagittal computed tomographic image of the cervical spine shows multiple coronal clefts, as well as a focal kyphosis at the C3 level. This child has Kniest dysplasia.

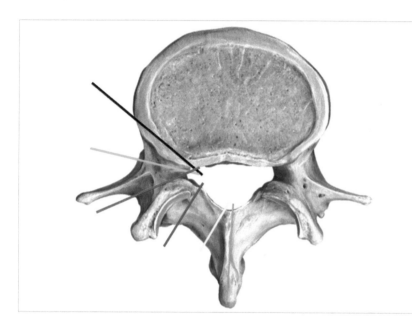

Fig. 26.3 Congenital clefts (pars, etc). Transverse diagram of the spine showing the locations of different congenital clefts, including persistent neurocentral synchondrosis (*black line*), a retrosomatic cleft (*green line*), a pars interarticularis defect (*red line*), a retroisthmic cleft (*blue line*), a paraspinous cleft (*yellow line*), and a spinous cleft (*orange line*). From Atlas of Anatomy, © Thieme 2012, Illustration by Karl Wesker.

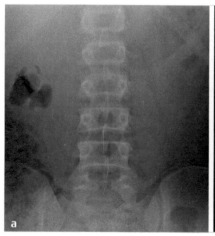 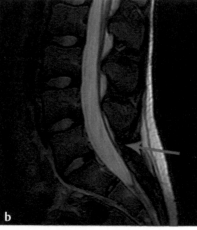

Fig. 26.4 Intraspinous cleft (S1). (a) Frontal radiograph of the lumbosacral junction of a 13-year-old boy shows incomplete closure of the posterior neural arch of a vertebra (*red arrowhead*). The patient had 12 pairs of ribs, and there were 5 non–rib-bearing vertebrae above a partially lumbarized vertebra at the lumbosacral junction; this transitional vertebra therefore probably represents a partially lumbarized S1. (b) Sagittal T2 W image of the lumbosacral junction shows absence of the spinous process at this level (*red arrow*).

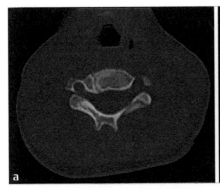
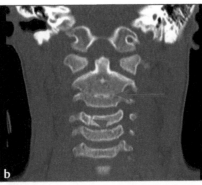

Fig. 26.5 Persistent neurocentral synchondrosis. (a) Axial computed tomographic image of the spine of a 4-year-old boy made for the evaluation of trauma shows a persistent right neurocentral synchdrosis in C4 (*red arrowhead*). (b) Coronal computed tomographic image of the cervical spine shows the right C4 neurocentral synchondrosis (*red arrowhead*). There is also incomplete segmentation of C2–C3 (*red arrow*).

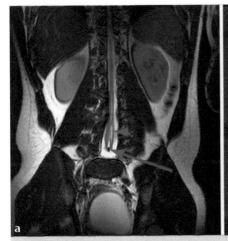
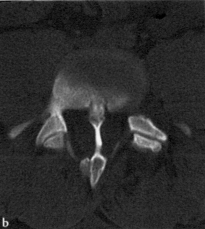
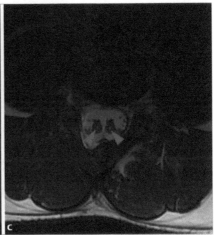

Fig. 26.6 Diastematomyelia. (a) Coronal T2 W image of the spine of a 17-year-old boy shows a focal area of signal abnormality in the spinal cord (*red arrowhead*), above a hypointense structure projecting within the lower cord (*red arrow*). (b) Axial computed tomographic image shows a midline osseous bar within the vertebral column, corresponding to the location of the hypointense structure in (a). (c) Axial T2 W image of the spine immediately above the osseous bar in (b) shows two separate hemicords (*red arrowheads*). This represents diastematomyelia.

generally used to describe an open spinal dysraphism, such as a myelomeningocele.

Following midline incomplete closure of the posterior neural arch of C1 and S1, the next most common vertebral cleft is a cleft of the pars interarticularis, also referred to as spondylolysis. This cleft, which may not be a congenital cleft, occurs in the posterior elements of the vertebra approximately between the level of the superior and inferior articulating facets, and is most common at L5. At L5 it can be unilateral or bilateral. When a cleft of the pars interarticularis is unilateral, there is sclerosis and thickening of the contralateral pedicle, probably as the result of increased stress on it. When such a cleft is bilateral, the patient may have an anterolisthesis (also known as a spondylolisthesis). It is therefore possible to have spondylolysis with or without spondylolisthesis. Although a cleft of the pars interarticularis can be congenital, most such clefts are probably chronic stress fractures. In the pediatric and adolescent populations, those at greatest risk for such fractures are athletes with excess stress at the lumbosacral junction, including gymnasts and cheerleaders, as well as punters in football. These fractures can be identified on radiography and computed tomography (CT). Magnetic resonance imaging may show adjacent marrow edema. When the diagnosis is uncertain, a nuclear medicine bone scan with single-photon emission computed tomography

(SPECT) can be used to look for signs of increased metabolism suggestive of abnormal stress.

Other, more rare vertebral clefts than those of the posterior neural arch or pars interarticularis include a persistent neurocentral synchondrosis (▶ Fig. 26.5), a retrosomatic cleft, a retroisthmic cleft, and a paraspinous cleft (▶ Fig. 26.3), all of which are more common in the setting of multifocal anomalies of osseous segmentation.

26.4 Diastematomyelia

A developmental anomaly that has a very interesting presentation both clinically and on imaging is diastematomyelia. This is a separation within the spinal canal that separates the thecal sac into two. The separation is typically partitioned by a septum, which may be fibrous or osseous. In diastematomyelia, the spinal cord is split into two, with each hemicord giving off a single ipsilateral pair of nerve roots (dorsal and ventral). A true cord duplication, in which each cord gives off right- and left-sided dorsal and ventral nerve roots, is exceedingly rare and is referred to as diplomyelia (▶ Fig. 26.6). Diastematomyelia can present with symptoms of a tethered cord and with hydromyelia, both of which are discussed later in this chapter.

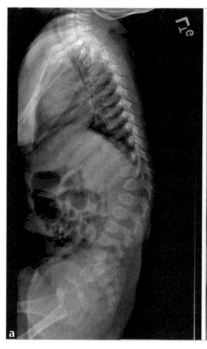 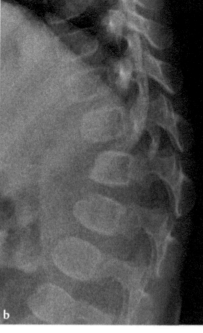

Fig. 26.7 Gibbus deformity. (a) Lateral radiograph of the thoracolumbar spine in a 2.5-year-old girl shows a focal kyphosis at the thoracolumbar junction. (b) Magnified view of the kyphosis shows a shortened anteroposterior dimension of the T12 vertebra, with an anterior-inferior beak. This represents a gibbus deformity related to a focal vertebral hypoplasia.

26.5 Sagittal Alignment

The sagittal alignment of the cervical vertebral column varies through childhood, starting with a kyphosis and progressing to a lordosis in young adulthood. Accordingly, a straightened alignment of the cervical vertebral column in an adolescent is normal, and should not be described as "loss of cervical lordosis," and when seen with trauma does not necessarily indicate muscle spasm. Most children have a mild kyphosis in the thoracic spine and a mild lordosis in the lumbar spine. Altered alignment in one vertebral section can result in compensatory alterations in the alignment of other segments.

A congenital focal kyphosis can be present in the spine, commonly at the thoracolumbar junction, with a dysplastic vertebral body that demonstrates ventral "beaking." This is known as a gibbus deformity and has both congenital and acquired etiologies (▶ Fig. 26.7).

26.6 Coronal Alignment: Scoliosis

Scoliosis is a term for a curved spine, particularly in the coronal plane, as opposed to kyphosis and lordosis, which refers to curvature of the spine in the sagittal plane (▶ Fig. 26.8). Adolescent idiopathic scoliosis (AIS) is encountered in young girls from approximately 8 to 15 years of age, and most commonly has a right-convexity curvature in the thoracic spine and a left-convexity curvature in the lumbar spine. Collectively, this double curvature is called a sigmoid scoliosis, and as the "I" in AIS implies, is typically idiopathic. Identification of AIS in the early stages of development is important because its progression can be prevented (and possibly even reversed) with physical therapy and the wearing of a back brace. Sigmoid scoliosis is best identified on physical examination, and any concerns brought up in such examination should be followed by subspecialist consultation and likely imaging. Because most subtle curvatures of the spine seen on imaging can be related to patient positioning, proper technique is crucial in obtaining radiographs for the identification and assessment of scoliosis. Complex scoliosis may have a rotatory component.

The atypical features of scoliosis are a reverse-sigmoid curvature, male patient, patients younger than 6 to 8 years of age, bowel/bladder dysfunction, and/or rapid progression of scoliosis. The finding of any of these features warrants further evaluation. Neuromuscular conditions, including cerebral palsy, can result in an atypical scoliosis, as can neurocutaneous syndromes, including neurofibromatosis type 1. The apex of scoliotic curvature in a patient with neurofibromatosis may be associated with a prominent neurofibroma.

Scoliosis is best evaluated with standing radiographs made with a posteroanterior beam direction. The reason for this is that a posteroanterior beam direction reduces the radiation dose to the breast by 90% of the dose with an anteroposteriorly directed beam. If scoliosis is associated with anomalies of segmentation, such as hemivertebrae, block vertebrae, or osseous clefts, CT may be helpful. Unexplained scoliosis may benefit from MRI for intradural pathology, such as a syrinx, a thickened filum terminale, or a neoplasm (see Chapter 27).

26.7 Skeletal Dysplasias and Osseous Developmental Abnormalities

Multiple skeletal dysplasias are associated with characteristic abnormalities of the spine, but these are too numerous to list and, for the most part, too rare to learn before an advanced level of knowledge is achieved. Achondroplasia, however, is a relatively commonly encountered dysplasia with features that are important to clearly recognize. Patients with achondroplasia can have stenosis of the foramen magnum, further discussed in the section of this chapter on the craniocervical junction.

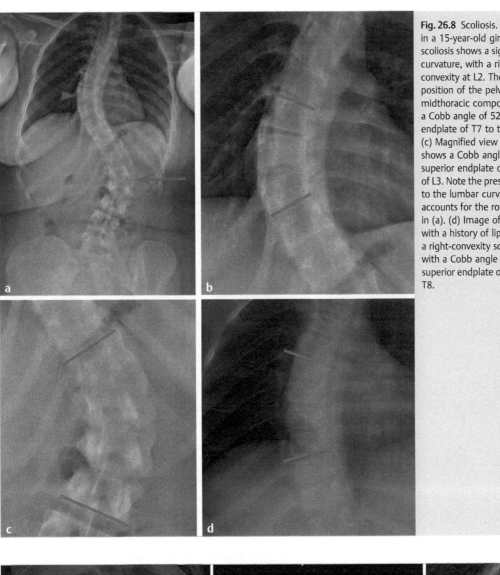

Fig. 26.8 Scoliosis. (a) Standing image of scoliosis in a 15-year-old girl with adolescent idiopathic scoliosis shows a sigmoid thoracolumbar scoliotic curvature, with a right convexity at T8 and a left convexity at L2. There is an asymmetric (rotated) position of the pelvis. (b) Magnified view of the midthoracic component of the scoliosis showing a Cobb angle of 52° measured from the superior endplate of T7 to the inferior endplate of T9. (c) Magnified view of the thoracolumbar region shows a Cobb angle of 57° measured from the superior endplate of T12 to the inferior endplate of L3. Note the presence of a rotatory component to the lumbar curvature (rotoscoliosis), which accounts for the rotated appearance of the pelvis in (a). (d) Image of the spine of a 7-year-old boy with a history of lipomyelomeningocele, showing a right-convexity scoliosis with an apex at T6–T7, with a Cobb angle of 32° as measured from the superior endplate of T5 to the inferior endplate of T8.

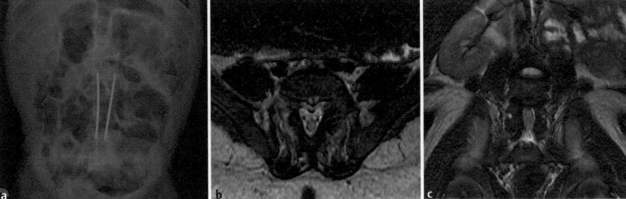

Fig. 26.9 Achondroplasia of the lumbar spine. (a) Frontal radiograph of the abdomen of a 7-month-old boy with achondroplasia. Although there is considerable overlying bowel gas, the pedicles in the lumbar spine have a progressively more medial position in a progressively caudal direction. (b) Axial and (c) coronal T2 W images at the L5 level of the patient in (a), made at 10 months of age, show a narrow transverse dimension of the spinal canal (*red line*).

Within the lumbar spine, patients with achondroplasia have a narrowing of the spinal canal between the pedicles of the lower vertebrae, resulting in a spinal stenosis in the transverse plane (▶ Fig. 26.9). Patients with achondroplasia will also often have straightening of the normal lumbar lordosis of the spine, and may have a thoracic lordosis.

Short and flattened vertebrae, known as platyspondyly, can be seen in a variety of disorders, including Morquio syndrome

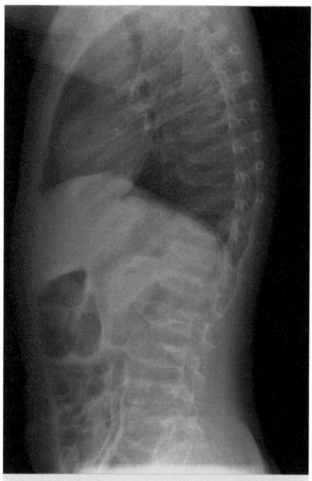

Fig. 26.10 Platyspondyly. Lateral radiograph of the lumbar and lower thoracic vertebral column of a 4-year-old girl shows a short and flattened appearance of all vertebrae, known as platyspondyly, in this patient with suspected Morquio syndrome.

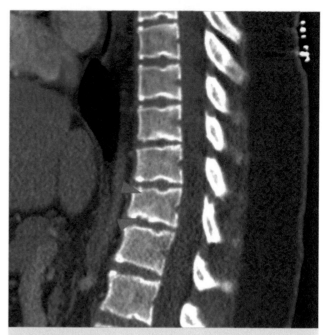

Fig. 26.11 Scheuermann disease. Sagittal computed tomographic image of the spine of a 13-year-old girl with a kyphosis shows ventral wedging of a vertebra (*red arrowheads*) at the thoracolumbar junction, with superior and inferior endplate abnormalities. Slight endplate abnormalities are noted at additional levels of the spine. These findings probably represents a mild case of Scheuermann disease, an osteochondrosis of the vertebral endplates that is typically associated with a kyphosis.

(▶ Fig. 26.10), thanatophoric dysplasia, Gaucher disease, and others. When present at a single level, this finding is known as vertebra plana, and has a differential diagnosis other than that including these disorders, and which includes, but is by no means limited to, Langerhans cell histiocytosis (LCH), which is discussed in further detail in Chapter 27.

Some patients have an osteochondrosis of the superior and inferior endplates of multiple adjacent thoracolumbar vertebrae with loss of height and a resulting kyphosis, a condition known as Scheuermann's disease (▶ Fig. 26.11). Appropriately recognizing this as a developmental condition and not a sequela of trauma is important.

26.8 Tethered Cord and the Filum Terminale

Cord tethering is a clinical constellation of symptoms that can present with dysfunction of the bowel and bladder and/or lower extremities, or with syringohydromyelia of the cord. Although it is difficult to definitively diagnose cord tethering through structural findings alone and without a neurologic

deficit, the finding of certain features in conjunction with neurologic dysfunction helps in making this diagnosis. Both a low position of the tip of the conus medullaris, below the superior endplate of L3, and thickening of the filum terminale to more than 1.5 mm, are associated with the eventual development of symptoms of tethered cord syndrome. However, it can be difficult to predict whether, or exactly when, a given patient with these features will become symptomatic.

The filum terminale is normally a thin, pial–ependymal extension from apex of the conus medullaris to the distal end of the thecal sac. If it is too thick, it is felt to "tether" the cord and thereby prevent it from moving during CSF pulsations or changes in patient position. The filum terminale may have internal fat, which can be seen on CT as fat density, on MRI as an area of T1 shortening with a chemical-shift artifact and suppression on fat-saturated imaging (▶ Fig. 26.12), and on ultrasonography as a thickened area of echogenicity.

Beyond the possibility of a fibrolipoma of the filum terminale, some patients have a cyst within the filum terminale. The cyst is more easily identified with ultrasound than with CT or MRI. It is not known whether a filar cyst carries an increased risk of cord tethering; however, in the absence of other features that raise the suspicion of cord tethering, such as a low conus, it is probably incidental (▶ Fig. 26.13).

26.9 Sacral Dimples

Patients with a sacral dimple have an increased risk of having a tethered cord. When a sacral dimple is present at birth,

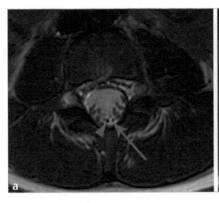
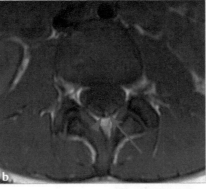

Fig. 26.12 Fibrolipoma. (a) Axial T2 W image of the lumbar spine of a 4-year-old girl shows a hyperintense appearance of the filum terminale (*red arrow*), with a hypointense appearance to the left of the filum representing a chemical shift artifact (*red arrowhead*). (b) Axial T1 W image shows T1 shortening in the filum terminale (*red arrow*) with a chemical shift artifact (*red arrowhead*). The chemical-shift artifact is in the frequency-encoding direction, and confirms that the T1 and T2 hyperintense signals in these magnetic resonance images are related to fat, in this case a fibrolipoma of the filum terminale.

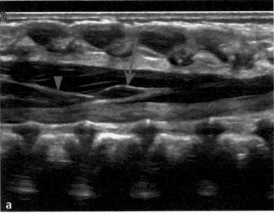
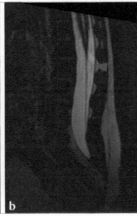

Fig. 26.13 Filar cyst. (a) Sagittal ultrasonographic image of the lumbar spine of a 1-month-old boy shows tapering of the conus medullaris (*red arrowhead*) and a cyst within the upper portion of the filum terminale (*red arrow*). (b) Sagittal image of the patient's spine made with fast imaging employing steady-state acquisition at 15 months of age shows persistence of the filar cyst (*red arrowhead*).

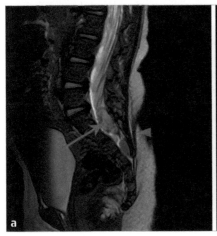
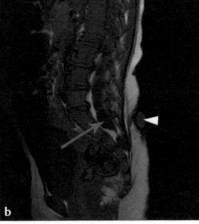

Fig. 26.14 Spinal dermoid cyst. (a) Sagittal T2 W image of the spine of a 16-month-old girl, made to evaluate a sacral dimple, shows a dermal sinus tract extending from the sacral dimple (*red arrowhead*) and an intradural lesion within the sacral portion of the thecal sac (*red arrow*). (b) Sagittal T1 W image shows a vitamin E capsule placed to mark the patient's sacral dimple (*white arrowhead*), allowing confirmation of its location on imaging, as well as showing the dermal sinus tract (*red arrowhead*) extending from the dimple. The intradural lesion is also seen (*red arrow*), which at surgery was confirmed to represent a dermoid.

ultrasonography can be done to evaluate the position of the conus medullaris and whether there is thickening of the filum terminale, possibly with echogenicity suggestive of a fibrolipoma. Ultrasonography also allows dynamic evaluation of the nerve roots of the filum terminale and the position of the conus medullaris, to determine whether there is gentle movement of the nerves due to CSF pulsations, the absence of which suggests cord tethering even more strongly than the structural findings that typically indicate its presence.

Most sacral dimples are not associated with cord tethering. They may be associated with a sinus tract extending to the thecal sac, which is in turn commonly associated with a congenital

inclusion cyst, such as a dermoid cyst (▶ Fig. 26.14). The presence of a sinus tract may increase the risk of spinal infection/meningitis. Sacral dimples may have sinus tracts, known as pilonidal tracts, that extend to the coccyx (▶ Fig. 26.15). These are typically incidental, but patients with them have an increased risk for later developing coccygeal osteomyelitis.

If MRI is used to evaluate a sacral dimple, it is important to ensure that the entire sacrum and coccyx are imaged, in contrast to the practice in many protocols for imaging the adult spine, which stop just below the L5–S1 disk space. It is very helpful to place a marker, such as a vitamin E capsule, on a sacral dimple, as an indicator of where to seek abnormalities.

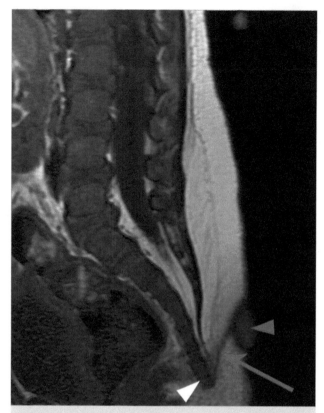

Fig. 26.15 Pilonidal tract. Sagittal T1 W image of the spine of a 15-month-old girl with a sacral dimple shows a pilonidal tract (*red arrow*) extending toward a retroflexed coccyx (*white arrowhead*). Note that the sacral dimple was marked with a vitamin E capsule (*red arrowhead*).

26.10 Defects of Neural Tube Closure

Abnormalities in neural tube closure can result in a variety of defects. Spinal defects in neural tube closure are nearly always encountered in the lumbosacral region, at the caudal end of the developing spinal canal. Rostral defects in neural tube closure,

such as anencephaly and encephalocele, are discussed in Chapter 3. Defects in closure of the midportion of the neural tube are rare, but when present are often associated with additional congenital malformations.

Neural tube defects are most commonly associated with impaired closure of the posterior neural arch. The protrusion of meninges and passage of CSF through a defect in closure of the posterior neural arch is known as a meningocele. The lesion in which neural elements are also present in a meningocele is referred to as a myelomeningocele (▶ Fig. 5.2). The lesion that contains both neural elements and fat as well as meninges and CSF is known as a lipomyelomeningocele (▶ Fig. 26.16).

During development, the open neural tube folds over and creates the spinal cord. The posterior margin of the open tube is lined by ependyma, and will eventually form the central canal of the spinal cord. This closes simultaneously with its pulling away from the posterior body wall in the process known as disjunction. A myelomeningocele is an open neural tube defect at the location of which disjunction does not occur normally, an abnormality known as nondisjunction. The neural tube that failed to close remains a vertically oriented, flat structure known as a neural placode. The exposed portion of the neural placode, which would have been the ependyma-lined central canal of the spinal cord, will leak CSF. This results in an increased concentration of alpha-fetoprotein in amniotic fluid, and in low CSF pressures. The low CSF pressures result in sagging of the contents of the posterior fossa, with a resulting Chiari type II malformation. For all practical purposes, there is a 100% association between a Chiari type II malformation and a myelomeningocele.

Because the surgical repair of a myelomeningocele takes place immediately after birth, the images made of this defect in cord developoment are typically either prenatal or postsurgical. Recent attempts have been made to repair myelomeningoceles in utero, with a consequently decreased severity of the Chiari type II phenotype and other neurologic abnormalities associated with these spinal defects. Patients with a history of myelomeningocele have a high incidence of neurogenic bladder. Historically, patients who have had a myelomeningocele have also had a high incidence of latex allergies, possibly as a result of sensitization during early surgery for this defect.

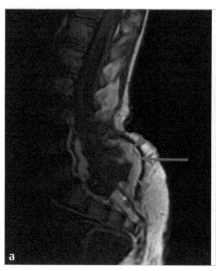
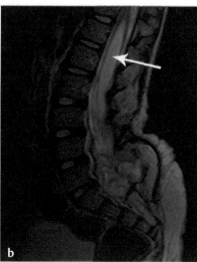

Fig. 26.16 Lipomyelomeningocele. (a) Sagittal T1 W image of the spine of a 5-year-old boy shows a skin-covered spinal dysraphism at the lumbosacral junction, with a thick dural covering (*red arrow*) and internal areas of T1-hyperintense signal representing fat (*red arrowheads*).
(b) Sagittal T2 W image shows syringohydromyelia (*white arrow*) within the lumbar portion of the spinal cord, which extends lower than typically expected. This represents a lipomyelomeningocele. Because this lesion is skin covered, and related to premature disjunction, there will be no associated Chiari type II malformation.

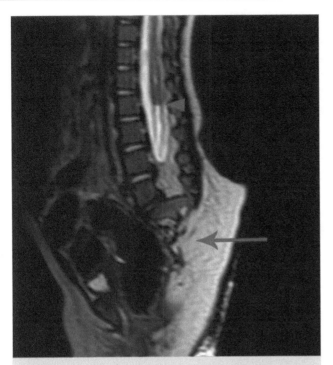

Fig. 26.17 Caudal agenesis type I. Sagittal T2W image of the spine of a 1-year-old girl shows partial agenesis of the sacrum and coccyx (*red arrow*). There is a blunted termination of the spinal cord (*red arrowhead*), as opposed to a tapered conus medullaris. This represents type I caudal agenesis, with a blunted, nontethered cord. Note that caudal agenesis is also referred to as caudal regression syndrome, although in formal terms the caudal vertebrae in this condition do not regress but in fact never develop.

If disjunction occurs too early, the neural tube pulls away with entrapped mesenchymal elements. The affected mesenchyme will often differentiate into fat, resulting in a lipomyelomeningocele, lipomyelocele, or an intradural lipoma, depending upon how early disjunction takes place. By definition, premature disjunction is therefore a skin-covered defect, and without loss of CSF pressure there is no associated Chiari type II

malformation. Stated in another way, whereas an open myelomeningocele is always associated with a Chiari type II malformation, a (skin-covered) lipomyelomeningocele has no association with a Chiari type II malformation.

Two further malformations are associated with defects of the caudal aspect of the neural tube. Agenesis of the caudal-most part of the tube (also known as "caudal regression syndrome") does not technically involve regression but only agenesis of this part of the tube. Caudal agenesis can be of varying severity, and involves two patterns of intradural abnormality. Patients with the first of these patterns, known as type I caudal agenesis, have a high termination of the spinal cord with a blunted tip of the cord rather than a conus medullaris (▸ Fig. 26.17). Patients with the second pattern, known as type II caudal agenesis, have a spinal cord that extends to the distal aspect of the thecal sac, possibly in association with a lipoma, and have a high likelihood of manifesting the symptoms of tethered cord syndrome (▸ Fig. 26.18).

An additional defect at the caudal aspect of the spinal column is a terminal myelocystocele, in which the spinal cord and meninges protrude through a defect in the vertebral arch, and the portion of the cord that protrudes through this defect has a dilated central canal. The primary differential consideration for a terminal myelocystocele is a sacrococcygeal teratoma, which is discussed further in Chapter 27.

26.11 Hydromyelia, Syringomyelia, and Syringohydromyelia

The spinal cord arises from a portion of the neural tube known as the myelencephalon, which is why an infectious/inflammatory process of the cord is known as a myelitis and dysfunction of the cord is known as a myelopathy. The central canal of the spinal cord is an ependyma-lined structure filled with CSF that extends superiorly to the base of the fourth ventricle, with its outflow known as the obex. With high-resolution MRI, the central canal can sometimes be seen, and a diameter of the canal of

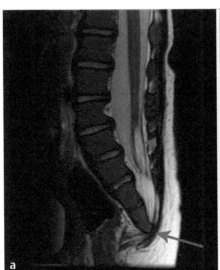
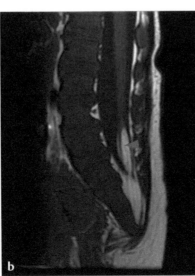

Fig. 26.18 Caudal agenesis type II. (a) Sagittal T2W image of the spine of an 11-month-old boy shows a blunted distal sacrum (*red arrow*). The spinal cord extends to the end of the thecal sac, and within the cord is a T2 hyperintense abnormality (*red arrowhead*). (b) Sagittal T1W image shows an area of T1 hyperintense signal within the distal aspect of the spinal cord (*red arrowhead*), representing a lipoma in the setting of a tethered cord and mild caudal agenesis. When present with a low termination of the cord, often with a lipoma/tethering, this is known as type II caudal agenesis.

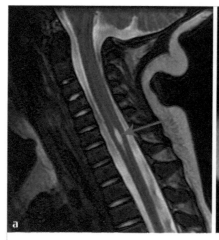
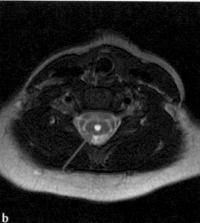

Fig. 26.19 Hydromyelia. (a) Sagittal T2 W image of the cervical spine of a 13-month-old boy shows a dilation of the central canal of the spinal cord (*red arrow*). (b) Axial T2 W image shows well-defined margins of this centrally located signal abnormality, representing hydromyelia (*red arrow*). This was identified as an incidental finding at the periphery of a magnetic resonance imaging (MRI) scan of the brain that was done to evaluate seizures. In the absence of a Chiari type I malformation or history of prior cord contusion at this level, hydromyelia is a finding that merits suspicion and warrants a contrast-enhanced MRI scan of the brain and entire spine to look for an obstructing lesion (such as a tumor) or for signs of cord tethering. No contrast-enhancing lesion was found, and the hydromyelia in this patient was presumed to be incidental; however, follow-up study is needed to document the stability of a hydromyelia, and any change may require further investigation.

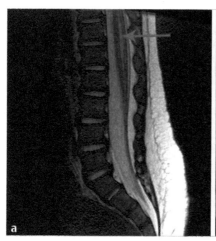
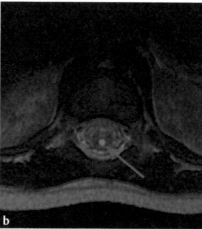

Fig. 26.20 Ventriculus terminalis. (a) Sagittal T2 W image of the spine of a 4-month-old boy shows a vertically oriented, linear hyperintense region in the lower cord (*red arrow*), just above the conus medullaris. (b) Axial T2 W image through region this shows a circumscribed hyperintense area in central cord (*red arrow*), centered slightly posteriorly within the conus medullaris. This represents a ventriculus terminalis ("fifth ventricle"), which is an incidental finding.

less than 1.5 mm is a normal finding. Dilation of the central canal to 1.5 mm or more is known as hydromyelia ("water in the cord"). The finding of hydromyelia is accompanied by the assumption that the central canal of the spinal cord has an intact ependymal lining. The condition in which the spinal cord contains fluid that is not within the central canal is known as syringomyelia. Sometimes the size of this fluid collection is so great that it cannot be determined whether or not the collection arose from the central canal, and there may be an edema-like signal surrounding the collection and making it difficult to estimate whether the ependymal lining of the central canal is intact, for which reason this condition is sometimes referred to as syringohydromyelia. Collectively, the conditions labeled syringomyelia encompass the condition described by the collo-quial term syrinx; however the term syringomyelia serves a more descriptive role (▶ Fig. 26.19).

Hydromyelia is in essence a "hydrocephalus" of the spinal cord, and can occur in the setting of a Chiari type I malformation. Hydromyelia in the absence of a Chiari type I malformation is a finding that merits suspicion and warrants a contrast-enhanced MRI examination of the entire neural axis (brain and total spine) for possible signs of a neoplasm. High-resolution MRI of the obex may be helpful in some cases of hydromyelia. A circumstance in which fluid prominence within the cord can be a normal variant is when the central canal in the region of the conus medullaris is cystically dilated, with smooth and well-defined margins. This is known as the ventriculus terminalis, sometimes described as the "fifth ventricle" (▶ Fig. 26.20).

26.12 Suggested Reading

[1] Rufener SL, Ibrahim M, Raybaud CA, Parmar HA. Congenital spine and spinal cord malformations—Pictorial review. AJR Am J Roentgenol 2010; 194(3) Suppl:S26–S37

27 Neoplasm

27.1 Spinal Neoplasm

Tumors of the spinal cord and vertebral column come in many varieties. The most common are primary tumors, but some metastatic lesions are also identified. In characterizing primary tumors, the differential considerations are based largely on location. The first differentiating feature is whether the origin of the tumor is intradural or extradural. Intradural tumors can be classified as being of intramedullary or extramedullary origin. Most tumors of the spinal cord and vertebral column can be put into one of these classifications, which allows a methodical approach to their characterization on imaging.

27.2 Intradural Intramedullary Neoplasms

Intradural intramedullary tumors are those arising from the spinal cord itself. However, because the spinal cord is a part of the central nervous system (CNS), tumors of the cord are identical to many of those seen intracranially. The most common intramedullary spinal cord neoplasm (IMSCN) in children and adolescents is pilocytic astrocytoma (▶ Fig. 27.1).

Pilocytic astrocytomas of the spinal cord can have features of cerebellar pilocytic astrocytomas, including contrast-enhancing

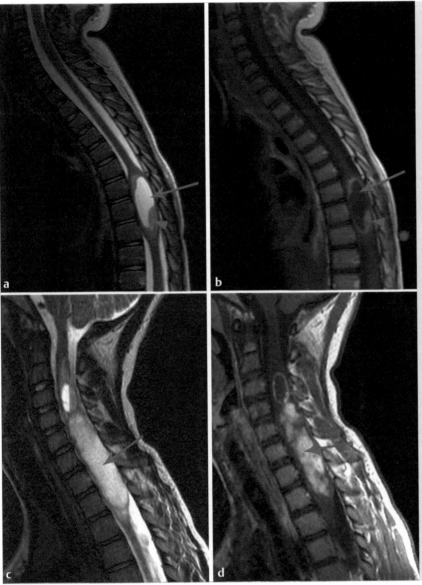

Fig. 27.1 Pilocytic astrocytoma of the spine. (a) Sagittal T2 W image of the spine of a 5-year-old boy with back pain shows an intramedullary tumor in the thoracic cord. The tumor is expansile and has a cystic component (*red arrow*) and a nodular component (*red arrowhead*). (b) Sagittal T1 W plus contrast image shows enhancement of the nodular component (*red arrowhead*) and the wall of the cyst, but not of the cystic-appearing area (*red arrow*). This represents an intramedullary pilocytic astrocytoma of the spinal cord. (c) Sagittal T2 W image of the cervical spine of a 12-year-old boy shows an expansile mass in the cervical cord (*red arrow*), with a cyst superior to this that has an internal fluid level (*red arrowhead*). (d) Sagittal T1 W plus contrast image shows heterogeneous enhancement within the solid portion of the mass (*red arrow*), and a slightly irregular peripheral rim of enhancement around cystic area (*red arrowhead*). This was a pilocytic astrocytoma. Note that although it is said that in adults, ependymomas are more likely to hemorrhage than astrocytomas, intramedullary pilocytic astrocytomas will not uncommonly hemorrhage.

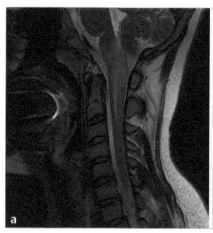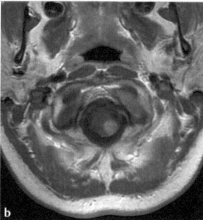

Fig. 27.2 Ganglioglioma. (a) Sagittal T2 W image of the cervical spine of a 14-year-old boy with neck and jaw pain shows an ill-defined area of expansile T2 hyperintense signal spanning the cervicomedullary junction. (b) Axial T1 W plus contrast image at the C1 level shows a more discrete enhancing lesion in the left dorsolateral aspect of the spinal cord. Biopsy demonstrated this to be a ganglioglioma with infiltration of the surrounding white matter tracts.

solid nodular components and cystic areas. As with some pilocytic astrocytomas intrinsic to the brainstem, however, some such lesions of the spinal cord are predominantly solid. Pilocytic astrocytomas of the spinal cord are more likely to hemorrhage than those in the cerebellum, which can result in diagnostic confusion. In the literature on adult neoplasms, it is stated that ependymomas of the spinal cord are more likely to hemorrhage than are astrocytomas of the cord, and in the adult population this is true. However, there are several differences in the characteristics of these tumors in the pediatric and adult populations. In adults, astrocytomas tend to be fibrillary or anaplastic astrocytomas, or glioblastoma. In children, astrocytomas are nearly always pilocytic. Additionally, ependymomas are very rare in children, especially those younger than 15 years of age, unless there is a history of neurofibromatosis type 2 (NF2) (▶ Fig. 7.10b).

Both ependymomas and pilocytic astrocytomas tend to be discrete lesions that displace nerve fibers of the cord, whereas the other types of astrocytomas (which are the only astrocytomas seen in adults) infiltrate such fibers. It is therefore possible to surgically resect pilocytic astrocytomas and ependymomas of the spinal cord, whereas astrocytomas that infiltrate the cord cannot be easily resected without disrupting neurologic functions. The relationship between a lesion and the fibers of the spinal cord has been suggested as a way in which diffusion tensor imaging (DTI) can be used to predict the histology of an IMSCN in adults; if an ependymoma is suspected, a resection may be done, whereas if an astrocytoma is suspected, biopsy may be preferred. In children, however, DTI likely plays an equally important role in determining the resectability of an IMSCN by revealing whether spinal cord fibers are displaced as opposed to being infiltrated by the IMSCN. But because pediatric astrocytomas are more commonly pilocytic astrocytomas, DTI is unlikely to be useful for predicting the histology of IMSCN in children. As noted earlier, age in the pediatric population generally predicts the histology of an IMSCN, which will only rarely be ependymoma. Nevertheless, ependymomas can occur in children, and particularly those who have NF2.

An additional IMSCN seen in children but not common in adults is ganglioglioma (▶ Fig. 27.2). Gangliogliomas are low-grade tumors that have a tendency to infiltrate spinal cord fibers, possibly limiting the ability to safely resect these lesions while preserving cord function. Gangliogliomas of the cord in children tend to have fewer cystic areas than intracranial gangliogliomas, and are more likely to be eccentrically located within the cord than are pilocytic astrocytomas or ependymomas. Because they may be difficult to safely resect, it is fortunate that intramedullary gangliogliomas of the cord respond well to radiation therapy. Pilocytic astrocytomas of the spinal cord also respond well to radiation therapy, for which reason subtotal resection of these tumors is sometimes planned if it is difficult to differentiate tumor from cord tissue at the periphery of some lesions. The theory is that the residual tumor can be observed, and if necessary can be treated with repeat surgery or radiation therapy.

Intramedullary spinal cord neoplasms in the upper cervical cord have a propensity to grow superiorly across the cervicomedullary junction. Their growth along the craniocaudal axis is less restricted than in the transverse axis because there are few transversely oriented fibers to restrict this growth. When a tumor extends superiorly into the medulla oblongata, it is obstructed from extending more superiorly by the pyramidal and lemniscal decussations, and the medulla will focally enlarge (▶ Fig. 27.3). From a treatment perspective, tumors of the craniocervical junction respond in the same way as IMSCN.[1]

Patients with IMSCN resected from the cervical cord are at risk for the subsequent development of a kyphosis as the result of osseous and neuromuscular destabilization.

Hemangioblastomas are IMSCN that are highly vascular and can occur in a multifocal manner in patients with von Hippel–Lindau syndrome. It is important to be aware that the multifocal nature of these tumors does not indicate metastatic disease, and that each of the lesions of these tumors is instead the result of genetic predisposition.

It is important to recognize that some non-neoplastic conditions can mimic IMSCN. This is particularly true of noninfectious inflammatory conditions, such as acute disseminated encephalomyelitis (ADEM) and Devic's syndrome/neuromyelitis optica, which are further discussed in Chapter 25.

27.3 Intradural Extramedullary Neoplasms

Another compartment of the spine in which pediatric spinal tumors occur is the intradural extramedullary space. The most

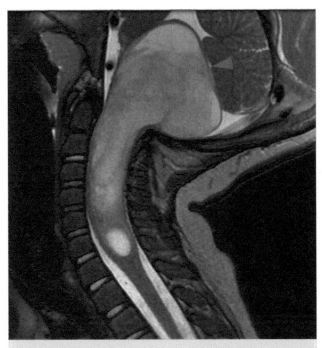

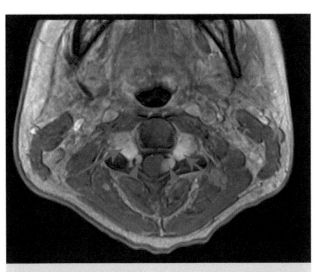

Fig. 27.4 Intradural neurofibroma. Axial T1 W plus contrast image of the cervical spine of a 16-year-old-girl with neurofibromatosis type 1 shows bilateral, intradural, extramedullary contrast-enhancing masses (*red arrowheads*), larger on the left than on the right. The patient also had masses extending through and expanding the neural foramina (*red arrows*).

Fig. 27.3 Pilocytic astrocytoma. Sagittal T2 W image of the lower head and spine of a 2.5-year-old boy shows an expansile, predominantly solid lesion spanning the cervicomedullary junction, with a small cyst at the caudal margin. There is expansion of the medullary component that results in posterior displacement of the foramen of Magendie (*red arrowhead*). This represented a pilocytic astrocytoma that peripherally splayed the surrounding white matter tracts.

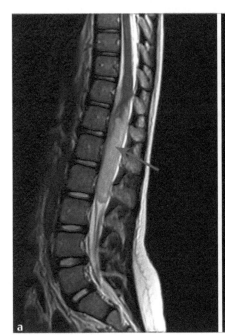

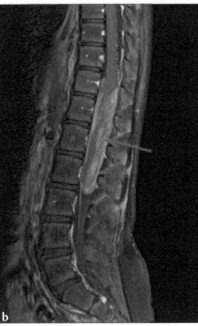

Fig. 27.5 Myxopapillary ependymoma. (a) Sagittal T2 W image of the spine of an 8-year-old girl with back pain shows an ill-defined intradural mass (*red arrow*) surrounding the region of the conus medullaris. (b) Sagittal T1 W plus contrast fat-saturated image shows heterogeneous enhancement within the lesion (*red arrow*), which was proven to be an intradural extramedullary myxopapillary ependymoma of the filum terminale.

common entities arising in this compartment are nerve sheath tumors, including both neurofibromas and schwannomas. Differentiating these two neoplasms can be difficult unless there is a condition predisposing to one or the other of them. Neurofibromas are seen in neurofibromatosis type 1 (NF1), whereas schwannomas are seen in NF2 (▶ Fig. 27.4). In adults, meningio-

mas can be difficult to differentiate from nerve sheath tumors, but are rare in children other than those with NF2.

Although primary ependymomas are typically intramedullary, a specific histologic subtype of primary ependymoma, known as a myxopapillary ependymoma, occurs in association with the filum terminale (▶ Fig. 27.5). These lesions tend to enhance and

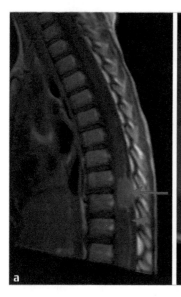
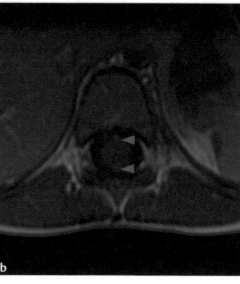

Fig. 27.6 Nodular metastatic deposit. (a) Sagittal T1 W plus contrast image of the lower thoracic spine of a 4-year-old girl with a mass in the posterior fossa shows a large dorsal intradural extramedullary mass pushing on the spinal cord (*red arrow*), as well as linear enhancement along the dorsal margin of the spinal cord below this (*red arrowhead*). The mass represents a metastatic deposit from a medulloblastoma. (b) Axial T1 W plus contrast image of the spinal cord below the mass shows enlarged vascular structures along the anterior and posterior margins of the cord (*red arrowheads*), corresponding to the finding in the sagittal image of the cord shown in (a), which represent congested veins rather than additional foci of metastatic disease.

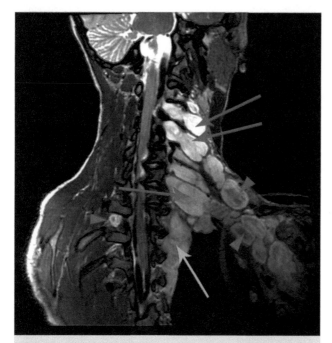

Fig. 27.7 Plexiform neurofibroma. Coronal oblique T2 W image of the left shoulder of a 9-year-old boy with neurofibromatosis type 1 demonstrates numerous enlarged tubular masses emanating from the neural foramina along the brachial plexus (*red arrows*). Several lesions have a targetoid appearance (*red arrowheads*), which is a feature more often seen in neurofibromas than in schwannomas. Note that there is posterior paraspinous/mediastinal extension of the lesions (*green arrow*). The masses in this patient represent plexiform neurofibromas in the setting of NF1.

results in leptomeningeal metastatic deposits of tumor cells. These can take the form of focal nodular areas (▶ Fig. 27.6) or diffuse, smooth coating ("sugar-coating").

27.4 Extradural Soft Tissue Neoplasms

Extradural spinal tumors include tumors of neural, soft tissue, and osseous origin. The most common among those of neural origin are nerve sheath tumors. These can be isolated nerve sheath tumors or, in some patients with NF1, plexiform neurofibromas, which are large tubular lesions that extend along the nerve plexus (▶ Fig. 27.7).

A congenital lesion specific to newborns and infants is a sacrococcygeal teratoma (▶ Fig. 27.8). Features of this tumor must be considered whenever a myelomeningocele, terminal myelocystocele, or presacral mass is encountered on fetal imaging. As its name suggests, a sacrococcygeal teratoma is a teratoma associated with the caud-almost aspect of the vertebral column. These lesions tend to be heterogeneous, having areas of fat and solid tissue, and may have variable degrees of maturity/differentiation. They can occasionally be predominantly cystic, in which case they provide the greatest diagnostic challenge. Sacrococcygeal teratomas are categorized by their location, with a larger percentage occurring on the inside than on the outside of the body. Sacrococcygeal teratomas of type I occur entirely outside the body and are attached to it by a narrow stalk. Sacrococcygeal teratomas of types II and III are located partly inside and partly outside the body, with type II lesions being largely outside and type III being largely inside the body. A sacrococcygeal teratoma of type IV is a presacral lesion located entirely inside the body.

27.5 Osseous Tumors

Osseous tumors of the spine fit into the category of extradural tumors. A multicystic expansile lesion with internal cystic areas that have layering of blood products is an aneurysmal bone cyst (ABC), which is an osteolytic neoplasm of bone (▶ Fig. 27.9).

have a very heterogeneous, multicystic appearance on imaging. Their appearance and location are highly characteristic, and although a paraganglioma can have an appearance similar to this, the most likely diagnosis for a lesion with this appearance and location is myxopapillary ependymoma.

Several pediatric intracranial tumors, in particular ependymomas and primitive neuroectodermal tumors (PNET)/medulloblastomas, have a tendency to disseminate in the CSF, which

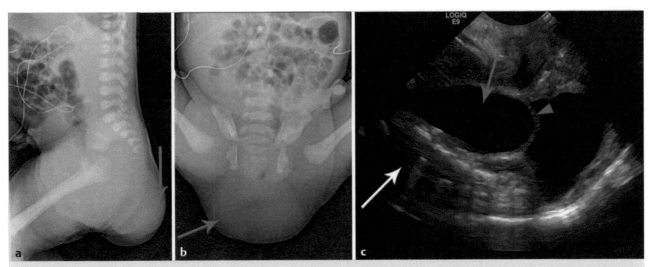

Fig. 27.8 Sacrococcygeal teratoma. (a) Lateral and (b) frontal radiographs of the pelvis of a newborn (0-day-old) girl shows a soft tissue mass (*red arrow*) below the sacrum. (c) Ultrasonographic image shows multiple cystic components (*red arrow*) with internal septae (*red arrowhead*). The ultrasonographic image also shows the relationship of the mass in this patient to the sacrum (*white arrow*). This represents a sacrococcygeal teratoma.

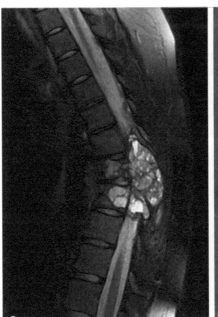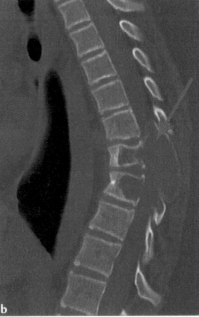

Fig. 27.9 Thoracic ABC. (a) Sagittal T2 W fat-saturated image of the spine of a 12-year-old girl with back pain and kyphosis shows a circumscribed heterogeneous lesion involving the bodies and posterior elements of two adjacent vertebrae at the apex of the kyphosis. There are multiple fluid levels within the lesion. (b) Sagittal computed tomographic image of the patient's spine at the level of the lesion shows it as having a lytic and expansile appearance (*red arrow*). This represents an aneurysmal bone cyst.

Chordomas are tumors of notochordal origin that can occur anywhere within the vertebral column and central skull base, although the two most common locations of these tumors' origin are the sacrum and the clivus, with the next most common location being the cervical spine. Chordomas can be heterogeneous mixed solid and cystic lesions, and often present as T2 hyperintense, enhancing masses at the locations of their occurrence. The origin of such a tumor is often the primary clue to its diagnosis.

Langerhans cell histiocytosis (LCH), also known as eosinophilic granuloma, is a multisystem histiocytic disease that can involve bones. When there is osseous involvement within the spine, patients may have pathologic compression fractures that result in a flattened vertebral body, or "vertebra plana."

(▶ Fig. 27.10) The differential diagnosis of vertebra plana is broad. Potential etiologies include: trauma LCH (eosinophilic granuloma), leukemia, neoplasm (metastasis), and infection (including tuberculosis). When vertebra plana is encountered, a radiographic skeletal survey should be done for other signs of LCH, such as circumscribed lytic lesions within long bones and the calvarium. Langerhans cell histiocytosis can also cause an interstitial lung disease, with small cysts having walls of intermediate thickness (as opposed to thin-walled cysts in conditions like lymphangioleiomyomatosis [LAM]).

Patients with hematopoietic malignancies can have visible changes in the bone marrow on magnetic resonance imaging (MRI). The fat in yellow marrow has a bright signal on T1 W and T2 W imaging, and any process that results in the proliferation

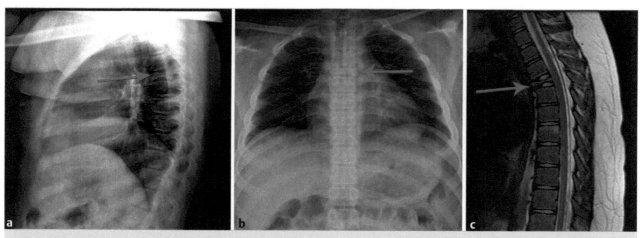

Fig. 27.10 Vertebra plana. (a) Lateral and (b) frontal radiographs of the thoracic spine of an 11-year-old boy show vertebra plana at T4 (*red arrow*). (c) Sagittal T2 W image shows no intrinsic mass, marrow abnormality, or destructive lesion in the flattened vertebra (*red arrow*). There is focal hyperintense marrow signal subjacent to the superior endplate of T7.

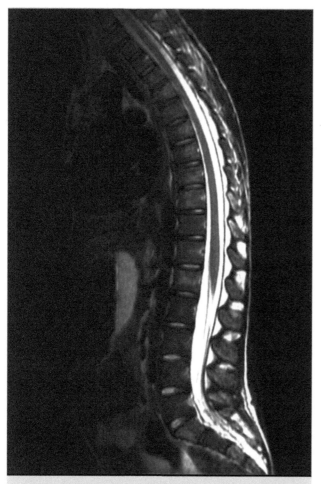

Fig. 27.11 Marrow infiltration. Sagittal T2 W magnetic resonance image of the spine of a 7-year-old male with back pain shows a diffusely hypointense appearance of the bone marrow, with heterogeneous areas of hyperintense signal. This is suggestive of infiltration of red marrow, and can be seen in leukemia as well as profound anemia (including sickle-cell anemia).

of red marrow will result in the marrow's having a more hypointense appearance on both T1 W and T2 W imaging than is normal. This finding is nonspecific, and can occur in hematopoietic malignancies (▶ Fig. 27.11). Chronic anemia, either from iron deficiency, chronic disease, or a hemoglobinopathy, such as sickle-cell disease or thalassemia, also results in the proliferation of red marrow and produces a similar appearance on T1 W and T2 W imaging. A finding of marrow with this appearance should prompt a complete blood count with a hematopathologic review of a blood smear, and may eventually necessitate a bone marrow biopsy.

Osseous metastases are much less common in children than in adults, although the one neoplastic entity that does commonly result in spinal osseous metastatic disease in children is neuroblastoma. In patients with neuroblastoma, heterogeneous bone marrow may be the primary clue to metastatic disease. Because neuroblastoma is a tumor characterized by small round blue cells having a high nuclear-to-cytoplasmic ratio, diffusion-weighted imaging (DWI) can aid in detecting its osseous (and soft tissue) metastatic spread (▶ Fig. 27.12).

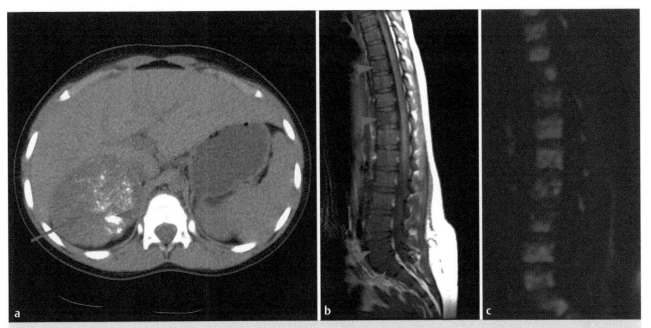

Fig. 27.12 Metastatic neuroblastoma of the spine. (a) Axial computed tomographic image of the spine of a 9-year-old boy shows a right-sided retroperitoneal mass (*red arrow*) with heterogeneous internal calcifications (*red arrowhead*). This was separate from the kidney, but no normal right adrenal gland was identified. (b) Sagittal T1 W image of the lumbar and lower thoracic spine demonstrates several areas of heterogeneous marrow (*red arrowheads*). (c) Sagittal diffusion-weighted image of the lumbar and lower thoracic spine shows numerous metastatic deposits and a heterogeneous marrow signal. This represents neuroblastoma, which is a small round blue cell tumor.

27.6 Suggested Reading

[1] Soderlund KA, Smith AB, Rushing EJ, Smirniotopolous JG. Radiologic-pathologic correlation of pediatric and adolescent spinal neoplasms: Part 2, Intradural extramedullary spinal neoplasms. AJR Am J Roentgenol 2012; 198(1): 44–51

[2] Smith AB, Soderlund KA, Rushing EJ, Smirniotopolous JG. Radiologic-pathologic correlation of pediatric and adolescent spinal neoplasms: Part 1, Intramedullary spinal neoplasms. AJR Am J Roentgenol 2012; 198(1):34–43

[3] Huisman TA. Pediatric tumors of the spine. Cancer Imaging 2009; 9 Spec No A:S45–S48

[4] Choudhri AF, Whitehead MT, Klimo P Jr, Montgomery BK, Boop FA. Diffusion tensor imaging to guide surgical planning in intramedullary spinal cord tumors in children. Neuroradiology 2014; 56(2):169–174

References

[1] McAbee JH, Modica J, Thompson CJ et al. Cervicomedullary tumors in children. J Neurosurg Pediatr 2015:1–10

28 Trauma

28.1 Spinal Trauma

Traumatic injuries to the spine, either alone or in conjunction with other injuries, are common reasons for visits to the emergency department. Not all injuries to the spine require imaging, and different imaging modalities and workups for spinal injuries are required, depending on the mechanism of injury and symptoms. At times, a high-impact injury may warrant imaging despite the absence of clinical symptoms (e.g., computed tomographic imaging for a patient ejected from a vehicle traveling at 80 mph), and at times neurologic symptoms may warrant further evaluation despite normal findings in other studies (e.g., numbness of an extremity after a motor-vehicle accident [MVA], with normal findings on a computed tomographic study being followed by magnetic resonance imaging [MRI]). Other injuries, which may interfere with the clinical exam, can make it difficult to clinically "clear" a spine as being free of injury. Special considerations exist with children, including the continued role of radiography for evaluation of spinal trauma, in contrast to the situation with adults, for whom computed tomography (CT) has supplanted radiography, and concern about radiation dose, the possibility of mistaking developmental findings for fractures, and the possible need for sedation with MRI (▶ Table 28.1). In the case of the cervical spine, ligamentous injuries are more common in children than in adults, and tend to occur in the upper cervical region, especially in children younger than 8 years of age, as opposed to adults, who more often have injuries of the lower cervical region. Approximately 60% to 80% of spinal injuries in children involve the cervical spine, in contrast to 30 to 40% of spinal injuries involving the cervical spine in adults.

Table 28.1 Considerations in developing protocols for imaging of the spine

Radiography	Typically, only anteroposterior and lateral radiographs of the spine section being evaluated are needed. Open-mouth odontoid views are not needed in radiography of the cervical spine in children under the age of 8 years. Oblique radiographs and coned-down lumbosacral views are rarely indicated in children.
Computed tomography	Helical acquisition, three-plane bone algorithm images (less than 3 mm and ideally 1–2 mm slice thickness); axial and sagittal soft tissue algorithm images.
Magnetic resonance imaging	Include sagittal short tau inversion recovery to investigate for marrow and soft tissue edema. Axial images should be contiguous and parallel (unlike many protocols for adult degenerative disease, which call only for images parallel to the disk space with skip sections).
Nuclear medicine bone scan	Frontal and lateral projections in whole-body scans. Narrow field-of-view evaluation and possible single-photon emission computed tomography of areas of uncertainty.

28.2 Anatomic Considerations

In addition to ligamentous laxity, anatomic considerations in interpreting images of the spine in pediatric trauma include the differences in vertebral shape from that in adults and incomplete ossification. In pediatric patients, the stage of ossification varies at different ages, which creates particular uncertainty in the case of C1 and C2 (▶ Fig. 24.2, ▶ Fig. 24.3, ▶ Fig. 24.4, ▶ Fig. 24.5). The alignment of the spine is also different in children, particularly in the cervical spine, which can have a mild kyphosis in young children, as well as "pseudosubluxation" of C1 with respect to C2 (▶ Fig. 24.6).

28.3 Imaging Modalities

28.3.1 Choice of Imaging: Plain Film, Computed Tomography, or Magnetic Resonance Imaging

Plain films and computed tomographic scans are the primary means of detecting fractures and abnormalities of alignment of the spine after traumatic injury. The optimal choice between these imaging modalities is a balance based on the mechanism of injury, symptoms, and concerns about radiation. It is important to keep in mind that although computed tomography (CT) involves greater radiation exposure than does plain radiography, missing a fracture is not an appropriate tradeoff for a lower radiation dose.

Many traumatic injuries warrant CT of the chest, abdomen, and pelvis for evaluating the state of visceral organs. With image acquisition through helical multidetector CT scanners, the thoracic and lumbar spine can be examined via the thin-section bone algorithm reformatting of source data without additional radiation exposure. This therefore constitutes a situation (assuming that CT was already being performed for other reasons) in which plain radiography would expose the patient to greater radiation than would CT. Perhaps the best way to reduce radiation exposure of the pediatric trauma patient is to avoid any imaging when there are no relevant indications for it. Research has shown that clinical examination can be effective in excluding cervical spine injuries,[1,2] even in children younger than 3 years of age.[3] The development and adoption of criteria for appropriateness of the use of imaging, and additional research on this, will be required, with specific attention to different age subgroups.[4,5,6]

Magnetic resonance imaging is ideal for evaluating ligamentous injury and seeking signs of cord compression or contusion. However, MRI of the spine may require 20 to 30 minutes per section of the spine, requiring a patient to be away from the patient's care unit or intensive care unit (ICU) for an extended period, and MRI may require sedation. Although fractures typically show signs of marrow edema on MRI, MRI should not be used as the primary means of detecting a possible fracture. Research has examined the role of diffusion tensor imaging (DTI) for evaluating the integrity of the spinal cord and possibly identifying subtle contusions of the cord, but its use is not yet

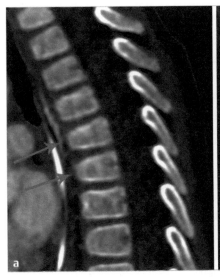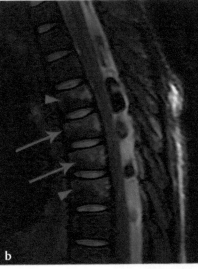

Fig. 28.1 Compression fracture. (a) Sagittal bone algorithm image from a computed tomographic study of the thorax of a 4-year-old boy after a motor-vehicle accident shows subtle wedging of two adjacent midthoracic vertebrae (*red arrows*). (b) Sagittal short tau inversion recovery image shows marrow edema within the two vertebrae (*red arrows*), which have slight superior endplate irregularities, consistent with acute compression fractures. There is also marrow edema within the adjacent vertebrae (*red arrowheads*), without significant endplate irregularity, representing bone contusions as opposed to very subtle compression fractures.

routine in clinical practice. Magnetic resonance imaging is typically an adjunctive technique, providing additional information in conjunction with CT and other imaging modalities.

Ultrasonography and nuclear medicine imaging are not commonly used in the setting of trauma. Ultrasonography can be used for evaluating a paraspinal hematoma, and radionuclide bone scans can be used for identifying or ruling out suspected compression fractures or acute defects of the pars interarticularis, particularly when there are contraindications to MRI. A nuclear medicine bone scan is sometimes used to investigate suspected abusive trauma.

Determining the appropriate diagnostic workup for a particular pediatric patient, including clinical examination, observation, and imaging, requires multidisciplinary input involving members of the radiology, neurosurgery, orthopaedic surgery, trauma, and pediatric emergency medicine staff.

28.4 Fractures

Traumatic fractures of the spine can result from hyperflexion, distraction, or compressive forces. Perhaps the most common type of fracture is a compression fracture. A compression fracture typically involves loss of height resulting from an irregularity in the vertebral superior endplate. If such a fracture is detected on radiographs, CT and MRI are typically performed. Computed tomography is done to fully characterize the fracture, and MRI is done to evaluate for ligamentous and cord injury. When a compression fracture is identified, the degree of height loss should be reported, as should any abnormality in spinal alignment, such as a focal kyphosis. Also important is whether there is retropulsion of the posterior cortex of the vertebral body into the central canal, and if so, a description of the degree of narrowing of the central canal and the effect of the vertebral retropulsion on the spinal cord. Sagittal short tau inversion recovery (STIR) imaging is highly sensitive to marrow edema, and in cases of traumatic injury of the spine typically identifies several adjacent levels of osseous injury. In the setting of trauma, marrow edema without loss of height is considered to represent a bone contusion, probably in the form of trabecular microfractures without cortical disruption (▶ Fig. 28.1).

Vertebral contusions will typically heal completely without loss of height if treated conservatively, particularly through the short-term avoidance of excessive weight-bearing and contact sports. They can, however, predispose to a delayed loss of height if the patient experiences a second traumatic event within a short period after the initial contusive event. For this reason, vertebral contusions may affect the time at which a patient can return to athletic activity.

In addition to their susceptibility to traditional osseous fractures, young children with incompletely ossified vertebrae are susceptible to synchondrosis fractures, which are the equivalent of Salter–Harris type I fractures. A particular site of proneness to synchondrosis fracture is the odontoid synchondrosis (▶ Fig. 28.2).

Fractures in adolescents with maturely ossified vertebrae tend to have features and patterns on imaging that resemble those in young adults. A three-column hyperflexion-distraction injury of the spine, known as a Chance fracture (▶ Fig. 28.3), is an unstable fracture that must be rapidly identified. This pattern of injury is most commonly seen when passengers in a car are restrained with a lap-belt alone, and its incidence has decreased in the era of child safety and three-point seatbelts.

28.5 Ligamentous Injury

Because of the greater ligamentous laxity of children, ligamentous stretch injuries are more common in this population than in adults, particularly in the cervical spine. A ligamentous injury will often lack an associated fracture, and may cause abnormality in spinal alignment, yet may result in injury to the spinal cord. Accordingly, a posttraumatic neurologic deficit in a child warrants further evaluation with MRI.

Stretch injury to the interspinous ligaments is perhaps the most common type of ligamentous injury of the spine, with clinical symptoms corresponding to those of whiplash injury (▶ Fig. 28.4). A stretch injury occurring as an isolated finding is managed conservatively, but close attention is required to exclude additional ligamentous injury that may require prolonged immobilization (▶ Fig. 28.5). A ligamentous injury does not typically require surgical management.

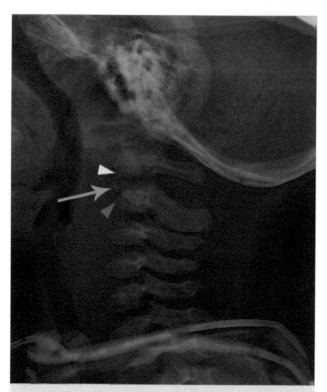

Fig. 28.2 Synchondrosis fracture. Lateral radiograph of the upper cervical spine of a 1-year-old girl with a history of trauma shows the odontoid process anteriorly displaced and angulated (*white arrowhead*) relative to the C2 vertebral body (*red arrowhead*). A tiny ossific fragment (*blue arrow*) is seen at the anterior aspect of the odontoid synchondrosis. This represents an odontoid synchondrosis subluxation/fracture, which was confirmed on magnetic resonance imaging as not representing pseudosubluxation.

Sagittal STIR imaging is helpful for identifying ligamentous edema and/or disruption. High-resolution imaging, such as constructive interference in steady state (CISS)/fast imaging employing steady-state acquisition (FIESTA) imaging, can provide additional detail in cases of ligamentous injury.

28.6 Cord Injury

Cord contusion represents injury to the spinal cord resulting from direct contact. Magnetic resonance imaging is the optimal method of identifying and characterizing a contusion of the cord, particularly in T2 W images, whereas a contusion will be occult on radiography and probably also on CT. A very mild contusion of the cord may be occult if MRI is done soon after the injury that causes it, whereas DTI of the cord in this setting may show subtle decreases in fractional anisotropy. However, the use of DTI in identifying cord injury, although an area of active research, is not currently applicable at the clinical level.

A contusion of the spinal cord will usually show up as a T2 W hyperintense area, and if the contusion is severe, the cord may be expanded by edema. Children can experience contusions even in the absence of fracture, acute disk herniation, or compressive hematoma. This is a result of the ligamentous laxity in children, which may allow a hyperflexion injury of the cord without a vertebral fracture, and with a posttraumatic return to normal alignment. Contusions can present clinically as numbness, weakness, or paralysis, depending on the portion(s) of the cord that they involve and the severity of the injury that causes them. Mild contusions of the cord cause transient neurologic symptoms with an eventual return of function. More severe contusions can cause permanent deficits.

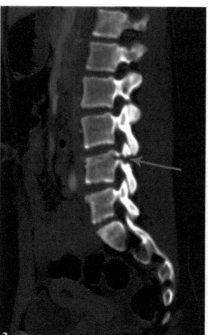
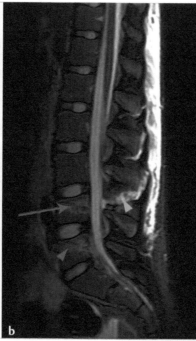

Fig. 28.3 Chance fracture. (a) Sagittal bone algorithm image of the lumbar spine from an abdominal/pelvic computed tomography examination of a 13-year-old female shows a fracture through the superior endplate of L4 (*red arrowhead*) that extends to the posterior elements (*red arrow*), with posterior splaying and subtle focal kyphosis. (b) Sagittal short tau inversion recovery image shows marrow edema throughout the L4 vertebra (*red arrow*), as well as in L5 (*red arrowhead*). There is edema throughout the disrupted L3–L4 interspinous ligaments (*green arrowhead*).

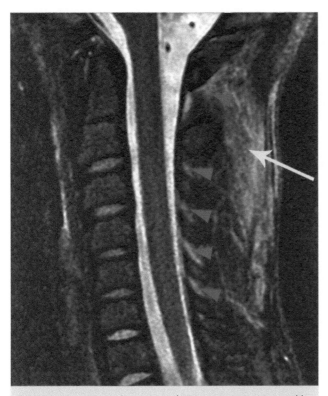

Fig. 28.4 Interspinous edema. Sagittal STIR image in an 11-year-old male after MVA shows hyperintense signal in the interspinous ligament throughout the mid and upper cervical spine (*red arrowheads*), consistent with interspinous ligamentous edema. Additional hyperintense signal is seen within and deep to the nuchal ligament (*white arrow*). This degree of injury typically resolves spontaneously with conservative therapy, and likely correlates with clinical signs of "whiplash."

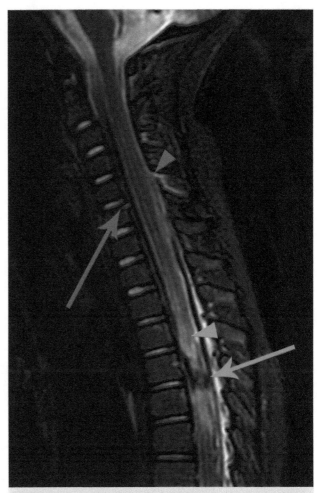

Fig. 28.5 Stretch injury. Sagittal short tau inversion recovery image of the cervical and upper thoracic spine of a 32-month-old female after a motor-vehicle accident shows that the alignment of the cervical vertebral column is within normal limits for this age. There is focal disruption of the ligamentum flavum at the C4–C5 level (*red arrowhead*) and injury to the posterior longitudinal ligament at the superior endplate of C6 (*red arrow*). There is no adjacent cord contusion, but in the upper thoracic cord there is cord edema (*blue arrowhead*), including areas of hypointense signal representing hematomyelia (*blue arrow*). The thoracic cord injury in this patient is probably a stretch injury related to a midcervical hyperflexion injury.

An additional pattern of injury to the spinal cord is hematomyelia, or blood within the cord. Hematomyelia will show up as an area of heterogenous signal, often with T2 hypointense areas, and generally indicates a low likelihood of full functional recovery.

Ligamentous laxity makes it possible for a cord stretch injury to occur in locations away from the location of a ligamentous injury (▶ Fig. 28.5). As in the case of hematomyelia, a stretch injury to the spinal cord may be associated with incomplete functional recovery.

The anteroposterior (AP) diameter of the central canal of the cervical spinal cord is typically greater than approximately 12 mm at the level of the inferior endplate of C2. A congenital stenosis (or borderline stenosis) of the cervical spinal canal can be diagnosed when there is narrowing of the canal as the result of short vertebral pedicles. Although this by itself may not be pathologic, it predisposes to cord contusion from minor trauma, in which a hyperflexion injury, minor ligamentous injury, or small disk herniation may impact on the cord. A narrowed cervical canal can easily be overlooked on CT if it is not considered and sought, and neurologic signs of cord injury in the presence of a normal result of CT scanning warrant an MRI of the cervical spine. A common scenario in which narrowing of the cervical canal is encountered is that of an adolescent male who, after a helmet hit while playing football, experiences paresthesias in

the upper extremity, an experience colloquially known as a "stinger" (▶ Fig. 28.6). Recognizing the factors that predispose to narrowing of the cervical canal and recommending an MRI to identify this abnormality may prevent further injury and allow the functional recovery of a patient.

28.6.1 Spinal Cord Injury Without Radiographic Abnormality

Spinal cord injury without radiographic abnormality (SCIWORA) is a term used to describe patients with neurologic signs of spinal cord injury in the setting of normal findings on a radiographic evaluation. The definition of this entity does not make clear what is indicated by "radiographic," since it is possible to have ligamentous injury and cord contusion with normal

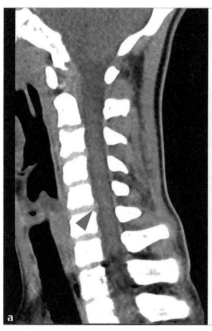
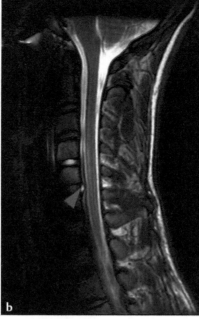

Fig. 28.6 "Stinger." (a) Sagittal computed tomographic image reconstructed with a soft tissue algorithm of the cervical spine of a 14-year-old boy with upper-extremity numbness and paresthesias of abrupt onset, known as a "stinger," after a forceful contact in a football game. Although there was no fracture, there are signs of a disk herniation at the C5–C6 level (*red arrowhead*), highlighting the role of soft tissue algorithm reconstructions as part of a computed tomographic protocol for imaging of the spine. (b) Sagittal T2 W image shows hyperintense signal within the herniated portion of the disk (*red arrowhead*), which in this setting represents an acute herniation. However, it is important to note that a hyperintense signal in a T2 W image does not always indicate an acute disk herniation.

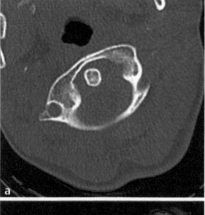
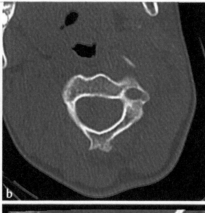
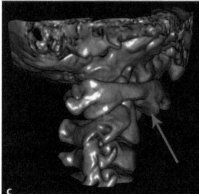
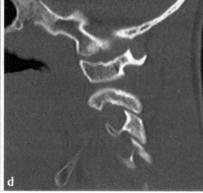

Fig. 28.7 Rotatory subluxation. (a) Axial computed tomographic image of C1 in a 10-year-old girl with fixed torticollis. (b) Axial computed tomographic image of C2 in the same patient, with the same orientation, showing a rotation of approximately 34° between C1 and C2. (c) Three-dimensional reconstruction from a computed tomographic examination showing uncovering of the right lateral mass of C2 (*red arrowhead*) and anterior subluxation of the left lateral mass of C1 (*red arrow*). (d) Sagittal computed tomographic image shows a convex inferior margin to the right lateral mass of C1 (rocker-bottom lateral mass), which predisposes to rotatory subluxation.

results on plain film and computed tomographic examination. The true nature of SCIWORA is probably a cord contusion of some type that occurs in the absence of a fracture or subsequent abnormality of spinal alignment. However, a detectible abnormality is often found on MRI in patients with SCIWORA. Therefore, SCIWORA is a diagnosis of exclusion, and is probably a soft tissue injury that might be detectable if MRI were performed, and therefore may not truly be a discrete disease entity.

It is not a radiologic diagnosis, but awareness of SCIWORA is important because the term may be used by other physicians.

28.7 Rotatory Subluxation

The normal function of the C1–C2 articulation is to provide the head with the capacity to rotate. The normal extent of its rotation is up to approximately 20° to the left and right (▶ Fig. 28.7).

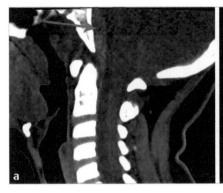
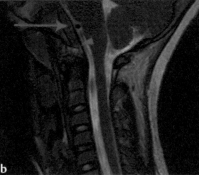

Fig. 28.8 Retroclival epidural hematoma. (a) Sagittal soft tissue algorithm computed tomographic image of the upper cervical spine of an 8-year-old girl, acquired after a motor-vehicle accident, shows a high-density retroclival collection (*red arrow*). (b) Sagittal T2 W image shows a heterogeneous retroclival collection (*red arrow*). The tectorial membrane and retroclival dura (*red arrowhead*) are uplifted from the dorsal cortex of the clivus but remain intact.

Although CT and MRI scans are typically done with the head in neutral position, a slight turn of the head can result in a rotated appearance of C1 with respect to C2. By itself, this finding does not indicate rotatory subluxation. Rotatory subluxation of C1 with respect to C2 is associated with a fixed or locked position of the vertebrae, typically of more than 20° to the right or left. When this is seen, it is important to exclude a possible fracture, and thin-section computed tomographic images are important for this. To evaluate the degree of rotation of which the head is capable, scans can be done with the head in the neutral position and in right and left turns. The neutral scan can be of the entire cervical spine, and the images made with the head turned can be of the section from the occiput to C3. When evaluating these studies, it is also important to evaluate for possible osseous developmental abnormalities, such as the fusion of a lateral mass of C1 to the occipital condyle. Also, a flattened or convex margin of the inferior cortex of either lateral mass of C1 ("rocker-bottom" C1 lateral mass) increases the risk for rotatory subluxation (▶ Fig. 28.7d).

28.8 Retroclival Epidural Hematoma

In the setting of high-impact trauma at the craniocervical junction, the tectorial membrane may get stripped away from the dorsal aspect of the clivus yet remain intact. This results in a retroclival epidural hematoma (▶ Fig. 28.8), and may be difficult to detect on CT of the head without the availability of sagittal soft tissue reformats.[7] When a retroclival epidural hematoma is found, the patient must be evaluated for signs of additional ligamentous injury at the craniocervical junction with an MRI of the cervical spine.

A mechanism of injury similar to that causing a retroclival epidural hematoma and that results in disruption of the tectorial membrane leads to atlanto-occipital dissociation, identified on the basis of an increased distance between the occipital condyles and the lateral masses of C1 on lateral radiography or sagittal CT.

28.9 Abusive Trauma and the Spine

Injuries from abusive trauma can involve both the osseous and soft tissue components of the spine. These injuries can include vertebral compression fractures, spinal subdural hematomas, ligamentous injuries with resultant focal abnormalities of alignment, and cord contusion. Fractures and abnormalities of alignment can be detected on radiographic skeletal surveys. Spinal subdural hematomas, ligamentous injuries without abnormalities of alignment, and cord contusion are best identified on MRI. In cases of suspected abusive trauma in which there are abnormalities of alignment, severe thoracoabdominal injuries, or unexplained neurologic deficits of the extremities, MRI of the spine should be considered in addition to MRI of the head. As with all aspects of evaluative imaging in cases of known or suspected abuse, a multidisciplinary assessment for identifying clinical findings before imaging is done will optimize the diagnostic yield.[8,9] Some institutions use a nuclear medicine bone scan to identify skeletal trauma in cases of suspected abuse, and this may be an additional way of detecting fractures of the spine. When fracture is identified on a bone scan, further evaluation of the specific area of concern with CT and/or MRI is warranted.

28.10 Clearance of the Spine

Clearing the spine, and particularly the cervical spine, of having possibly sustained an injury is a clinical process with established guidelines. It is important to note that imaging does not "clear" the spine, although the absence of abnormality on imaging is supportive information for possible clearance in the clinical decision-making process. Therefore, in response to the question, "Is the cervical spine CT clear?" it is never appropriate to say "Yes." An appropriate response to this question, in the setting of a normal study, is "There are no fractures." If this accords with the findings on clinical examination, the treating physician may deem the cervical spine cleared. If the patient has a persistent neurologic deficit that is not explained, an MRI may be indicated. Therefore, although CT may show no spinal fractures, this alone cannot "clear" the spine of having an injury. This distinction may not result in confusion at a large academic medical center with dedicated specialists in spinal trauma, but one should not make assumptions about how the reported information will be interpreted.

28.11 Injury to the Brachial Plexus

The brachial plexus is a network of nerves arising from the C5 through T1 nerve roots that provides innervation to the upper extremities. The nerve roots themselves send fibers back and forth as they progress outward in segments known as trunks, divisions, cords, and branches. Traumatic impairment of the brachial plexus can result from direct injury, including blunt injury causing a hematoma that affects the components of the brachial plexus, and penetrating injury that partly or fully transects some of the fibers of the nerve roots. More common, however, is a traction or stretch injury from a rapid application of force to the nerves arising from the spine. This force can be related to trauma, such as from rapid abduction of the arms while trying to stop oneself from falling (rapid deceleration), or from an episode in athletics (athletic events can have traumatic components). Stretch injuries to the brachial plexus in the acute setting are best seen on fluid-sensitive sequences with some method of suppressing the hyperintense signal of fat, either T2 fat-saturated (FS) imaging or STIR. Thin-section coronal imaging, possibly with volumetric acquisition, improves the ability to detect abnormalities of the brachial plexus.

28.12 Perinatal Injury to the Brachial Plexus

A subtype of brachial plexus injury that is unique to the pediatric population is perinatal brachial plexopathy (▶ Fig. 28.9). In the peripartum period, the brachial plexus can sustain a stretch injury. Factors predisposing to this include shoulder dystocia and fetal macrosomia. Injury to the brachial plexus can be transient or permanent, and may involve parts of, or the entirety of, the brachial plexus. Perinatal injury to the brachial plexus is typically unilateral, and knowledge of the side on which it occurs, and which nerve roots are suspected of being involved, is critical for protocoling and interpreting imaging studies done for identifying such injury. Historically, myelography with post-myelographic CT has been called the gold standard for evaluating brachial plexus injury. More recently, high-resolution MRI has been used for this because it permits much better evaluation of the spinal cord and extraforaminal segments than does myelography, as well as allowing evaluation of the intradural and foraminal segments of the cord to a degree probably equal to that with myelography.[10] However, although MRI has the benefit of not requiring an invasive procedure and does not involve ionizing radiation, myelography remains the preferred method of imaging for possible brachial plexus injury at many institutions because of the anxiety that accompanies such injury and because MRI does not have as long a track record for this purpose as does myelography.

The most commonly encountered pattern of perinatal injury of the brachial plexus is isolated injury to an upper nerve root, such as C5 or C6, which results in the impairment of shoulder abduction known as Erb's palsy. A less common injury is isolated involvement of the lower nerve roots, of C8 and T1, which

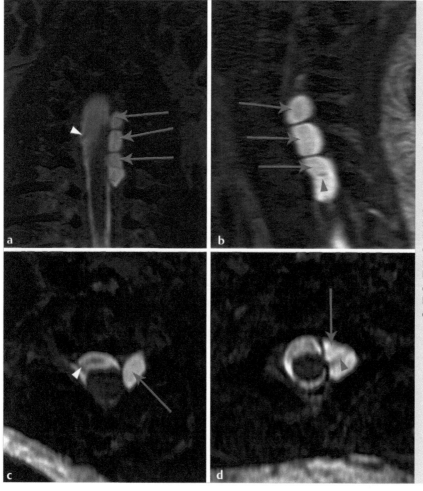

Fig. 28.9 Brachial plexus avulsion. (a) Coronal-oblique image and (b) sagittal image made with fast imaging employing steady-state acquisition (FIESTA) of the cervicothoracic junction in a 1-month-old infant male shows three left-sided perineural cysts/pseudomeningoceles (*red arrows*), including a thin nerve coursing through the caudal-most cyst, probably representing the T1 nerve root (*red arrowhead*). Normal right-sided nerve roots can be seen (*white arrowhead*). (c) Axial-oblique FIESTA image of the lower cervical spine shows the intradural segment of the right C8 nerve root (*white arrowhead*); however, there is a perineural cyst/pseudomeningocele on the left (*red arrow*) that is in contact with the spinal cord, although no nerve root is seen. This finding suggests a left-sided neurotmesis. (d) Axial FIESTA image at the cervicothoracic junction shows a left-sided perineural cyst/pseudomeningocele (*red arrow*); however, a nerve is seen (*red arrowhead*) coursing through the cyst, suggesting that it may be intact, possibly indicating axonotmesis as opposed to neurotmesis at this level.

can result in a Klumpke's palsy, in which there is impairment of forearm and hand muscles. Occasionally, there will be injury to the entirety of the brachial plexus, a condition known as panplexopathy.

When imaging an injury of the brachial plexus, it is important to know that such injury can be of differing severities. Peripheral nerve injury is sometimes described by the Seddon classification, in which the most mild form of injury is known as neurapraxia. Neurapraxia is an injury in which the nerves are stretched without being disrupted, with results that typically include a transient functional deficit and spontaneous recovery. The next most severe type of injury to the brachial plexus is known as axonotmesis. This involves axonal disruption, but the nerve bundle overall (including the supportive perinerium) remains intact, and because the two ends of disrupted axons remain in close proximity owing to the integrity of the environment surrounding the axon, there may be some degree of spontaneous recovery. The complete transection of axons and the structures supporting them is known as neurotmesis. The chance of spontaneous recovery in neurotmesis is much lower than that in axonotmesis because the nerve fibers in this type of injury may move apart from one another. The absence of nerve roots arising from the spinal cord at the expected location of the root-exit zone is a special subset of neurotmesis related to avulsion. The presence of a perineural cyst and/or pseudomeningocele in a given neural foramen of the spine is suggestive of neurotmesis in the particular nerve root that passes through that foramen.

If neurotmesis is identified, microsurgical techniques can be used to bring the ends of the separated nerve fibers together in the hope of facilitating healing. Identification of the presence and location of neurotmesis is one of the goals of imaging in perinatal brachial plexopathy. In examining a particular case of neurotmesis, it is important to carefully identify the nerve root and neural foramen it involves, in order to help the surgeon plan the nerve-repair procedure. In this context it is important to remember that the numbering of nerve roots in the cervical spine is different than in the thoracic and lumbar spine, and that the C4–C5 neural foramen contains the C5 nerve root (and that C8 is a nerve without a bone!). I recommend that MRI images used for evaluating nerve-root injuries be examined during acquisition to ensure that they yield the maximum possible information before the imaging is completed. The protocols for the age at which to perform such a study, and whether to use myelography or MRI, should be addressed ahead of time in conjunction with the relevant surgeons, who may be plastic surgeons or neurosurgeons.

28.13 Suggested Reading

[1] Holmes JF, Akkinepalli R. Computed tomography versus plain radiography to screen for cervical spine injury: A meta-analysis. J Trauma 2005; 58(5): 902–905

References

[1] Stiell IG, Wells GA, Vandemheen KL et al. The Canadian C-spine rule for radiography in alert and stable trauma patients. JAMA 2001; 286(15):1841–1848

[2] Hoffman JR, Wolfson AB, Todd K, Mower WR. Selective cervical spine radiography in blunt trauma: Methodology of the National Emergency X-Radiography Utilization Study (NEXUS). Ann Emerg Med 1998; 32(4):461–469

[3] Pieretti-Vanmarcke R, Velmahos GC, Nance ML et al. Clinical clearance of the cervical spine in blunt trauma patients younger than 3 years: A multi-center study of the American Association for the Surgery of Trauma. J Trauma 2009; 67(3):543–549, discussion 549–550

[4] Daffner, RH, Weissman BN, Wippold FJ, et al. ACR Appropriateness Criteria® Suspected Spine Trauma. Available at http://www.acr.org/~/media/ACR/Documents/AppCriteria/Diagnostic/SuspectedSpineTrauma.pdf, American College of Radiology, Accessed February 20, 2015

[5] Silva CT, Doria AS, Traubici J, Moineddin R, Davila J, Shroff M. Do additional views improve the diagnostic performance of cervical spine radiography in pediatric trauma? AJR Am J Roentgenol 2010; 194(2):500–508

[6] Jimenez RR, Deguzman MA, Shiran S, Karrellas A, Lorenzo RL. CT versus plain radiographs for evaluation of C-spine injury in young children: Do benefits outweigh risks? Pediatr Radiol 2008; 38(6):635–644

[7] Meoded A, Singhi S, Poretti A, Eran A, Tekes A, Huisman TAGM. Tectorial membrane injury: Frequently overlooked in pediatric traumatic head injury. AJNR Am J Neuroradiol 2011; 32(10):1806–1811

[8] Kemp A, Cowley L, Maguire S. Spinal injuries in abusive head trauma: Patterns and recommendations. Pediatr Radiol 2014; 44 Suppl 4:S604–S612

[9] Barber I, Perez-Rossello JM, Wilson CR, Silvera MV, Kleinman PK. Prevalence and relevance of pediatric spinal fractures in suspected child abuse. Pediatr Radiol 2013; 43(11):1507–1515

[10] Somashekar D, Yang LJS, Ibrahim M et al. High-resolution MRI evaluation of neonatal brachial plexus palsy: A promising alternative to traditional CT myelography. AJNR Am J Neuroradiol 2014; 35:1209–1213

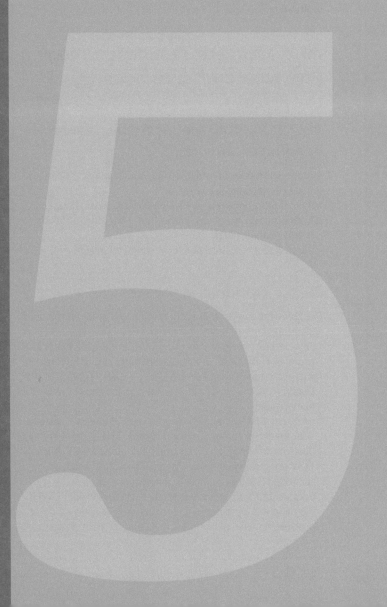

Part 5

Appendices

29 Appendix 1. Protocols

29.1 General Considerations

An organized approach to establishing the protocol for an imaging study is required, especially if radiation is used, as in computed tomography (CT), or if a patient is sedated, as often is the case with magnetic resonance imaging (MRI). Disease/symptom–optimized protocols can improve the diagnostic yield, but it is important to be aware that having a wide variety of protocols creates the risk of confusion among technologists and referring physicians. A reasonable middle ground is to have a least-common-denominator series of sequences that is the foundation for a majority of protocols. When possible, it is ideal to prospectively prescribe a protocol for a given patient's clinical symptoms after examining the available clinical information and prior imaging studies on that patient. Also, evaluating images before the completion of a study can show whether additional sequences are needed to troubleshoot areas of uncertainty; this is especially helpful in children who are sedated. For computed tomographic scans, determining that imaging parameters appropriate to patient size and age are used is very important to minimize radiation dosage, although excessively low doses may prevent obtaining optimal diagnostic information.

29.2 Magnetic Resonance Imaging Protocols for Neuroradiology of the Brain

29.2.1 Routine Magnetic Resonance Imaging of the Brain

- Sagittal and axial T1-weighted (T1 W) images
- Axial T2-weighted (T2 W) images
- Axial fluid-attenuated inversion recovery (FLAIR) images
- Axial diffusion-weighted images (DWI) (consider diffusion tensor imaging [DTI])
- Coronal short tau inversion recovery (STIR) images

29.2.2 Optional Sequences

The following can be added to a routine MRI study of the brain, depending on the circumstances:

- Susceptibility-weighted imaging (SWI) if there is a history of trauma, stroke, or severe prematurity and also in known or suspected tuberous sclerosis or Sturge–Weber syndrome. Double-check the retina in these images for signs of retinal hemorrhage.
- Contrast enhancement: To identify signs of infection, cranial neuropathy, or tumor. Axial and coronal T1-weighted (T1 W) postcontrast imaging can be added to routine MRI. Sagittal T1 W images should be considered if a midline lesion is suspected (such as a pineal or pituitary mass).
- Coronal diffusion-weighted imaging (DWI): Consider DWI if the patient is a premature infant and there is concern about possible hypoxic–ischemic encephalopathy (HIE). At our

institution, coronal DWI is done at a 3-mm slice thickness and can confirm questionable signal abnormalities seen on axial DWI/DTI. These images also allow direct comparison of the cerebral hemispheres with the cerebellum in suspected "superscans."

- Axial cranial nerve imaging (constructive interference in steady-state [CISS], fast imaging employing steady-state acquisition [FIESTA]) of brainstem/internal auditory canal (IAC): Consider if the patient has hearing loss and/or signs of cranial neuropathy. These sequences also aid in the evaluation of complex cysts by identifying thin membranes.
- Axial and coronal T1 W thin-section imaging: Consider if the patient has hearing loss and/or signs of cranial neuropathy. Thin-section T1 imaging is also routinely applied to imaging protocols evaluating the pituitary and pineal glands.
- Cerebrospinal-fluid (CSF) flow studies: Consider the use of CSF flow studies in patients with a Chiari type I malformation or in any circumstance in which there is effacement of the CSF spaces surrounding the foramen magnum. A CSF flow study is usually done as a sagittal flow study through the foramen magnum. Consider also an axial CSF flow study through the foramen magnum. Cerebrospinal-fluid flow studies can be used to evaluate aqueductal stenosis and to investigate the patency of an endoscopic third ventriculostomy.

29.2.3 Special Considerations

Consider developing dedicated imaging protocols for patients with the following disorders/indications.

Seizure/Epilepsy

Add coronal thin-section STIR imaging of the temporal lobes and coronal T2 FLAIR imaging. If signs of a congenital malformation are present, consider a volumetric T1 W image for cortical evaluation (fast spoiled gradient echo (FSPGR) MRI, magnetization-prepared 180-degree radio-frequency-pulse and rapid-gradient-echo (MP-RAGE), etc.). Pay close attention to the temporal lobes, hippocampi, and other brain structures and features.

Pituitary

Sagittal and coronal T1 W thin-section imaging of the pituitary gland before and after the administration of contrast material. T1-weighted thin-section images should be the first images made after gadolinium administration.

Internal Auditory Canals

High-resolution CISS/FIESTA and T1 W images through the left and right IAC in the axial and coronal planes before and after the administration of contrast material. Dedicated sagittal-oblique CISS/FIESTA can also be acquired perpendicular to the course of the facial, cochlear, and vestibular nerves within the IAC. This type of study is ideal for a patient undergoing evaluation for placement of a cochlear implant because the implant will not work unless the cochlear nerve is present.

Neurocutaneous Syndromes

- All: Postcontrast imaging.
- Neurofibromatosis type 1: Consider MRI of the orbit without and with contrast material.
- Neurofibromatosis type 2: Thin-section postcontrast T1 imaging of the brainstem/IAC.
- Tuberous sclerosis complex: Use the imaging protocol for seizures with high-resolution postcontrast T1 imaging, thin-section FLAIR, and susceptibility-weighted imaging.
- Sturge–Weber syndrome: Seizure protocol with high-resolution T1 plus contrast weighted imaging and susceptibility-weighted imaging.

Headaches

Use susceptibility-weighted imaging if the patient has a history of trauma. If the patient has vascular migraine headaches, consider magnetic resonance angiography (MRA). If available, consider the use of arterial spin-labeled (ASL) perfusion in patients with a history of vascular migraine headaches or acute neurologic symptoms.

Vascular Abnormality

If the patient has signs of a vascular abnormality, such as moyamoya and/or sickle-cell disease, consider ASL perfusion and MRA with and without a contrast agent.

Arteriovenous Shunting Lesion

If the patient has signs of an arteriovenous shunting lesion, including an arteriovenous malformation (AVM), arteriovenous fistula (AVF), or vein of Galen aneurysmal malformation (VGAM), consider using dynamic contrast-enhanced MRA. Imaging in the sagittal plane works best for a VGAM. Imaging in the sagittal or coronal plane may be appropriate for an AVM/AVF, depending upon its location.

29.2.4 Additional Considerations

Add imaging modalities and techniques as needed.

Mass/Tumor

For the postcontrast imaging of a mass or tumor, consider adding sagittal postcontrast imaging and/or volumetric T1 W imaging (e.g., MP-RAGE or FSPGR). Ensure that there are apparent diffusion coefficient (ADC) maps to allow the quantitative assessment of diffusion characteristics. Consider perfusion imaging. Magnetic resonance spectroscopy may or may not have a role, in particular if it is unclear whether or not a lesion is a tumor. Postcontrast FLAIR imaging can be helpful for detecting leptomeningeal metastatic deposits. If a postoperative follow-up is done, preoperative imaging should be examined to identify sequences that made a tumor maximally conspicuous.

Evaluation of Hydrocephalus

If the patient has a pattern of aqueductal stenosis (triventricular), consider sagittal CISS/FIESTA imaging of the aqueduct. If the patient has a history of prematurity, trauma, or prior tumor, consider SWI. Consider an axial and/or sagittal CSF flow study of the sylvian aqueduct. If the patient has a history of endoscopic third ventriculostomy, sagittal CISS/FIESTA imaging of the floor of the third ventricle should be done, as should an axial and/or sagittal CSF flow study of the floor of the third ventricle.

Evaluation of Rapid Hydrocephalus

Three-plane, single-shot T2 W imaging and axial DWI. Imaging should be repeated until at least two planes of single-shot T2 W imaging are obtained without significant motion artifact. Imaging with these modalities is typically done as a follow-up examination, and not as the first MRI of the brain in a child.

Skull/Scalp Lesion

T2 fat-saturated (FS) imaging, T1 + FS postcontrast imaging, and coronal DWI should be considered for abnormalities of the head and neck. If a calvarial defect (such as a possible meningocele) is suspected, CISS/FIESTA imaging should be considered for evaluating it. Consider CT for osseous detail; CT can often be complementary to MRI.

Magnetic Resonance Angiography

Axially acquired 3D time-of-flight (TOF) MRA is typically done in conjunction with MRI of the brain. Indications for it include vascular migraine headaches, stroke, sickle-cell disease, and unexplained intracranial hemorrhage, among others. Coverage typically extends from the midvertebral arteries to the level of the body of the lateral ventricles. If symptoms of a posterior-fossa tumor are present, starting imaging at the level of the foramen magnum should be considered. If MRA of the neck is also being done, it is important to ensure that it overlaps coverage of the brain. Magnetic resonance imaging does not usually require contrast enhancement, but the latter can help in troubleshooting areas of turbulent flow, suspected stenosis, and vascular malformation, and in evaluation of the venous system. Dynamic MRA done during the administration of contrast material can be helpful in investigating vascular malformations and stenosis (including moyamoya syndrome).

Magnetic Resonance Venography

Options in imaging the brain and spine with magnetic resonance venography (MRV) include two-dimensional (2D) time-of-flight (TOF) imaging (typically done in two separate planes, such as the axial and coronal planes) and phase-contrast imaging (often done in the sagittal plane). Both of these types of imaging are done without intravenous contrast material. The optimal scanning sequences available on a particular scanner must be confirmed. Postcontrast 2D or 3D TOF imaging has fewer flow-related artifacts than does unenhanced MRV and can be helpful in differentiating turbulence and/or thrombus from flow-related artifacts.

29.3 Neuroradiology Protocols for Magnetic Resonance Imaging of the Head and Neck

29.3.1 Soft Tissues of the Neck (Face, Floor of Mouth, etc.)

- Coronal T2 + FS imaging
- Axial fluid-sensitive imaging (T2, T2 + FS, or STIR)
- Axial or coronal DWI
- Axial T1 imaging
- Coronal T1 + FS imaging
- Axial and coronal T1 + FS postcontrast imaging. (In addition to the axial T1 and coronal T1 + FS precontrast, this allows at least one set of T1 images that have FS both before and after the administration of contrast material.)
- If a base-of-tongue lesion (thyroglossal duct cyst) or prevertebral/retropharyngeal lesion exists, sagittal T2 + FS imaging and sagittal T1 + FS postcontrast imaging should be considered.

29.3.2 Orbits

- Axial and coronal T2 + FS imaging of the orbits (at a 3-mm slice thickness).
- Axial and coronal pre- and postcontrast T1 imaging (3 mm); postcontrast imaging should include fat saturation. Coronal imaging should be extended posteriorly to the optic chiasm.
- High-resolution CISS/FIESTA imaging, to evaluate the cisternal segments of the oculomotor and abducens nerve, can be added to this protocol. Such imaging is usually done in addition to an MRI of the brain rather than as an isolated study.

29.3.3 Brachial Plexus

- The protocol for imaging of the brachial plexus is similar to that for imaging of the soft tissue of the neck, but with thin-section imaging and sagittal T2 and T1 + FS postcontrast imaging extending from the midline to the shoulder on the affected side. The use of a volumetric coronal T2 + FS sequence should be considered.
- In the case of possible nerve-root avulsion (e.g., perinatal injury), consideration should be given to coronal CISS/FIESTA imaging of the spinal cord.
- In many cases, two studies will be done, such as a study of the cervical spine and another of the shoulder, or of the soft tissue of the neck and of the shoulder, or of the soft tissue of the neck and of the chest, depending on the exact location of the pathology in a particular patient. Thus, for instance, if a nerve-root avulsion is suspected, a study of the cervical spine and either a study of the soft tissue of the neck or a study of the shoulder will be done. If there is an apical mass in the lung, a soft tissue examination of the neck and an examination of the chest will be done.

29.3.4 Horner Syndrome

- If Horner syndrome is suspected, MRI should be done of the brain, neck/orbits, and upper chest, to evaluate the entire sympathetic pathway. If the patient's symptoms arise after trauma, or in the setting of a known connective tissue disorder, MRA of the head and neck should also be considered.

29.3.5 Magnetic Resonance Angiography of the Neck

Magnetic resonance angiography of the neck should be done with axial 2D TOF imaging. If dissection is a concern, consideration should be given to axial T1 W imaging (plus or minus FS imaging, depending upon the interpreting physician's comfort level in detecting intramural hemorrhage).

29.3.6 Neck Mass

If MRI reveals a mass in the neck, a study should be done with DWI. If signs of a vascular lesion are found, such as a capillary hemangioma, dynamic contrast-enhanced MRA should be considered (with sagittal acquisition if the lesion is in the midline and coronal acquisition if the lesion is located laterally).

29.4 Neuroradiology Protocols for Magnetic Resonance Imaging of the Spine

29.4.1 Routine Magnetic Resonance Imaging of the Spine

- Protocols for routine MRI of the spine should call for axial and sagittal T1 and T2 W imaging.
- If scoliosis or signs of congenital abnormality are present, a coronal T2 W sequence should be considered.
- If the patient has experienced trauma, a sagittal STIR scan should be added.
- If there are signs of an intradural infectious or inflammatory process, axial and sagittal T1 plus contrast imaging should be done.
- If concern exists about a possible extradural infectious process (osteomyelitis, epidural abscess), axial and sagittal T1 + FS postcontrast imaging should be done.
- If signs of syringohydromyelia are found, examination should be done for a Chiari type I malformation. If a Chiari type I malformation is found, sagittal (and possibly axial) CSF flow studies should be done of the foramen magnum. If there is syringohydromyelia ("syrinx") without Chiari type 1 malformation, postcontrast MRI of the entire neural axis (brain and total spine) is indicated to rule out a tumor.
- If signs of an intradural tumor are present, axial and sagittal postcontrast T1 W imaging should be done. If an intramedullary tumor is suspected, axial and sagittal DTI at a 2-mm slice thickness should be done. If an extradural tumor is suspected, CISS/FIESTA imaging should be considered (with axial and sagittal imaging if the tumor is below the conus medullaris, and axial and coronal imaging if it is above the conus medullaris).
- Coronal T2 + FS and coronal T1 + FS postcontrast imaging can be helpful in a patient with neurofibromatosis type 1 and suspected plexiform neurofibromas.

29.4.2 Magnetic Resonance Angiography of the Spine

Magnetic resonance angiography of the spine is typically done only for a suspected vascular malformation or some other lesion that requires troubleshooting. Dynamic contrast-enhanced MRA of the spine can also be done, usually in the sagittal plane. The conditions for image acquisition, imaging plane, and field of view for targeting the specific area of clinical concern must be optimized for the specific concerns on a given study. Magnetic resonance angiography can be used to identify the artery of Adamkiewicz before retroperitoneal surgery, although this vessel is difficult to find when it is not dilated.

29.5 Computed Tomography

29.5.1 Brain

Unenhanced computed tomographic imaging of the head for trauma, headache, hydrocephalus, and other conditions can be done when the patient's symptoms warrant it. Contrast-enhanced CT of the brain is rarely helpful when done in addition to unenhanced CT, and where there is concern, MRI should be done if possible. Contrast-enhanced CT may be appropriate if there is a contraindication to MRI or if MRI will be unavailable for a patient who has signs of an infection and an unexplained fluid collection on unenhanced CT.

When possible, a CT scanner should be used to make separate images with bone and soft tissue algorithms. When possible, the scanner should be used to create these images in both the sagittal and coronal planes.

When a patient has a history of significant trauma, 3D images should be made of the skull. Such images should be considered for all children under 2 years of age, even if they have minor trauma and particularly if they have scalp swelling or an abnormality in the shape of the head. Three-dimensional images of the calvarium make subtle fractures and craniosynostosis much more conspicuous.

Computed Tomographic Angiography

Three-plane, 1-mm reconstructions of CT angiograms (CTA) should be evaluated. Thick-section reconstructions of maximum-intensity-projection (MIP) images may be helpful, but only in addition to standard thin-section reconstructions, and not instead of them. Three-dimensional rendering of vessels should be evaluated. Images should be acquired in the arterial phase after the administration of contrast material. Timing should be based off a readily identifable artery, such as the carotid bifurcation.

Computed Tomographic Venography

Performed as a poorly timed CTA (i.e., the same imaging parameters as a CTA, but with images acquired later than the intended arterial phase of the CTA). The same bolus injection and bolus tracking should be used as are used for CTA, but with the addition of a delay of approximately 12 seconds.

29.5.2 Face and Neck

Computed tomography of the face or orbits (for trauma) should be performed with helically acquired images without contrast. The imaging data should be used to create three-plane bone algorithm images of 1-mm slice thickness, as well as three-plane soft tissue algorithm images of 2- to 3-mm slice thickness. If the patient has facial trauma, imaging should include the entire mandible. If the patient has only orbital trauma and there is no concern about the possible existence of other facial injuries, imaging should include only the orbits. Three-dimensional images should be considered if fractures are present.

Sinuses

Images of the sinuses should be helically acquired and made without contrast material. Three-plane bone algorithm images of 1-mm thickness, as well as three plane soft tissue algorithm images of 2- to 3-mm thickness, should be created from the CT dataset.

Orbits or Face for Infection

Helically acquired postcontrast images of the orbits or face should be made to investigate for infection. (There is almost never any reason to perform CT of the orbits/face both without and with contrast enhancement, which entails an excessive dose of radiation and is unlikely to provide any significant additional information.) Imaging should be done to create three-plane bone algorithm images of 1-mm slice thickness, as well as three-plane soft tissue algorithm images of 2- to 3-mm slice thickness.

Soft Tissues of the Neck

The soft tissues of the neck should be examined with helically acquired postcontrast images made from the level of the upper mediastinum to the level of the orbits, and with three-plane soft tissue algorithm images of the same region. The creation of bone algorithm reconstructions should also be considered.

Computed Tomographic Angiography of the Neck

CT angiography of the neck should be obtained as helically acquired images from the aortic arch to the carotid canal (in the petrous temporal bone), during the arterial phase after contrast administration. The scan should be begun at the time of appearance of the maximal blush of contrast material in the aortic arch. Three-plane 1 mm images should be created from the CT dataset, as well as three-dimensional reconstructions.

Temporal Bone

Imaging of the temporal bone should be done in the axial plane. The imaging can be thinly collimated axial imaging or helical imaging. Axial and coronal thin-section (1 mm or less) bone algorithm images of the temporal bones should be created from the CT dataset, as well as axial soft tissue algorithm reconstructions. With high-resolution multidetector imaging, direct coronal imaging is not typically required.

Computed Tomography of the Head and Face

For facial dysmorphism and cranoisynostosis, CT should be done of the head and face (through the mandible) in one helical acquisition. Multiplanar soft tissue reconstructions of the brain and facial soft tissues should be made with a slice thickness of approximately 3 mm, together with a multiplanar bone algorithm reconstruction of the entire head and face. Three-dimensional images should be strongly considered. If a 3D printed model is to be created, axial 1-mm soft tissue algorithm images should be saved.

29.5.3 Spine

Imaging of the spine should be done with helical acquisition. Three-plane bone algorithm reconstructions of 1- to 2-mm slice thickness should be made. Axial and sagittal soft tissue algorithm reconstructions should also be made, again with a slice thickness of 1 to 2 mm. Postcontrast computed tomographic imaging of the spine is rarely indicated unless there is a suspicion of infection in a patient with a contraindication to MRI. Computed tomographic angiography of the spine is rarely indicated unless there is a suspected spinal vascular malformation and MRI is contraindicated, or unless the higher spatial resolution of CT is required over that of MRA.

29.6 Ultrasonography

29.6.1 Brain

The brain should be imaged with sagittal and coronal grayscale images through the anterior fontanelle, made with a linear-array transducer. Doppler ultrasonography of the midline vessels (anterior cerebral artery [ACA]/pericallosal artery) should be considered. Transverse images through the mastoid fontanelle should also be considered, for evaluation of the posterior fossa.

29.6.2 Head and Neck

Investigation of the head and neck should be done with grayscale imaging of the area of concern, possibly with Doppler imaging to confirm the positions of vessels and/or to look for hyperemia in the setting of suspected infection. Doppler imaging of a suspected mass helps to identify features suggestive of a vascular lesion, such as a capillary hemangioma. Any mass or lesion (including lymph nodes) that is evaluated should be imaged in at least two orthogonal planes. Information obtained by ultrasonography is often complementary to information obtained with CT and MRI, and should not be overlooked as a potential further step in evaluating complex superficial masses of the head and neck.

29.6.3 Spine

Ultrasonography of the spine is typically done to evaluate for signs of a low conus medullaris and/or cord tethering, and it is usually successful for this only in first 2 to 3 months of life. Sagittal gray-scale imaging should also be done from the tip of the coccyx superiorly to above the level of the conus medullaris, ideally with stitched-together images of the lumbar spine if the ultrasound machine supports this. Axial images throughout this region should also be obtained.

If signs of a sacral dimple are present, the patient should be closely evaluated for a possible sinus tract extending to the thecal sac or to the coccyx (pilonidal tract). However, these features are better seen on MRI than with ultrasonography.

30 Appendix 2. Thoughts on Dictation with Sample Templates

30.1 General Considerations

The dictation of a report is a critical component in the communication of findings of an imaging study. Person-to-person communication of findings is very important for the consultative role of a radiologist. Ultimately, however, it is the report that is the permanent documentation of the study and is likely to be kept on file longer than the images themselves. Accordingly, it is important to approach the dictation of a report in a careful manner, with the goal of being appropriately descriptive in a consultative manner, yet not unnecessarily verbose. Those goals may not always be simultaneously achievable.

Reporting styles are very personal and are shaped by local practice environments. Robotlike structured reporting methods have been adopted in many locations, with both merits and limitations. My reporting style is summarized by the following examples of reports of normal (or nearly normal) findings on imaging. The descriptions of findings in many of the figure legends in this book also follow my descriptive style. There are no universally correct or incorrect methods of reporting the findings in an imaging procedure, but I present my thought process on reporting in a manner that I hope will be helpful and consultative.

With regard to the wording of a report, I have some recommendations. They are not mandatory unless you are a trainee working with me, but I present my rationales for them in the following sections.

First, I strongly advise that you never use the words "clinical correlation is recommended" or "please clinically correlate." Although often meant to be helpful, these words may or may not be helpful, and they are almost certainly received with frustration. If there is a specific clinical finding that may affect the implications of a given finding on imaging, state that. It is here that I suggest using a grammatical structure used in computer programming, the "if/then" statement (or its companion, the "if/then/else" statement). For instance, instead of saying "There is a linear lucency in the (bone), which could be a fracture or vascular groove, please clinically correlate," I believe that a more clear way to convey the possible implications of these findings is to say "There is a linear lucency in the (bone). If there is focal tenderness, this may represent a subtle nondisplaced fracture; otherwise this is most likely a vascular groove." Or (I know that these are nonneurologic examples) "There is a focal opacity in the right lower lobe; if the patient has fever, this could represent pneumonia, otherwise this probably represents atelectasis." Perhaps this is what some people are thinking when they suggest clinical correlation, but that does not come across.

Also, as I mentioned earlier, the radiology report is a permanent record of an imaging procedure. For this reason, I believe that open-ended questions within the report are out of place. For instance, at the end of the impression of a study, questions like "Does the patient have any pain in this location?" or "Was there prior surgery?" are open-ended and unhelpful unless there are plans to follow up on such issues and provide an addendum describing what was determined and how it may affect the interpretation of various findings. By contrast, an example of a potentially helpful statement might be "There is a metallic foreign body in the (location), which may represent a surgical implant. However it is unknown at the time of interpretation of the patient has had prior surgery in this location."

Many trainees in radiology learn to make clinical decisions and gain autonomy through on-call experiences. Accordingly, statements along the lines of "no acute disease" or "no acute process" are commonly used in reporting imaging studies. Although a statement like "no acute disease" is likely to address the concerns of an emergency physician attempting to differentiate a headache from a herniation or a fracture from a sprain, to state that there is "no acute process" is not a particularly helpful summary of an elective/outpatient study. In the case of an elective study in which no abnormalities are found, one shouldn't feel uncomfortable in interpreting the results as "normal" or "within normal limits."

30.2 Communication of Findings

It is important to remember that the radiologist's interpretation of the findings in a study reflect a consultation with the referring physician as well as with the patient. Any emergent or unexpected findings should be communicated to the referring physician. Many hospitals and departments have lists of findings that mandate communication with the referring physician or the physician's representative and require documentation of such communication. Although the findings mandating such communication may vary from one institution to another, some examples of findings to which this commonly applies are:

- New or increasing intracranial blood products
- New or increasing pneumocephalus
- A new or increasing mass effect or midline shift
- New or increasing hydrocephalus
- Fracture
- New or worsening stroke (or signs suspected of indicating a stroke)
  (note that small amounts of blood products or pneumocephalus after a known craniotomy are not unexpected findings)

When documenting a finding, it is important to state the name of the physician with whom the reporting radiologist spoke, and not merely that the "findings were discussed with the patient's covering physician." The date and time of the communication should also be documented, rather than simply that the finding was communicated "at the time of dictation." Likewise, it is helpful to specify the means by which the communication was made, such as, "Findings were discussed by telephone with Dr. Smith of the emergency department at 2:56 on 3/14/15. Findings were reviewed in person with Dr. Jones of neurology at 5:42 on 3/14/15." If findings are sent in a (secure) text message, by e-mail, or by facsimile transmission, the radiology report should not state that the findings were sent unless there was confirmation of their receipt and review by the receiving individual.

Sometimes it is necessary to recommend a follow-up study. If so, the recommendation should be made and communicated. In some cases, a follow-up study may be helpful in a specific circumstance and not in others, in which case it is important to be aware that the word "recommend" may make the referring physician feel a need to follow up or be seen as ignoring a recommendation. In such circumstances, it can be helpful to state, for example, that "If the patient has continued pain, MRI of the lumbar spine may be able to further characterize its origin." There are no perfect answers. It is important to speak with one's referring physicians and learn how they speak and think, and let them learn how you speak and think, to ensure that everyone is on the same page. It is also important to know that excessive or unneeded recommendations for follow-up study can impair one's credibility without helping the patient.

At times, however, the workup of a finding will be complex and will require subsequent studies. It may be helpful to state this up front, to alert the referring physician (and possibly the patient) to the finding and the thought process on which the need for further studies is based. This may also allow the radiologist interpreting the follow-up study to understand the rationale for it. If, for instance, an imaging study reveals a hyperemic mass in a patient's neck that cannot be definitively identified as a resolving infection or a hemangioma, a follow-up ultrasound examination may seem appropriate. If the mass does not resolve, an MRI may seem needed. To avoid having the referring physician (and patient) wonder whether the recommendation for multiple scans in such a case represents a haphazard approach, the initial report of the mass can state that it is an atypical finding and that a follow-up ultrasound examination in 4 to 6 weeks is recommended, and specify that if the mass does not resolve, MRI may be indicated for its further characterization. This is the way in which most consulting physicians write a consultation note, and a radiology report should be no different.

It may be appropriate to communicate certain nonemergent findings to a nurse or administrative assistant (this should be confirmed with local guidelines), as in the case of a renal mass found incidentally and which is not acutely life threatening but requires follow-up study. On the other hand, the finding, for example, of signs of herniation or acute hydrocephalus, should be communicated directly to a physician whenever possible. Nor does the communication of findings in an imaging study transfer the responsibility for their follow-up to the recipient of this information; the radiologist's work is not done until there is reason to believe that the patient is receiving appropriate care for any potentially important finding in an imaging study.

30.3 Describing a Finding

When describing a finding, both the number of the image and the plane in which it appears should be conveyed as part of a radiology report. Thus, for instance, a mass in the cerebrum should be described in the following manner: "There is a 2.2 × 1.5 × 1.8 cm ovoid, circumscribed mass in the left cerebellar hemisphere (oblique anteroposterior x oblique transverse x cra-

niocaudal dimensions in series 3, image 14, and series 15, image 9)." Providing the numbers of the series and image containing a finding is particularly helpful when the finding is anatomically relatively small and when the study in which it was found included multiple sequences. This is helpful both to the referring physician and to the radiologist who examines a follow-up examination of a patient, both in facilitating their ability to read the original report and to use it for comparison with their own findings. Nor should saving measurements as key-images be the sole means of documenting the way in which the images were made because this information is often not transmitted with the study containing the images if the patient transfers to another institution, and also because, in contrast to their inclusion in an original radiology report, they may not be made a part of the patient's permanent medical record.

If the findings were being compared to a prior study, and you feel they are unchanged, but the numbers you list are different than on the prior report, it is important to be clear. If in January there is a 1.5 × 1.3 cm mass, and on follow-up there is a mass that is 1.7 × 1.2 cm and described as unchanged, it can appear confusing. However, it can be helpful to state "The left inferior frontal mass measures 1.7 × 1.2 cm, which is unchanged from the January 2015 study when measured using similar measurement landmarks."

30.4 Structure of the Report

Ease in reading a radiology report makes it more helpful. It is therefore a good idea to simplify the grammatical structure of a report and clearly describe the findings it contains. Ideally, it is best if an entire practice group follows this pattern. Thus, for instance, I find benefit in a standardized report format. This must include a clearly identified indication for the imaging study described in the report. A list of the findings in an earlier study or other data for comparison should also be included. Additionally, all cross-sectional studies should include a distinct section on the techniques used in them. In the case of MRI, this should include a list of the imaging sequences used, and not merely a statement like "multiplanar multisequence MRI was performed." If you are unable to quickly and clearly describe the imaging sequences being interpreted, you should not be interpreting them.

If in CT and MRI an intravenous contrast material was administered, it is important to state the volume administered and to specify the identity of the contrast material. If administration of the contrast material caused no complications, this too should be stated. Such a statement might read, "The intravenous administration of 10 mL of [Brand of gadolinium] contrast material was uneventful and was followed by axial and coronal T1 W imaging of the brain."

If there is additional information that would seem useful to convey, it too should be included, as in the case of "Several sequences were repeated because of patient motion."

When a report is long, it should be broken into multiple paragraphs, each dealing with specific topics. If, for example, a patient is found to have three masses, each should be described in a separate paragraph. This avoids a monolithic report in which it is difficult to find specific information.

30.5 Sample Reports

30.5.1 Magnetic Resonance Imaging

Routine MRI of the Brain

There is no evidence of extra-axial fluid collection, abnormal intracranial mass effect, or midline shift. The ventricular system is normal in size and configuration. The basal cisterns are patent. There is an age-appropriate myelination pattern. The brainstem and cerebellum are within normal limits. There is no abnormal intracranial diffusion restriction. There is no significant sinus mucosal disease. The orbits are unremarkable. There are no focal suspicious calvarial lesions.

Modifications

The following are examples of statements that should be used as modifications/additions to the standard description of findings for an MRI of the brain.

- For a postcontrast scan: There is no abnormal intracranial enhancement.
- In the case of a protocol for MRI of the internal auditory canal (IAC): The cisternal and canalicular segments of cranial nerves VII and VIII are within normal limits bilaterally. There is no abnormal enhancement within the internal auditory canals or cerebellopontine angles bilaterally. The appearance of the inner-ear structures is within normal limits bilaterally.
- For a protocol involving the pituitary: There is a normal morphology of the adenohypophysis and neurohypophysis, with a physiologic enhancement pattern. The pituitary stalk is midline and normal in appearance. The hypothalami are within normal limits. The optic chiasm is normal in position and appearance. The cavernous sinuses are within normal limits.

Magnetic Resonance Angiogram of the Head

- The distal cervical, petrous, and intracranial portions of the internal carotid arteries are within normal limits. The bilateral anterior and middle cerebral arteries are within normal limits, as is the anterior communicating artery. The V4 segments of both vertebral arteries, the basilar artery, and both posterior cerebral arteries are within normal limits. The bilateral posterior communicating arteries are within normal limits.

Magnetic Resonance Venogram of the Head

- The bilateral internal cerebral veins, vein of Galen, and straight sinus are patent. The superior sagittal sinus is patent. The bilateral transverse sinuses, sigmoid sinuses, jugular bulbs, and cephalad portions of the internal jugular veins are within normal limits.

Seizure Protocol

In addition to the routine MRI of the brain report, studies done for evaluation of seizures should comment on the hippocampi. A sample description is: The hippocampi demonstrate a normal volume and morphology, without associated signal abnormality.

Cerebrospinal Fluid Flow Study/Chiari Type I Malformation

- Normal: There is pulsatile bidirectional flow of CSF dorsal and ventral to the brainstem/cervicomedullary junction through the plane of the foramen magnum.
- Mild impairment: There is narrowing of the ventral CSF space at the level of the foramen magnum but with bidirectional pulsatile flow of CSF. No significant flow of CSF is seen dorsal to the cerebellar tonsils through the foramen magnum.
- Moderate impairment: There is narrowing of the ventral CSF space at the level of the foramen magnum with high-velocity flow. No significant flow of CSF is seen dorsal to the cerebellar tonsils through the foramen magnum.
- Severe impairment: There is no significant pulsatile flow of CSF dorsal or ventral to the brainstem through the level of the foramen magnum. There is hyperdynamic flow of CSF ventrolateral to the cervicomedullary junction through the foramen magnum, seen on axial CSF flow study.

Head and Neck

Orbits

- The globes are normal in appearance bilaterally. There is a normal appearance of the extraocular muscles bilaterally. The intraconal and extraconal fat is within normal limits bilaterally, as are the lacrimal glands. There is no abnormal orbital enhancement. The optic nerves are normal in appearance bilaterally, without abnormal enhancement.

Soft Tissues of the Neck

(The emphasis in reporting the findings of a study of the soft tissues of the neck varies in accord with the indication for the study; since MRI of the soft tissues of the neck is usually done to evaluate a specific lesion, and not for a primary screen, the findings in such an examination are rarely normal.)

The parotid and submandibular glands are within normal limits. The nasopharynx, oropharynx, and hypopharynx are patent. The glottic and infraglottic structures are unremarkable. There is no deep or superficial soft tissue swelling. There is no prevertebral soft tissue swelling.

There is no abnormal enhancement identified. The major vascular structures within the neck are grossly intact.

There is no significant paranasal sinus disease. The thyroid gland is within normal limits. The orbits are within normal limits. The osseous structures are unremarkable.

Magnetic Resonance Angiography of the Neck

- There is a (three-vessel) branching pattern to the aortic arch. The innominate artery is within normal limits. The bilateral subclavian arteries are within normal limits. The bilateral common carotid arteries and carotid bifurcations are within normal limits. The cervical segments of the bilateral internal and external carotid arteries are within normal limits. The V1 through V4 segments of the vertebral arteries are within normal limits bilaterally.

Spine

Routine Study of the Cervical Spine

- The alignment of the cervical vertebral column is within normal limits. The vertebral body heights and intervertebral disk spaces are preserved. There is no MRI evidence of vertebral segmentation anomaly. There are no focal suspicious marrow lesions. The cervical cord is normal in volume and signal. The imaged portions of the posterior cranial fossa are within normal limits.

Routine Study of the Thoracic Spine

- The alignment of the thoracic vertebral column is within normal limits. The vertebral body heights and intervertebral disk spaces are preserved. There is no MRI evidence of vertebral segmentation anomaly. There are no focal suspicious marrow lesions. The thoracic cord is normal in volume and signal. The imaged portions of the posterior thoracic contents and mediastinum are within normal limits.

Routine Study of the Lumbar Spine

- The alignment of the lumbar vertebral column is within normal limits. The vertebral body heights and intervertebral disk spaces are preserved. There is no MR evidence of vertebral segmentation anomaly. There are no focal suspicious marrow lesions. The imaged portions of the spinal cord are within normal limits. The conus terminates at the level of the (BLANK). In reporting the level of termination of the conus medullaris, it should be based on axial T2 W images, as referenced to a sagittal image. The level of termination should be reported as being at a given disk space, at the superior endplate of a specific vertebra, at the midbody of a vertebra, or at the inferior endplate of a specific vertebra. Thus, for example, instead of stating that the conus terminates "at an appropriate level" or "at L1," I recommend stating that the conus terminates "at the level of the inferior endplate of L1."
- There is no evidence of thickening of the filum terminale. The nerve roots of the cauda equina are normally distributed throughout the thecal sac without focal thickening or clumping. The imaged portions of the posterior abdominal and retroperitoneal contents are within normal limits.

Variations

- Contrast: There is no abnormal enhancement.
- Trauma: There is no abnormal edema signal within the marrow. The anterior longitudinal ligament, posterior longitudinal ligament, and ligamentum flavum are intact.
- Evaluation of a sacral dimple: A cutaneous marker is in place corresponding with the clinically reported sacral dimple.

There is no dermal sinus tract connecting the sacral dimple to the thecal sac. There is no associated mass lesion to suggest a dermoid/epidermoid inclusion cyst.

30.5.2 Computed Tomography

Brain

Routine

- There is no evidence of acute intracranial hemorrhage*, extra-axial fluid collection, mass effect, or midline shift. The ventricular system is normal in size and configuration. The basal cisterns are patent. There is no focal obscuration of the gray-white differentiation. There is no significant sinus mucosal disease. The orbits are unremarkable. There are no focal calvarial lesions**.
- If for head-shape abnormality, I state (assuming it is a valid statement) there is an age-appropriate suture maturation pattern.

*I specifically state no evidence of *acute* intracranial hemorrhage. Many patients with susceptibility-weighted imaging of prior hemorrhage have no abnormality on CT.
**If evaluation was for trauma, I state "there are no fractures."

Follow-up Examination of a Patient with a Shunt for Hydrocephalus

- I describe the approach of the catheter and location of the tip, and whether the ventricles are the same, bigger, or smaller than in the prior examination of the patient. Thus: "There is a ventriculostomy catheter inserted through a right frontal approach with its tip in the anterior body of the right lateral ventricle adjacent to the foramen of Monro, which is unchanged since the prior study. There is an unchanged decompressed appearance of the ventricular system."

Computed Tomographic Angiogram

Vascular

- The distal cervical, petrous, and intracranial portions of the internal carotid arteries are within normal limits. The bilateral anterior and middle cerebral arteries are within normal limits, as is the anterior communicating artery. The V4 segments of both vertebral arteries, the basilar artery, and both posterior cerebral arteries are within normal limits. The bilateral posterior communicating arteries are within normal limits.

Nonvascular

Describe nonvascular findings in a manner similar to the way in which they would be described in a CT study of the head.

Head and Neck

Orbits

- The globes are normal in appearance bilaterally. There is a normal appearance of the extraocular muscles bilaterally. The intraconal and extraconal fat is within normal limits bilaterally, as are the lacrimal glands. The optic-nerve sheath complex is normal in appearance bilaterally. The imaged portions of the paranasal sinuses are clear. There is no significant sinus mucosal disease.

If a study is done for trauma and without contrast enhancement, I add: "There are no orbital fractures."

If the study is a postcontrast study done for infection, I add: "There is no abnormal orbital enhancement." In the body of the report, and in the impression, I add: "There is no evidence of orbital cellulitis or abscess."

If there is preseptal cellulitis, my impression will read: "There is right infraorbital/premaxillary swelling, consistent with preseptal cellulitis. There is no evidence of abscess, and there is no evidence of postseptal extension." (Note: "preseptal" is the same as "periorbital," and "postseptal" is the same as "orbital.")

Sinuses

- The maxillary sinuses are clear bilaterally. The frontal sinuses are clear bilaterally*. The ethmoid sinuses are clear bilaterally. The sphenoid sinuses are clear bilaterally. The bilateral osteomeatal complexes are patent. The frontal recesses are patent bilaterally. The sphenoethmoidal recesses are patent bilaterally. There are no fluid levels. There are no osseous erosions. The nasal septum is midline. The cribriform plate and fovea ethmoidalis are symmetric and intact. The lamina papyracea is intact bilaterally. There is no facial soft tissue swelling. The orbits are within normal limits. The imaged portions of the intracranial contents are within normal limits.

*Note that, in many children, the frontal and sphenoid sinuses may have not yet developed. If this is the case, describe that the given sinus is hypoplastic or has not yet formed.

Soft Tissues of the Neck

- The imaged portions of the intracranial contents and orbits are within normal limits. There is no significant sinus mucosal disease. The parotid, submandibular, and sublingual glands are within normal limits. The nasopharynx, oropharynx, and hypopharynx are patent. The larynx and paraglottic soft tissues are within normal limits. The thyroid is normal in appearance. The imaged portions of the lung apices are within normal limits. The osseous structures are within normal limits.

Computed Tomographic Angiogram of the Neck

- There is a (three-vessel) branching pattern to the aortic arch. The innominate artery is within normal limits. The bilateral subclavian arteries are within normal limits. The bilateral common carotid arteries and carotid bifurcations are within normal limits. The cervical segments of the bilateral internal and external carotid arteries are within normal limits. The V1 through V4 segments of the vertebral arteries are within normal limits bilaterally.

Temporal Bone
Right Ear

- The external auditory canal is patent. The mesotympanum and epitympanum are clear. The ossicular chain is intact. The cochlea and modiolus are normal in appearance. The vestibule and semicircular canals are nondilated. The vestibular aqueduct is nondilated. The internal auditory canal is normal in caliber. There is a normal osseous course of the facial nerve. The mastoid air cells are clear.

Left Ear

(The entries used in reporting findings are the same as for the right ear, but note that, in temporal-bone studies for hearing loss, the findings for each ear should be reported separately, even if the findings for both ears are normal.)

Other

- The imaged portions of the intracranial contents, orbits, and paranasal sinuses are within normal limits.

Spine
Computed Tomogram of the Spine

- The alignment of the (cervical, thoracic, lumbar) vertebral column is within normal limits. The heights of the vertebral bodies and intervertebral disk spaces are preserved. There are no (cervical, thoracic, lumbar) factures (a CT of the spine is almost always performed to evaluate for trauma). The prevertebral and paravertebral soft tissues are within normal limits. (For the thoracic spine, mention whether the imaged portions of the chest are within normal limits; for the lumbar spine, mention whether the imaged portions of the posterior abdomen and retroperitoneum are within normal limits. Always remember to look at and comment on the prevertebral and paravertebral soft tissues, especially on the cervical spine.)

30.5.3 Ultrasonography
Brain

- The ventricular system is symmetric and nondilated. There is no evidence of subependymal or intraventricular hemorrhage. There is no abnormal parenchymal echogenicity.

Head and Neck

There is no standard template for reporting findings in the head and neck, because they vary considerably according to the area being evaluated. The most common indications for studies are the evaluation a palpable finding or swelling.

Spine

- The conus medullaris has a normal morphology and terminates with its tip at the level of the (superior endplate of L2). There is no evidence of thickening of the filum terminale. There is a normal pulsatile movement of the nerve roots of the cauda equina. (If a study was performed for a sacral dimple, add: "There is no evidence of a dermal sinus tract subjacent to the clinically reported sacral dimple. There is no cyst or other abnormality associated with the dimple.")

31 Appendix 3. Quick Reference

31.1 Introduction

This appendix, which focuses predominantly on topics more commonly encountered in pediatric than in adult neuroradiology, is meant to serve as a practical resource with which readers can ensure that they evaluate the relevant clinical, anatomic, and pathologic features of a patient's imaging study. Thus, for example, what type of imaging study should be done for a patient with a sacral dimple, or a patient with hearing loss? What items require detailed investigation in the imaging study and in the patient's history? What specific pertinent positive and/or negative findings are important to the physician who requests the imaging study? Further information about disease- and symptom-specific pathways for the diagnosis of various diseases can be found in the neuroradiology and pediatric sections of the American College of Radiology Appropriateness Criteria, which represent evidence-based guidance, developed by expert multidisciplinary panels, toward disease diagnoses: < https://acsearch.acr.org/list > .

31.2 Outline

1. Brain
   a) Myelination
   b) Headache
   c) Seizure
      • Neonatal seizure
   d) Cutaneous abnormalities and neurocutaneous disorders
   e) Movement disorders
   f) Short stature
   g) Precocious puberty
   h) Tumor or intracranial mass
   i) Prematurity
   j) Hydrocephalus
   k) Macrocephaly
   l) Microcephaly
   m) Head-shape abnormality
   n) Hemispheric asymmetry
   o) Metabolic disorders
   p) Cyst of the posterior fossa
   q) Corpus-callosum abnormality
2. Head and Neck
   a) Eye-movement abnormalities
   b) Optic-nerve hypoplasia
   c) Hearing loss
3. Spine
   a) Sacral dimple
   b) Scoliosis
   c) Spina bifida
4. Areas of Uncertainty
   a) Mild Chiari malformation vs. cerebellar tonsillar ectopia
   b) Prominent central canal vs. hydromyelia vs. syrinx
   c) Pineal cysts: Normal or abnormal?

31.3 Brain

31.3.1 Myelination

Evaluation

Either in a routine study or in patients with delayed developmental milestones.

Studies to Perform

Brain myelination is typically evaluated through magnetic resonance imaging (MRI), with axial T1-weighted (T1 W) and T2-weighted (T2 W) images being the mainstays for assessing myelination. If the patient has a history of prematurity, susceptibility-weighted imaging (SWI) can help in seeking signs of germinal matrix hemorrhage.

Important Clinical Information

The patient's estimated gestational age at birth is very important. A premature infant born at 32 weeks' gestational age (i.e., approximately 8 weeks early) and who is 2 months of age at the time of examination should have a myelination pattern similar to that of a full-term infant rather than that of a 2-month-old infant.

Know whether the patient has delays in developmental milestones, which can be caused by many forms of brain injury, or the absence of achieving milestones. Milestones whose development is delayed may eventually catch up, especially with appropriate therapy. The absence or loss of milestones is worrisome and raises the possibility of leukodystrophies or other progressive disorders.

Where to Double-Check

The most important structure to evaluate for myelination in the central nervous system (CNS) is the posterior limb of the internal capsule (PLIC). This can be done in T1 W images, in which, if myelination is normal, the PLIC should be hyperintense at birth. Other important landmarks are visualization of myelination of the splenium at 4 months and myelination of the genu by approximately 6 months. A T2-hypointense signal represents mature myelin, a T1-hyperintense signal represents myelin proteolipids. The corpus callosum will normally myelinate, predominantly in a posterior to anterior manner, from approximately the third to the tenth month postnatally (▶ Fig. 2.11).

Careful examination should be done for signs of a prior hemorrhage of the germinal matrix or injury to white matter, which can be difficult to detect if there is a symmetric abnormality.

Pertinent Positives and Negatives

Confirm whether the myelination pattern is appropriate for chronologic age. If not, confirm whether the myelination pattern is appropriate for corrected age.

Follow-up Recommendations

If the patient experiences a regression of developmental milestones, a follow-up study with MRI may be needed, as also may consideration of a workup for leukodystrophy.

31.3.2 Headache

Studies to Perform

First and foremost, confirm whether any imaging study is needed for a particular patient. If there is a history of recent trauma or neurologic deficit, CT may be the most appropriate modality for a first study, with the possibility that MRI will ultimately provide more information. If MRI is performed and there is history of trauma, add SWI. If there is a history of acute migraine, consider adding an arterial spin-labeling perfusion study.

Important Clinical Information

Find out if the patient has a history of trauma. Find out if headaches are new or persistent and where they occur (e.g., frontal headaches). Find out if there are provoking features of headache or other symptoms. Find out if the patient has had a recent clinical or diagnostic procedure, such as a lumbar puncture. Find out if the patient has any neurologic symptoms, and if so whether they are permanent or transient.

Where to Double-Check

Look for punctate foci of signal hyperintensity in T2/fluid-attenuated inversion recovery (FLAIR) images of the juxtacortical white matter, particularly subjacent to the superior frontal gyri, which are a common finding in the setting of chronic migraine headache. Double check the paranasal sinuses for signs of mucosal disease. Also check the cerebellar tonsils to determine if there is a Chiari I malformation.

Pertinent Positives and Negatives

Similar to those in a routine study, as named above.

Follow-up Recommendations

If CT is negative for CNS pathology and the patient has neurologic symptoms, MRI may be appropriate. Otherwise, no specific follow-up imaging is indicated, although clinical evaluation by a physician who has practical experience with the diagnosis and treatment of headaches can be helpful.

31.3.3 Seizure

Other Terms

Epilepsy, spells, infantile spasms.

Studies to Perform

Magnetic resonance imaging of the brain. If the patient shows signs of infection, or a tumor-predisposing condition (such as tuberous sclerosis), postcontrast imaging can be helpful. Use SWI if there is a history of trauma. If there are focal abnormalities on electroencephalography (EEG) in the setting of a normal MRI, consider ictal–interictal subtraction perfusion imaging with single-photon emission computed tomography (SPECT). Use CT if seizures are seen after recent trauma or if there are signs of dystrophic mineralization. Functional magnetic resonance imaging (fMRI) has a role in many cases of seizure before surgical intervention is undertaken.

Important Clinical Information

1. New onset or longstanding.
2. Clinical features of a particular seizure (e.g., tonic–clonic, absence, laughing spells, etc.).
3. History of trauma?
4. Any known syndrome or other disease condition? Any clinical features (e.g., cutaneous findings) that may be associated with a given condition?
5. History of prematurity?

Where to Double-Check

Scrutinize the hippocampi, as well as the fornices and mamillary bodies. If a left-sided extremity moves during a seizure, look closely at the right hemisphere, and vice versa. If there are gelastic seizures (laughing spells), double check the hypothalami. Make sure to look for heterotopia and other abnormalities of neuronal migration on diffusion-weighted imaging (DWI).

Pertinent Positives and Negatives

Comment on hippocampal morphology and signal characteristics.

Follow-up Recommendations

Follow the recommendations of an epileptologist. If there are EEG or other clinical features suggesting a more localized origin of a particular patient's seizures, double-check the studies in patients showing these clinical features for possible subtle abnormalities that may have been missed on initial review. Consider high-resolution imaging to further scrutinize areas of the brain from which seizures are suspected to arise in a given patient.

31.3.4 Neonatal Seizure

Studies to Perform

Magnetic resonance imaging of the brain without contrast material and with SWI. If signs of infection are present, consider postcontrast imaging. If MRI/SWI shows atypical features or findings raising concern about leukoencephalopathy, consider magnetic resonance spectroscopy (although this is usually a troubleshooting tool). If there is a possible history of a hypoxic event, consider thin-slice coronal DWI. Thin-slice coronal DWI may also help confirm hippocampal edema, which may be hard to differentiate from artifact on axial diffusion sequences.

Important Clinical Information

Birth history, including gestational age of the patient.

Where to Double-Check

Double-check the status of the patient's myelination. Scrutinize SWI for signs of possible hemorrhage (such as germinal matrix hemorrhage).

Pertinent Positives and Negatives

Similar to those in a routine study.

Follow-up Recommendations

Follow the recommendations of an epileptologist.

31.3.5 Cutaneous Abnormalities and Neurocutaneous Disorders

Studies to Perform

Magnetic resonance imaging, typically with intravenous contrast material. Use SWI and/or CT for conditions in which intracranial mineralization may occur, such as tuberous sclerosis complex and Sturge–Weber syndrome. Use CT to look for fibrous dysplasia and associated complications in McCune–Albright syndrome. Internal auditory canal protocol study, including cranial nerve imaging and postcontrast thin-section T1 W imaging, in neurofibromatosis type 2 (NF2).

Important Clinical Information

Type and location of cutaneous findings (▶ Table 31.1). Associated clinical features (e.g., seizures, developmental delay). Family history.

Where to Double-Check

Tuberous sclerosis complex: Evaluate the size(s) of subependymal nodule(s). Large (> 10 mm) or rapidly enlarging nodules are likely to be subependymal giant-cell astrocytomas (SEGA). Look for calcified areas of cortical dysplasia ("tubers"), which may be more likely to be epileptogenic.

Table 31.1 Skin findings and associated neurocutaneous disorders

Skin finding	Associated neurocutaneous disorders
Ash-leaf spots	Tuberous sclerosis complex
Angiofibroma (facial)	Tuberous sclerosis complex
Adenoma sebaceum	Tuberous sclerosis complex
Café au lait spots	Neurofibromatosis type 1, McCune–Albright syndrome
Capillary hemangiomas (multiple)	Posterior-fossa malformations, hemangiomas, arterial anomalies, cardiac defects and coarctation of the aorta, eye abnormalities, and sternal abnormalities (PHACES)
Hypopigmented patches	Hypomelanosis of Ito
Nevus flammeus ("port-wine stain") in the distribution of the trigeminal nerve	Sturge–Weber syndrome
Multifocal nevi	Blue rubber bleb nevus syndrome
Shagreen patches	Tuberous sclerosis complex

Neurofibromatosis type 1: Look for signs of abnormal enhancement, abnormal T2 signal, or abnormal thickening of the optic nerves, chiasm, or tracts. Look for asymmetry of the sphenoid wings and evaluate the extracranial soft tissues for signs of neurofibromata. Look at the T2 flow voids in the region of the carotid terminus and lentiform nuclei to determine whether there is any concern for moyamoya-type disease.

Neurofibromatosis type 2: Evaluate cranial nerves [CN] III–XII for signs of neurofibromas. Look closely for any signs of possible meningiomas. Evaluate the spine for possible ependymoma.

Sturge–Weber syndrome: Look for hemispheric asymmetry, asymmetry in the size of the choroid plexus in the atria of the lateral ventricles, dystrophic mineralization, asymmetric retinal enhancement, and asymmetry in the depth of the anterior chambers of the globes.

Pertinent Positives and Negatives

Tuberous sclerosis complex: Report whether or not there are dominant or enlarging subependymal nodules that suggest SEGA.

Neurofibromatosis type 1: Report whether there are any enhancing lesions. Report whether there are any optic pathway abnormalities. Report whether or not there is evidence of sphenoid-wing dysplasia.

Neurofibromatosis type 2: Describe the locations of the facial and cochlear nerves relative to vestibular schwannomas.

Sturge–Weber syndrome: Comment on the extent of dystrophic mineralization and distribution of leptomeningeal enhancement.

Follow-up Recommendations

Cutaneous findings without signs of neurocutaneous disorder: Follow up according to clinical features. If there is a neurocutaneous syndrome, each particular condition has specific follow-up recommendations, often calling for annual follow-up during childhood and shifting to follow-up in alternate years in late childhood and adolescence.

31.3.6 Movement Disorders

Myoclonus vs. hemiparesis vs. spasticity vs. ataxia.

Studies to Perform

Magnetic resonance imaging of the brain, typically without contrast material. Susceptibility-weighted imaging is helpful, especially if there are signs of prematurity. Consider following the protocol for seizures if the abnormalities are not well characterized. If the patient has ataxia or unexplained spasticity, consider MRI of the spine.

Important Clinical Information

Find out whether the abnormality is of new onset or congenital, if there are any predisposing factors or syndromic associations, and if there is a history of prematurity/cerebral palsy (CP) (especially for hemiparesis and spasticity). Find out if the symptoms are bilateral and symmetric, bilateral and asymmetric, or unilateral. Find out if the symptoms involve the upper extremities, lower extremities, or both. Find out if there is involvement of the face in addition to (or instead of) the body and extremities. Find out if the patient is meeting appropriate developmental milestones.

Where to Double-Check

Scrutinize in a manner similar to that in a seizure study, including the hippocampi. Pay close attention to the morphology of the brainstem and cerebellum. Look for abnormalities in the deep gray nuclei.

Pertinent Positives and Negatives

Similar to those in a routine study for seizure.

Follow-up Recommendations

If the study is performed prior to completion of myelination, approximately the first 2 years, consider follow-up when the myelination pattern is more mature to improve detection of subtle abnormalities. Consider magnetic resonance spectroscopy, as well a MRI of the spine, when performing follow-up studies in patients with persistent symptoms but without an identified diagnosis.

31.3.7 Short Stature, Abnormal Growth

Studies to Perform

Magnetic resonance imaging according to the protocol for imaging of the pituitary gland without and with contrast material.

Important Clinical Information

Determine whether there are signs of a congenital malformation of the pituitary gland or hypothalami. Ectopic neurohypophysis is associated with anterior pituitary dysfunction, most commonly growth-hormone deficiency.

Where to Double-Check

Beyond evaluation of the pituitary gland, evaluate all structures as in a routine MRI of the brain.

Pertinent Positives and Negatives

Comment on whether there is an orthotopic neurohypophysis.

Follow-up Recommendations

Follow the recommendations of an endocrinologist. The need for and frequency of follow-up studies may be indicated by the duration of the patient's growth-hormone therapy.

31.3.8 Precocious Puberty

Studies to Perform

Pituitary protocol for MRI of the brain without/with contrast material.

Important Clinical Information

Age of the patient. Precocious puberty in an 8-year-old girl is early, but is becoming more common in the setting of childhood obesity, and the MRI in such cases will often be normal (apart from cases of perimenarchal glandular hyperplasia). Precocious puberty in any 3-year-old. Precocious puberty in a 3-year-old is always a concern and likely requires evaluation of the pituitary and adrenal glands.

Where to Double-Check

As in a routine pituitary study.

Pertinent Positives and Negatives

Similar to those in a routine study of the pituitary.

Follow-up Recommendations

Follow the recommendations of an endocrinologist.

31.3.9 Tumor or Intracranial Mass

Studies to Perform

Magnetic resonance imaging of the brain without and with contrast material and MRI of the cervical, thoracic, and lumbar spine without and with contrast material. Consider dedicated thin-slice T1 and T2 imaging of the lesion. Diffusion-weighted imaging with apparent diffusion coefficient (ADC) mapping is very important for the evaluation of a mass. If signs of vascular encasement are found, consider magnetic resonance angiography (MRA).

Important Clinical Information

Age of the patient. Any known syndromic associations.

Where to Double-Check

Examine the patient's entire body for metastases. Realize that some metastatic deposits may not enhance significantly, and could be better seen on DWI or on postcontrast FLAIR imaging than on conventional MRI. Evaluate the entire spine, to the caudal end of the thecal sac, for possible metastatic disease. Even if the mass does not touch the surface of the brain, look for (and, if present, comment on) overlying venous structures that the surgeon may encounter en route to the mass.

Pertinent Positives and Negatives

Describe the size, location, mass effect, signal characteristics, enhancement characteristics, and ADC values of the mass. Describe whether the margins are infiltrative or discrete. Comment on the relationship of the mass to adjacent vasculature and major structures, including the optic pathway and PLIC. Determine whether there are signs of metastatic disease.

Follow-up Recommendations

Most tumors are treated with surgery. Postoperative follow-up is determined by the extent of resection and histology of a tumor.

31.3.10 Prematurity

Studies to Perform

In infants younger than 32 weeks of age, a screening ultrasound (US) examination of the head can be done for signs of germinal-matrix hemorrhage, with this examination typically done in the first 2 weeks of life. Prematurity alone is not typically an indication for a study, although such a study provides critical information in the evaluation of other neurologic symptoms. When performing an MRI on a child with a history of prematurity, particularly a child born earlier than 36 weeks' gestation, SWI can be helpful in examining for signs of prior germinal matrix hemorrhage.

Important Clinical Information

The extent of prematurity is very important because the pattern and severity of injuries will be different in a child born at 26 weeks compared to one born at 36 weeks of gestation.

Where to Double-Check

Along the lateral margins of the body of the lateral ventricles for signs of germinal matrix hemorrhage. When MRI is performed after the perinatal period in a child with a history of prematurity, residual hemosiderin staining along the dependent margins of the occipital horns of the lateral ventricles may be the only clear sign of prior hemorrhage.

Pertinent Positives and Negatives

For MRI, comment on the patient's myelination pattern, even if it is appropriate for age.

If SWI is done on MRI, commenting on whether there are signs of prior parenchymal/germinal matrix hemorrhage is helpful, even if none is seen.

Follow-up Recommendations

For very premature infants, a US study done shortly after birth and at least one follow-up study at 36 weeks corrected gestational age may be warranted; establish a local standard of practice to avoid inconsistent workups.

31.3.11 Hydrocephalus

Studies to Perform

Acute exacerbation of known hydrocephalus: CT of the head without contrast material, or if available, rapid-sequence MRI (e.g., three-plane, single-shot T2 W images).

New hydrocephalus: CT for rapid evaluation, MRI for more detailed evaluation. With MRI, consider SWI to look for signs of hemorrhage. If the patient has triventricular hydrocephalus, add sagittal CISS/FIESTA and axial + sagittal CSF flow study of the aqueduct of Sylvius. If there are any signs of an obstructing mass, postcontrast MRI is recommended (as with the protocol for a tumor).

Neonatal hydrocephalus, posthemorrhagic: Serial US examinations of the head. Computed tomography and/or MRI before surgical intervention.

Neonatal hydrocephalus in the absence of a history of prior hemorrhage: MRI with SWI.

Loculated hydrocephalus with a failed shunt: Consider computed tomographic ventriculography with the neurosurgeon injecting iodinated contrast material (using an agent and preparation approved for intrathecal use) through the shunt. Consider MRI with CISS/FIESTA imaging to characterize the fluid loculations/membranes involved by hydrocephalus.

Important Clinical Information

Was the patient premature? Are there signs of current or prior infection? Where are the shunts located? Have they been recently manipulated? If an MRI is to be performed, does the patient have a programmable shunt? If so, do not start the MRI (or do not let the patient leave the MRI area) until and unless follow-up with the neurosurgery team is coordinated to reinterrogate the programmable shunt.

Acute exacerbation study: On what basis is it believed that the patient may have a shunt malfunction (e.g., emesis, headache)? Is the patient obtunded? Are there signs of infection?

Where to Double-Check

Pay close attention to the morphology of the third ventricle, including the chiasmatic and infundibular recesses, the lamina terminalis, and the floor of the third ventricle. Look for flow voids of the aqueduct of Sylvius.

Look at white-matter volume to see if the patient's ventriculomegaly could represent ex-vacuo dilation due to volume loss. If there is aqueductal stenosis, particularly in the absence of prior hemorrhage or infection, double-check to see if the patient has rhombencephalosynapsis. If the patient is a candidate for an endoscopic third ventriculostomy, scrutinize the sagittal CISS/FIESTA imaging to see if the basilar apex and posterior communicating arteries are in close proximity to the floor of the third ventricle (and if they are, communicate this directly to the neurosurgeon).

Pertinent Positives and Negatives

Acute exacerbation study: (1) Indicate whether or not the ventricles are unchanged in size; (2) describe the locations of the shunt catheters, whether their positions are unchanged, and whether the visible portions of the catheters are intact; (3) for purposes of comparison, comment about the time elapsed since a prior study was done (e.g., a minimal change in ventricular size may be less clinically relevant if the comparison study is several years, rather than several weeks, old).

Magnetic resonance imaging study: Is the aqueduct of Sylvius patent?

After endoscopic third ventriculostomy (ETV) study: Is the ETV patent (or is it not possible to determine this)?

Follow-up Recommendations

When an instance of hydrocephalus has been characterized and treated, follow-up examinations done with a radiation-reduced CT protocol or with a rapid-sequence MRI scan should be considered. If the patient has a programmable shunt, it must be interrogated/reprogrammed shortly after an MRI scan.

31.3.12 Macrocephaly

Studies to Perform

Macrocephaly can be the presenting feature of hydrocephalus, or it may be related to a brain tumor or to a growing subdural hematoma. None of these conditions is typically the cause of hydrocephalus, but because of concerns for conditions that may require acute management, CT is often performed to obtain rapid information. In a nonemergent situation, MRI can also be of help.

Important Clinical Information

The age of the patient constitutes critical information in macrocephaly because benign enlargement of the subarachnoid spaces most commonly presents at approximately 6 months of age, and children outgrow this at some time between 12 and 24 months of age. If there are imaging features that can be seen in benign enlargement of the subarachnoid space in infancy (BESSI), this latter diagnosis can be made only if there is also macrocephaly (i.e., normal brain, large cranium). If the patient is normocephalic, and the cranium is normal in size, then prominent subarachnoid space may indicate that the brain may be too small. It is important to note that it can be difficult on CT to differentiate BESSI from a subdural hygroma.

Trajectory of growth in head circumference: A child who is at the 90th percentile for head circumference, but has been at that level for 6 months, may be less of a subject for concern than a child whose head circumference has progressed from the 50th percentile to the 90th percentile over the course of several months.

Family history: Some patients with macrocephaly come from families whose members have relatively large heads.

Where to Double-Check

Determine whether there are signs of hydrocephalus. Investigate beyond ventriculomegaly to see if there is periventricular interstitial edema (particularly adjacent to the frontal horns of the lateral ventricles), and evaluate whether there is splaying of the chiasmatic and infundibular recesses of the third ventricle, which will not be splayed in ex vacuo dilation of the ventricles.

If there is ventriculomegaly, determine whether it is unchanged or new, and whether it is thought to be of an ex vacuo origin in relation to parenchymal volume loss.

Double-check for whether there is a normal volume of the subarachnoid spaces.

Pertinent Positives and Negatives

Comment on ventricular caliber as well as calvarial morphology (given that the study may be done to evaluate for hydrocephalus).

Follow-up Recommendations

Should be based on the patient's symptoms and the recommendations of the neurosurgery team.

31.3.13 Microcephaly

Studies to Perform

Microcephaly can occur when the brain is smaller than expected, often for unknown reasons. An MRI study without contrast material and with SWI, to seek signs of prior parenchymal injury, is ultimately the best study for microcephaly.

Important Clinical Information

Estimated gestational age: Microcephaly is more common in premature infants, especially those who have had injuries related to prematurity, such as germinal matrix hemorrhage and white-matter injury.

Trajectory of growth in head circumference: A child who is in the 20th percentile for head circumference, but who has been at that level for 6 months, may be less a subject of concern than a child whose head circumference has progressed from the 50th percentile to the 20th percentile over the course of several months.

Family history: Some patients with microcephaly come from a families whose members have relatively small heads.

Where to Double-Check

Look for signs of prior germinal matrix hemorrhage, in particular on SWI.

Look for signs of white-matter volume loss, especially in the parieto-occipital area; be aware that bilaterally symmetric abnormalities can be difficult to detect.

If there is loss of brain-parenchymal volume, double-check to see whether the gray matter is normal. Volume loss predominantly of white matter is more common in prematurity than is volume loss predominantly of gray matter.

Double-check to see if the cerebellum and brainstem are normal.

Pertinent Positives and Negatives

Comment on whether there are signs of focal parenchymal injury.

Follow-up Recommendations

Follow up according to clinical requirements.

31.3.14 Abnormalities of Head Shape

Studies to Perform

Any abnormality of head shape raises concern about possible craniosynostosis (▶ Fig. 15.3). Plagiocephaly, or focal flattening of the skull, raises such concern, although this finding is most often related to positional molding. Therefore, the first imaging study to be done on a patient with an abnormality of head shape is a careful clinical examination by a physician familiar with the features that differentiate positional plagiocephaly from craniosynostosis and vice versa. If there is uncertainty, CT of the head with three-dimensional (3D) reconstructions provides the best information about the patency of the calvarial sutures.

Radiographs have traditionally been used to evaluate for craniosynostosis, but their sensitivity and specificity are lower than those of CT, which can be a particular problem if the interpreting physician does not have substantial clinical experience with radiographs of the skull.

Important Clinical Information

Find out whether any additional clinical findings or syndromic associations have been made about the patient.

Family history: Head shape may be a familial characteristic. Brachycephaly is more common in some individuals of East Asian descent than in other population groups, and it can be a normal feature if not associated with osseous or cerebral abnormalities.

Where to Double-Check

Look for abnormalities in the skull base, including stenosis of the foramen magnum (which is common in achondroplasia). Also look for stenosis of the jugular foramen, which can be seen in various developmental abnormalities of the skull base, such as achondroplasia, possibly resulting in intracranial venous hypertension and hydrocephalus.

Pertinent Positives and Negatives

The age-appropriateness and symmetry of the cranial-suture maturation pattern are critical to assess and report.

Follow-up Recommendations

Other than isolated sagittal craniosynostosis, which is typically sporadic, craniosynostosis should prompt a genetic evaluation. Patients with most of the findings described above, other than the normal variants (brachycephaly, isolated bathrocephaly) and positional plagiocephaly, may benefit from a radiographic skeletal survey.

31.3.15 Hemispheric Asymmetry

Sturge–Weber syndrome vs. Rasmussen's syndrome vs. hemimegalencephaly vs. prior injury.

Studies to Perform

If there is asymmetry of the cerebral hemispheres, both CT and MRI can be helpful. This is something that will often first be identified on CT and then further characterized on MRI. Susceptibility-weighted imaging will be helpful on MRI, and in some cases postcontrast imaging can be helpful.

Important Clinical Information

Determine whether the patient has seizures and whether there are any cutaneous findings to suggest Sturge–Weber syndrome.

Where to Double-Check

Determine which lateral ventricle is larger, since it will typically be in the abnormal hemisphere. If the larger hemisphere is abnormal, there is probably hamartomatous overgrowth in the setting of hemimegalencephaly. If the abnormal hemisphere is smaller, which is more often the case, it should be determined whether this finding involves the hemisphere globally, which in the setting of profound seizures raises the possibility of Rasmussen's encephalitis, or whether the volume loss is more focal. Focal volume loss can be a result of prior stroke or trauma. Regional volume loss with abnormal cortical venous drainage is seen in Sturge–Weber syndrome, in which there will nearly always be an ipsilateral facial port-wine stain. Double-check for calvarial thickening overlying an area of volume loss, which likely indicates a Dyke-Davidoff-Masson phenomenon and confirms that the volume loss is chronic.

Pertinent Positives and Negatives

Determine whether the larger hemisphere is the normal or abnormal hemisphere.

Follow-up Recommendations

If there are signs of Sturge–Weber syndrome, postcontrast MRI and CT may be helpful. Otherwise, no specific follow-up recommendations exist beyond what is clinically required.

31.3.16 Metabolic Disorders, Known or Suspected

Studies to Perform

Magnetic resonance imaging of the brain, typically without contrast. Susceptibility-weighted imaging may help. Consider magnetic resonance spectroscopy, with short- and long-echo single-voxel spectroscopy of the deep gray nuclei and deep white matter (either frontal or parieto-occipital).

Important Clinical Information

Does the patient have any other systemic or biochemical disorders? Is the patient macrocephalic, microcephalic, or normocephalic? Does the patient have delayed developmental milestones? Is the patient losing milestones?

Where to Double-Check

The distribution and gradients are important to evaluate, as they will significantly focus the differential diagnosis. Determine whether the abnormality is white-matter predominant, gray-matter predominant, or both. Is there an anterior-predominant, posterior-predominant, or global involvement? Is there cerebellar involvement? Is there more central involvement, peripheral/juxtacortical involvement, or are there both types of involvement? If there is a comparison study, carefully examine both it and the current/immediate studies for subtle changes in distribution of signal abnormality and brain-parenchymal volume.

Pertinent Positives and Negatives

The presence or absence of abnormalities in the deep gray nuclei is important to document because these are often present in mitochondrial disorders. If spectroscopy is performed, confirming the absence of a lactate peak is important because the presence of lactate suggests anaerobic metabolism (which can be seen in conditions including mitochondrial disorders).

Follow-up Recommendations

It may help to repeat imaging studies if the patient has progression of symptoms. Consider imaging of the spine in atypical cases.

31.3.17 Cyst of the Posterior Fossa

Mega cisterna magna vs. Blake's pouch vs. arachnoid cyst vs. Dandy–Walker-spectrum disorder (▶ Fig. 4.9).

Studies to Perform

If there is concern about an abnormality of the posterior fossa, MRI is the diagnostic study of choice.

Important Clinical Information

History of prematurity, neurologic and developmental abnormalities, syndromic findings, and systemic abnormalities.

Where to Double-Check

Perhaps the most important finding is the morphology of the vermis. If the vermian morphology is normal, there is no malformation within the Dandy–Walker spectrum. Double-check for supratentorial abnormalities, such as dysgenesis of the corpus callosum.

Pertinent Positives and Negatives

Normal vs. abnormal volume and morphology of the cerebellar vermis as well as of the brainstem. A normal vs. abnormal position of the torcula, normal vs. abnormal corpus callosum, and normal vs. abnormal ventricular morphology.

Follow-up Recommendations

None specific.

31.3.18 Abnormality of the Corpus Callosum

Studies to Perform

Magnetic resonance imaging of the brain without contrast material. If there are signs of a possible pericallosal lipoma, consider sagittal T1 W without and with fat-saturation (FS) imaging. If signs exist of a prior acquired injury, such as focal callosal thinning related to Wallerian degeneration, SWI can be helpful.

Important Clinical Information

Age and clinical presentation. Note whether there are other midline abnormalities, such as a cleft lip and/or palate, single central incisor, or endocrine abnormalities.

Where to Double-Check

Look carefully at all midline structures, including the pituitary gland. Evaluate whether other commissures, particularly the anterior commissure, are normal. If the corpus callosum is abnormal, evaluate the structures of the posterior fossa and for any calvarial asymmetry.

If there is agenesis of the corpus callosum, look for and comment on an interhemispheric cyst. If there is agenesis of the corpus callosum in a female patient, look for abnormalities of the eye, which can be seen in Aicardi syndrome.

Pertinent Positives and Negatives

Is the corpus callosum present in its entirety? If not, name the parts that are present and those that are absent. Determine whether the parts that are present have a normal or abnormal morphology. Is the anteroposterior (AP) dimension of the corpus callosum normal?

Follow-up Recommendations

None specific.

31.4 Head and Neck

31.4.1 Abnormalities of Eye Movement

Nystagmus vs. strabismus vs. esotropia vs. exotropia vs. myopia vs. meiosis, etc.

Studies to Perform

Typically, MRI of the brain, and possibly also of the orbits. Studies without and with contrast material are preferred for most patients. Consider axial CISS/FIESTA imaging for cranial-nerve evaluation, especially for esotropia (palsy of CN VI).

If a pediatric patient has opsoclonus as an abnormality of eye movement, evaluation of the adrenal glands with US, CT, or MRI is mandatory; this can be more important than imaging of the brain and orbits because opsoclonus can be a paraneoplastic manifestation of neuroblastoma.

Important Clinical Information

Find out whether the abnormality is of new onset or chronic. Are there unilateral or bilateral abnormalities? Are there also problems with vision?

Where to Double-Check

Look closely at the brainstem, clivus, and petrous apices, as well as the cavernous sinuses. If there is no dedicated orbital imaging, it is important to closely examine brain images for possible orbital abnormalities; remember that strabismus can be caused by ocular tumors, such as retinoblastoma, and orbital tumors, such as rhabdomyosarcoma.

Pertinent Positives and Negatives

If imaging is done only of the brain, ensure that the evaluator's statement about the orbits specifies that they were evaluated only in nondedicated imaging.

Follow-up Recommendations

None specific.

31.4.2 Hypoplasia of the Optic Nerve

Studies to Perform

Magnetic resonance imaging of the brain without contrast. Consider MRI of the orbits. Consider thin-section sagittal T1 images of the pituitary gland as well as thin-section T1 W images of the brain.

Important Clinical Information

Determine whether the patient has developmental delay and/or seizures.

Where to Double-Check

Determine whether the septum pellucidum is present or absent. Determine whether there is an orthotopic (vs. ectopic) neurohypophysis. Look closely to determine whether there is a subtle closed-lip schizencephalic cleft. Look for optic-nerve hypoplasia; this can be more difficult if dedicated orbital imaging is not done in addition to brain imaging.

Pertinent Positives and Negatives

Specify whether or not the septum pellucidum is present. Specify whether there is an orthotopic neurohypophysis.

Follow-up Recommendations

Nothing specific beyond what is clinically indicated.

31.4.3 Hearing Loss

Conductive vs. sensorineural, congenital vs. acquired, sudden onset vs. progressive onset.

Studies to Perform

Sensorineural hearing loss: Congenital. CT of the temporal bones is probably the best imaging modality, although MRI with cranial nerve imaging of the internal auditory canals can help. Cranial-nerve imaging is especially helpful if there is a narrowed cochlear aperture and/or if cochlear implantation is contemplated.

Sensorineural hearing loss: Acquired. Consider both CT and MRI. Consider contrast-enhanced MRI.

Conductive hearing loss: CT of the temporal bones.

Important Clinical Information

Specify the ear that is involved. This information should be actively sought and reported.

Determine whether the hearing loss is conductive, sensorineural, or mixed. Is the hearing loss congenital or acquired? Is the hearing loss progressive? Does the patient have any known syndrome or other clinical abnormalities? Was the hearing loss determined by audiologic examination (as is most commonly

the case, particularly for a patient referred by an otolaryngologist) or clinical evaluation?

Where to Double-Check

The patient's clinical information is the most important thing to double-check. On CT for sensorineural hearing loss (SNHL), double-check the caliber of the vestibular aqueducts as well as the cochlear aperture. If the patient is a candidate for a cochlear implant, double-check for the presence of the modiolus.

If a CT of the temporal bones is done for sensorineural hearing loss, double-check the size of the cochlear aperture because a narrowed aperture (< ~1 mm) is associated with cochlear nerve hypoplasia/aplasia.

If a CT of the temporal bones done for a conductive hearing loss appears normal, double-check the entire study.

Pertinent Positives and Negatives

Comment on the morphology of the cochlea, vestibule, and semicircular canals. Comment on the caliber of the vestibular aqueduct. On MRI with cranial nerve imaging, comment on whether the cochlear nerve is present.

Follow-up Recommendations

If a cochlear implant is planned and the cochlear aperture is narrowed or obstructed, MRI with axial and sagittal oblique CISS/FIESTA imaging of the internal auditory canals (IACs) can help confirm the presence and caliber of the cochlear nerve.

31.5 Spine

31.5.1 Sacral Dimple

Specify the position of conus, filum, dermal sinus tract, cyst, lipoma, pilonidal tract, etc.

Studies to Perform

Ultrasound in the first few months of life, otherwise MRI. If there is concern about a possible osseous abnormality, subsequent CT may be helpful for troubleshooting. If there are signs of inflammation or infection, fat suppressed imaging, both T1 post-contrast and T2, can be helpful.

Important Clinical Information

The location of the dimple should be marked before MRI with something such as a vitamin E capsule. A dimple above the gluteal cleft is more likely to be associated with a congenital defect than is a dimple within the gluteal cleft.

Determine the depth and size of the dimple. Larger and deeper dimples are more likely to be associated with abnormalities.

Determine whether a skin discoloration or hairy patch is associated with the dimple, since these are features that increase the probability of an underlying congenital defect.

Determine whether there is any drainage or signs of infection/inflammation.

Determine whether the patient has any neurologic deficit, such as a limp, ataxia, bowel/bladder dysfunction.

Where to Double-Check

Confirm the location and morphology of the conus medullaris. Look for bladder thickening to suggest neurogenic bladder. Evaluate the integrity and morphology of the sacrum and coccyx (note that a retroflexed coccyx can be seen more often in the setting of a pilonidal tract).

Pertinent Positives and Negatives

Confirm the location and morphology of the conus medullaris. Comment on whether there is a dermal sinus tract connecting the sacral dimple to the thecal sac. If there is a dermal sinus tract, comment on whether there is any cyst or mass (such as a dermoid cyst or lipoma) associated with it. Comment on the caliber and signal of the filum terminale. Note that tethered cord is a clinical determination, and that although certain findings on MRI increase the risk of development of manifestations of tethered cord syndrome (e.g., a low conus, thickened filum), the specific diagnosis cannot be made without knowledge of the clinical symptoms. It is also not possible on MRI to completely exclude the existence of a tethered cord.

Follow-up Recommendations

If the ultrasonographic evaluation of a sacral dimple reveals atypical features, follow-up MRI may be indicated. Otherwise, follow-up should be determined by the clinical requirements in a particular case.

31.5.2 Scoliosis

Cross-sectional imaging evaluation.

Studies to Perform

Radiographs alone are typically used for investigating adolescent idiopathic scoliosis (AIS). Cross-sectional imaging helps if there are atypical features, including onset before 8 years of age, male gender, rapid progression, presence of a vertebral segmentation anomaly, neurologic deficits, and a curvature that does not follow the typical sigmoid (S-shaped) pattern of AIS.

If MRI is performed, coronal T2 W images are very helpful for evaluating AIS. If there is very severe scoliosis, it may be helpful to acquire axial and sagittal images relative to the plane of the vertebral column and not the long-axis of the patient, although this increases the image-acquisition time. If there is unexpected hydromyelia/syrinx, or if the scoliosis is associated with a neurocutaneous syndrome, contrast-enhanced MRI is beneficial. With CT, consider three-dimensional reformats of the imaging data.

Important Clinical Information

Determine whether the scoliosis has progressed and whether the patient has neurologic symptoms. Determine the age of onset of the scoliosis, gender of the patient, and any known syndrome (including neurocutaneous syndromes) diagnosed in the patient.

Where to Double-Check

If MRI is done, confirm the location of the conus medullaris. If anomalies of segmentation are present, ensure that there are no extra or missing vertebrae. Look for a syrinx. If the cervical spine is included, confirm whether or not there is a Chiari malformation or other abnormality in the imaged portions of the posterior cranial fossa. Look at all available comparison studies; prior chest and/or abdominal radiographs may provide additional information about the patient's bony anatomy and provide additional time points with which to assess any progression of scoliosis.

Pertinent Positives and Negatives

Comment on whether imaging reveals any anomalies of segmentation. Comment on the location of the conus medullaris and whether there is any thickening or fibrolipoma of the filum terminale. For CT and MRI, comment on whether the severity of the scoliosis is approximately similar to that in standing radiographs of the patient's spine.

Follow-up Recommendations

None specific beyond clinical follow-up.

31.5.3 Spina Bifida

Studies to Perform

Magnetic resonance imaging of the spine is the best means of identifying possible spinal dysraphism, including meningocele, myelomeningocele, lipomyelomeningocele, etc. If there is a suspected lipomatous component, T1 W imaging both without and with FS can be helpful. For examination after the treatment or correction of scoliosis, sagittal FIESTA/CISS imaging can help in seeking possible pseudomeningocele. If osseous information is needed beyond the detail provided by plain-film radiography, CT can be helpful. In the neonatal period, US of the spine can be considered. If there is a profound scoliotic curvature, consider acquiring magnetic resonance images with scan planes parallel and perpendicular to the axis of the spine in the affected region of the spine, which may require image acquisition in multiple separate segments of the spine.

Important Clinical Information

It is most important to clarify why spina bifida is suspected in a particular patient, and what the referring physician means by this term. The term "spina bifida" classically refers to a myelomeningocele, but in practice, people may use this term in requesting a study for many reasons. If a study is being done to evaluate incidental spina bifida occulta at S1, seen on an abdominal or pelvic radiograph, consider a discussion with the referring physician and other involved practitioners to see whether there is any other indication for a workup, since "spina bifida occulta" does not require further evaluation.

Where to Double-Check

Use FS imaging to confirm the location and extent of an intradural lipoma. Look for pelvic and retroperitoneal abnormalities, and particularly a thickened bladder wall suggestive of spinal dysraphism. Look for a syrinx.

Pertinent Positives and Negatives

Comment on whether imaging has revealed any segmentation anomalies. Comment on whether there is a conus medullaris, and if so at which level. If there is no conus medullaris, describe whether the cord terminates abruptly, whether it extends to the caudal end of the thecal sac, and whether there is a neural placode. If there is a lipoma, describe its relationship to the spinal cord and nerve roots of the cauda equina. Describe whether there are signs of a dermal sinus tract or other such connection. Comment on the coronal alignment (i.e., whether scoliosis is present).

Follow-up Recommendations

None specific.

31.6 Clarifying Areas of Uncertainty

31.6.1 Mild Chiari Malformation vs. Cerebellar Tonsillar Ectopia

Elongated cerebellar tonsils that extend below the foramen magnum and obstruct normal pulsatilve CSF flow are a feature of a Chiari type I malformation. In adults, tonsillar ectopia exceeding 5 mm is said to represent a Chiari type I malformation, but ectopia of 6 or 7 mm can sometimes be physiologic in children if there is a normal tonsillar morphology and patent CSF spaces around the cervicomedullary junction at the level of the foramen magnum.

31.6.2 Prominent Central Canal vs. Hydromyelia vs. Syrinx

The central canal of the spinal cord is an ependyma-lined CSF channel that is usually not visualized in standard imaging sequences. Mild prominence of the central canal, to approximately 1.5 mm in maximum axial dimension, can be physiologic if there are smooth margins without signal abnormality of the adjacent cord. Dilation of an ependymal-lined central canal beyond an axial dimension of 1.5 mm is known as hydromyelia. A fluid collection within the cord that is not within the ependyma-lined central canal (and is therefore not perfectly centrally located) is known as syringomyelia. When an abnormality is sufficiently large as to make it difficult to exactly characterize its location, or appears to be hydromyelia but with surrounding edema suggesting that the ependymal lining is no longer intact, the term "syringohydromyelia" is used to describe it.

31.6.3 Pineal Cysts: Normal or Abnormal?

Pineal cysts are physiologic findings seen in approximately 50% of individuals of all ages. They may contain proteinaceous material and occasionally contain layering debris. There is no formal consensus on how to address pineal cysts. In the absence of focal mural nodularity or other suspicious features, the following rough guideline is reasonable: Pineal cysts smaller than 5 mm do not typically require description in an imaging report; cysts between 5 and 10 mm in diameter are reasonable to mention in the body of the report but do not typically require description in the impression section of the report; cysts of more than 10 mm diameter are reasonable to mention in the impression section of a report, but it is unclear whether all such cysts require follow-up. A 12 month follow-up contrast-enhanced study is not unreasonable for cysts larger than 10mm, however the diagnostic yield of this will likely be low.

Index

Note: Page numbers set **bold** or *italic* indicate headings or figures, respectively.